ANTIOXIDANTS
and
Disease
Prevention

ANTIOXIDANTS
and
Disease
Prevention

edited by

Harinder S. Garewal, M.D., Ph.D.

CRC Press
Boca Raton   New York

Publisher/Life Sciences:	Robert B. Stern
Project Editor:	Carrie L. Unger
Editorial Assistant:	Carol Messing
Marketing Manager:	Susie Carlisle
Direct Marketing Manager:	Becky McEldowney
Cover design:	Dawn Boyd
PrePress:	Kevin Luong
Manufacturing:	Sheri Schwartz

Library of Congress Cataloging-in-Publication Data

Antioxidants and disease prevention / edited by Harinder S. Garewal.
      p. cm.
      Includes bibliographical references and index.
      ISBN 0-8493-8509-1 (alk. paper)
      1. Antioxidants—Therapeutic use. 2. Medicine, Preventive. 3. Free Radicals
(Chemistry)—Pathophysiology I. Garewal, Harinder S. II. Series: Modern nutrition (Boca
Raton, Fla.).
      [DNLM: 1. Antioxidants—therapeutic use. 2. Antioxidants—adverse effects. QV 800 A632
      1997]
RB170.A58 1997
616.07—dc21
DNLM/DLC
  for Library of Congress
                                            96-45089
                                                CIP

No claim to original U.S. Government works
International Standard Book Number 0-8493-8509-1
Library of Congress Card Number 96-45089
Printed in the United States of America   3 4 5 6 7 8 9 0
Printed on acid-free paper

MODERN NUTRITION

Edited by Ira Wolinsky and James F. Hickson, Jr.

Published Titles

Manganese in Health and Disease, Dorothy Klimis-Tavantzis
Nutrition and AIDS: Effects and Treatment, Ronald R. Watson
*Nutrition Care for HIV Positive Persons: A Manual for Individuals
    and Their Caregivers*, Saroj M. Bahl and James F. Hickson, Jr.
Calcium and Phosphorus in Health and Disease, John J. B. Anderson and
    Sanford C. Garner

Forthcoming Titles

Nutrients and Foods in AIDS, Ronald R. Watson
Nutrition and Women's Cancer, Barbara C. Pence and Dale M. Dunn

Edited by Ira Wolinsky

Published Titles

Handbook of Nutrition in the Aged, Ronald R. Watson
Practical Handbook of Nutrition in Clinical Practice, Donald F. Kirby and
    Stanley J. Dudrick
Handbook of Dairy Foods and Nutrition, Gregory D. Miller, Judith K. Jarvis and
    Lois D. McBean
Advanced Nutrition: Macronutrients, Carolyn D. Berdanier
Childhood Nutrition, Fima Lifshitz
Antioxidants and Disease Prevention, Harinder S. Garewal
Nutrition and Cancer Prevention, Ronald R. Watson and Siraj I. Mufti
Nutrition and Health: Topics and Controversies, Felix Bronner
Nutritional Concerns of Women, Ira Wolinsky and Dorothy Klimis-Tavantzis
Nutrients and Gene Expression: Clinical Aspects, Carolyn D. Berdanier

Forthcoming Titles

Laboratory Tests for the Assessment of Nutritional Status, 2nd Edition,
    H. E. Sauberlich
Nutrition: Chemistry and Biology, 2nd Edition, Julian E. Spallholz,
    L. Mallory Boylan and Judy A. Driskell
Advanced Nutrition: Micronutrients, Carolyn D. Berdanier and Mark L. Failla
Child Nutrition: An International Perspective, Noel W. Solomons
Handbook of Nutrition for Vegetarians, Rosemary A. Ratzin
Melatonin in the Promotion of Health, Ronald R. Watson
Nutrition and the Eye, Allen Taylor

SERIES PREFACE

The CRC Series in Modern Nutrition is dedicated to providing the widest possible coverage to topics in nutrition. Nutrition is an interdisciplinary, interprofessional field par excellence. It is noted by its broad range and diversity. We trust that the titles and authorship in this series will reflect that range and diversity.

Published for a broad audience, the volumes of the CRC Series in Modern Nutrition are designed to explain, review, and explore present knowledge and recent trends, developments, and advances in nutrition. As such, they appeal to professionals as well as to educated laymen. The format for the series will vary with the needs of the author and the topic, including, but not limited to, edited volumes, monographs, handbooks, and texts.

Contributors from any bona fide area of nutrition, including the controversial, are welcome.

We would like to welcome the contribution *Antioxidants and Disease Prevention*, edited by Harinder S. Garewal, M.D., Ph.D., to this series. In recent years, this topic has probably generated more research effort, hope, speculation, and controversy than any other topic in nutrition science.

Ira Wolinsky
Series Editor

THE EDITOR

Harinder S. Garewal, M.D., Ph.D., is the Assistant Director for Cancer Prevention and Control at the Tucson Veteran Affairs Medical Center and at the University of Arizona Cancer Center. He is Professor of Medicine at the University of Arizona Health Sciences Center and is Chief of the Section of Hematology–Oncology at the Tucson Veteran Affairs Medical Center

Dr. Garewal graduated in 1968 from St. Xavier's College (Calcutta University, India) with a major in chemistry. He completed graduate work for his doctorate at McGill University (Montreal, Canada) in 1972 and received a medical degree in 1977 from Harvard Medical School (Boston, Massachusetts). Following three years of residency training in internal medicine at the University of Oregon Health Sciences Center, he was selected as the Chief Medical Resident from 1980 to 1981. He did his fellowship training in hematology–oncology from 1981 to 1984 at the University of Arizona Health Sciences Center, after which he joined the Section of Hematology–Oncology at the same institution. He also holds appointments in the Section of Gastroenterology. Included among his numerous institutional appointments are Chair of the Research and Development Committee and Director of the Hematology–Oncology Fellowship Training Program. Dr. Garewal is a member of the American Association for Cancer Research, American Society of Preventive Oncology, American Society for Clinical Oncology, Western Society for Clinical Investigation, American Federation of Clinical Research, American Association for the Advancement of Science, American Gastroenterological Association, American Institute for Nutrition, and American Society of Clinical Nutrition. He is a member of the Southwest Oncology Group (SWOG) and serves on the Executive Committee of the Cancer Prevention and Control Committee of SWOG. He also served as a member of the Cancer Prevention and Control Committee of the American Society for Clinical Oncology.

Dr. Garewal has served as a reviewer for numerous scientific and medical journals. He has been a regular member of the National Cancer Institute/National Institutes of Health (NCI/NIH) grant review groups and presently serves on the Cancer Centers Review Committee.

Dr. Garewal has been a recipient of a National Science Talent Scholar Award from the government of India and a Medical Research Council of Canada scholarship for graduate and postdoctoral research. He has also received an American Cancer Society Career Development Award, and his research has been selected for presentation on two occasions at the Science Writers' Symposium organized by the American Cancer Society. He has received grant support from the National Cancer Institute, Veteran Affairs Administration, State of Arizona as well as from the pharmaceutical industry.

Dr. Garewal has been an invited speaker at numerous national and international meetings in addition to lectures at universities and academic institutions. He has published more than 170 articles and more than 150 meeting abstracts. His major research interests involve the prevention and treatment of cancers, especially those of the aerodigestive tract.

PREFACE

There is little doubt that successful prevention will be the key to controlling morbidity and mortality from chronic diseases affecting humankind. Equally evident is the realization that prevention will involve contributions from a number of interventions. In other words, there will be no magic bullet that will singly prevent all cases of a disease. Diet plays a crucial role in health maintenance, but it would be silly to hope for a "super-preventive" diet that would allow us to continue smoking and living a sedentary life while successfully preventing, for example, heart disease. For decades now, it has been appreciated that oxidative pathways can lead to tissue damage and contribute to disease causation. Fortunately, nature has provided us with mechanisms to defend against such injury. The so-called antioxidant nutritional agents have consequently attracted major attention and rightfully deserve to be studied carefully for possible beneficial roles.

At the onset, I would like to emphasize that quibbling about terminology is not the goal of this book. Yes, it is true that there is no such thing as a universal antioxidant, for the same chemical can behave as an oxidant or antioxidant under different circumstances. This is very true for vitamin agents which are the mainstay of this discussion. My goal is to study these agents scientifically and rationally with the objective of identifying potential diseases and populations where they may be beneficial, rather than debating forever whether they should be called antioxidants or not.

One of the main reasons for the interest in these agents is their virtual complete lack of harmful side-effects. This stands in stark contrast to many other agents that are promoted and studied for possible disease preventive activity. A recent example of this is in my own area of expertise, which is prevention of oral cavity and lung cancer. An intensely studied and heavily promoted group of compounds is the synthetic retinoids. Without a doubt, retinoids are extremely interesting compounds and produce biologic effects that are profoundly important in understanding carcinogenesis. Nevertheless, even a cursory glance at these agents immediately reveals that their potential for actual use in preventing disease is virtually nonexistent. This is because their toxicity profile is such that they cannot be safely administered without close monitoring for side-effects. Such a requirement negates widespread use, the latter being a prerequisite if an agent is going to make a significant impact on any disease in the world. Admittedly, there are some very high risk situations, such as many familial syndromes, where toxicity can be accepted because of the high risk of disease occurrence. However, such familial situations only account for a tiny fraction of that disease and even if all such cases were eradicated, the "bump" on the disease incidence and mortality graph would not be noticeable. This is not to say that such agents are not important at all, because they clearly are very important to the people affected by familial syndromes. Their significance to the overall spectrum of chronic disease prevention, though, is vanishingly small.

The subject of antioxidant or other nutritional agents in disease prevention is often associated with strong emotional responses, one way or another, which are totally uncharacteristic and unacceptable in a rational, scientific inquiry. I am a practicing medical oncologist who entered this field with considerable skepticism.

In other words, how could agents that "do nothing" be of any use? By "doing nothing" I am referring to the near absence of any side-effects, something that medical oncologists rarely, if ever, encounter in a compound. It was only through the gradual observation of results, our own as well as of other groups, that my interest in the subject increased, leading to its broadening to diseases outside the oncologic arena. Studies were being conducted by respected scientists in a number of important disease entities, ranging from cancer to heart disease to eye disease and eventually to general health maintenance such as infection prevention in the elderly. Yes, there are valid criticisms of many of these trials. Nevertheless, if one looks at the studies with an unbiased attitude, it becomes quite clear that many of these criticisms stem from unavoidable factors that the authors and scientists are perfectly familiar with, but cannot, in the proverbial "real world," do anything about. Thus, it is important to study all of the evidence, for and against, in order to reach a conclusion. This is something each of us will need to do because the subject is such that there will never be a single, perfect study that will determine once and for all whether these agents prevent heart disease or cancer or any other entity. Some of the reasons for this are touched upon in several of the chapters that follow.

In this context, it is interesting to study what conclusions have been arrived at by many physicians and scientists themselves. For example, what do cardiologists tell their patients concerning vitamin E and heart disease prevention? To go one step further, what do these cardiologists themselves do or what do they recommend to their own families? Similar questions could be posed to other healthcare providers, such as general physicians, nurses, etc. Although conclusive polling data are not available on this subject, last year we analyzed the response to a questionnaire survey addressing this issue. These questionnaires were mailed to a randomly selected sample of physicians, cardiologists, family practitioners, and general internists across the country. Interestingly, well over 50% of doctors surveyed use these agents themselves or recommend them to their patients or families. The figure was much higher for questions such as the use of vitamin E in heart disease prevention. Clearly, these physicians have made the decision as it affects themselves and their patients. Although this is not to say that their decision is the correct one, it points to the difficulty of trying lengthy, perfectly designed, randomized, blind-controlled trials with a placebo arm under these circumstances.

My goal in putting this book together was to provide wide coverage of the subject as it relates to many different disease states. In my efforts to familiarize myself with the literature over the past few years, I realized that a single collection of articles by leading investigators in their field would be very useful, not only to researchers, but to practicing physicians, health professionals, students, and other individuals interested in the subject. It is my hope that readers will find such a resource to be useful. Perhaps the researcher, whose work is focused in one or two areas, will find the information contained in other chapters to be of interest in helping to understand the breadth and depth of this area of research. As in any scientific endeavor, research moves at such a pace that, if not periodically updated, information soon becomes obsolete. With any luck, the chapters in this book will continue to serve as stepping stones for additional reading for many years to come. It should be possible to use these chapters as background material onto which to add new research findings as they become available.

Finally, I would like to thank each and every author who made a tremendous effort to produce truly excellent overviews. Clearly, without their cooperation and help, this would not have been possible.

Harinder S. Garewal, M.D., Ph.D.

CONTRIBUTORS

Sussan K. Ardestani
Institute of Biochemistry and Biophysics
University of Tehran
Tehran, Iran

Gerald F. Combs, Jr.
Division of Nutritional Sciences
Cornell University
Ithaca, New York

Anthony T. Diplock
International Antioxidant Research
  Centre
Division of Biochemistry and Molecular
  Biology
UMDS Guy's Hospital
London, England

Cindy J. Fuller
Food, Nutrition and Food Service
  Management
University of North Carolina
Greensboro, North Carolina

Harinder S. Garewal
Section of Hematology — Oncology
Arizona Cancer Center and
  Veteran Affairs Medical Center
Tucson, Arizona

Richard M. Hoffman
General Internal Medicine
Veteran Affairs Medical Center
University of New Mexico School of
  Medicine
Albuquerque, New Mexico

Paula F. Inserra
Department of Family and
  Community Medicine
University of Arizona
Tucson, Arizona

Paul F. Jacques
Epidemiology Program
Jean Mayer U.S. Department of
  Agriculture Human Nutrition Research
  Center on Aging
Tufts University
Boston, Massachusetts

I. Jialal
University of Texas
Southwestern Medical Center
Dallas, Texas

Susan T. Mayne
Department of Epidemiology and Public
  Health
Yale University School of Medicine
New Haven, Connecticut

Jerry W. McLarty
Department of Epidemiology
University of Texas Health Sciences
  Center
Tyler, Texas

Ronald Ross Watson
Department of Family and
  Community Medicine
University of Arizona
Tucson, Arizona

Zhen Zhang
Department of Family and
  Community Medicine
University of Arizona
Tucson, Arizona

Regina G. Ziegler
Nutritional Epidemiology Branch
National Institutes of Health/National
  Cancer Institute
Bethesda, Maryland

TABLE OF CONTENTS

Chapter 1
Introduction 1
Harinder S. Garewal

Chapter 2
The Safety of β-Carotene and the Antioxidant Vitamins C and E 3
Anthony T. Diplock

Chapter 3
Antioxidants and Immune Function 19
Paula F. Inserra, Sussan K. Ardestani, and Ronald Ross Watson

Chapter 4
Antioxidants and AIDS 31
Zhen Zhang, Paula F. Inserra, and Ronald Ross Watson

Chapter 5
Antioxidants and Cancer: The Epidemiologic Evidence 45
Jerry W. McLarty

Chapter 6
Antioxidant Nutrients and Lung Cancer 67
Susan T. Mayne and Regina G. Ziegler

Chapter 7
Antioxidant Nutrients and Oral Cavity Cancer 87
Harinder S. Garewal

Chapter 8
Selenium and Cancer Prevention 97
Gerald F. Combs, Jr.

Chapter 9
Antioxidants and LDL Oxidation 115
Cindy J. Fuller and I. Jialal

Chapter 10
Antioxidants and Coronary Artery Disease Prevention 131
Richard M. Hoffman and Harinder S. Garewal

Chapter 11
**Nutritional Antioxidants and Prevention
of Age-Related Eye Disease** 149
Paul F. Jacques

Index 179

Chapter 1

INTRODUCTION

Harinder S. Garewal

Emphasis on nutrition for health maintenance is backed by a large body of evidence accumulated over decades. The term "antioxidant" nutritional agent has been applied to a number of specific nutrients, most notably β-carotene, vitamin E, vitamin C, and more recently, selenium. From a purist's viewpoint, one can critique this nomenclature because it is admittedly a "loose" term. There is no such thing as an "antioxidant" that behaves as such under all circumstances. However, our goal is to prevent disease and promote health, rather than debate terminology. Oxidative pathways have been implicated in a variety of disease producing mechanisms.

Recognizing the importance of prevention as the most viable strategy for reducing morbidity and mortality from chronic diseases, the field of chemoprevention has blossomed in the recent past. Chemoprevention refers to the use of specific chemicals, either alone or in combinations, to decrease the incidence of disease. Antioxidant nutritional agents have been the focus of major attention in this effort, one of the primary reasons for this being their lack of significant toxicity and their ease of supplementation in large sections of the populations. Although this may sound trivial, it is a key property from the standpoint of prevention that is not uniformly shared by numerous agents that have been proposed and are being tested as putative chemopreventive compounds. Any significant side effect will preclude application of the agent for actual reduction in disease incidence in a population, regardless of how active that agent may be in any model system or intervention trial. Clearly, the amount and level of toxicity acceptable for preventive applications is dictated by the risk and severity of the disease being prevented. Although there are a few especially high risk populations in which some side effects can be justified, they constitute only a small minority of cases of chronic diseases. For example, familial polyposis of the colon, a genetic condition associated with a high rate of colon cancer, accounts for a tiny percent of colon cancer in the population. Consequently, agents that can be justified for use in this condition, but which are precluded by toxicity from general population use, will only have a very modest, if any, impact on colon cancer incidence in general.

In addition to their suitability for preventive use, another property of these antioxidant agents is the number and breadth of diseases in which a possible role has been hypothesized. One of my own areas of interest is prevention of oral cavity cancer, but I recognize that if an agent had activity in preventing oral cavity cancer only, it would have very limited, if any, beneficial impact on morbidity reduction and longevity in western populations. Even if a compound prevented half of all cases of this disease with no appreciable toxicity it would still be difficult to justify everyone taking such an agent, since the impact of this single disease is rather small. Clearly, if a significant preventive activity was found in a more prevalent condition, justification for use could be made. Nevertheless, a truly attractive chemopreventive agent would be one with activity in a number of disease entities. As evidenced by the diverse group of diseases discussed in this book, an attractive feature of the antioxidant agents lies in their potential role in various conditions, such as heart disease, cancer, and eye disease. In addition, recent work has implicated oxidative processes in more general settings such as infections in the elderly or the aging process itself.

Why is it that one cannot provide a definitive answer regarding a role for these compounds in preventing one disease or another? The answer lies in the very nature of the problem being posed. No one would argue that the definitive way to demonstrate whether a drug works against a disease is to do a properly controlled, randomized, blinded trial. Furthermore, the trial should be done in the right population, i.e., the population in which the drug will eventually be used. Clearly, if this was a simple matter, such trials would have been accomplished long ago. The problem, however, is that such perfectly designed studies are virtually impossible to carry out when one is dealing with compounds such as the antioxidant nutritional agents. These compounds are readily available, nontoxic, and the usual intake varies greatly from individual to individual in the population. Furthermore, when a disease entity is the endpoint in an otherwise healthy population, the number of subjects required in a study increases exponentially when compared with the usual straightforward, clinical efficacy trials. Consequently, the answer is not going to come from a single, definitive study. Even the large clinical trials that have been accomplished suffer from criticisms primarily relating to the population enrolled in these studies. These populations are selected, not because they represent the general target population, but because it is feasible to complete these studies in the selected populations. Overall, then, our conclusions regarding putative roles for these agents will depend upon examining all the evidence derived from laboratory, animal, and clinical studies.

The goal of this book is to present an up-to-date review of the field. An attempt was made to discuss the major diseases in our population, i.e., cancer, heart disease, eye disease, and immune dysfunction, with the hope that the reader will be able to appreciate the breadth of information that exists in this field. This is an evolving field where new data will need to be considered in the context of available information. I am grateful to each of the authors who have done an outstanding job producing chapters that will be of use to readers with many different backgrounds, ranging from students and researchers to clinicians who must answer questions regarding these agents for their patients. It is my hope that a single reference that provides information on a number of disease entities will be of wide interest and benefit.

Chapter 2

THE SAFETY OF β-CAROTENE AND THE ANTIOXIDANT VITAMINS C AND E

Anthony T. Diplock

Contents

I. Introduction 3

II. β-Carotene 4

III. Vitamin C 8

IV. Vitamin E 10

References 15

I. INTRODUCTION

The possibility has arisen within the past decade that major diseases that afflict humankind worldwide may be preventable by the simple expedient of improving the dietary intake of those nutrient substances that have become called "antioxidant nutrients." The quality of diet with respect to the intake of fresh fruits and vegetables may be improved by voluntary means so that there may be a consequent decrease in the risk of disease; among the factors of these foods that may be of special benefit are the antioxidant nutrients, and a large number of other factors, for example the flavonoids, which are not regarded as nutrients (they are sometimes referred to as "non-nutrient antioxidants") but which are currently of special interest. In the present context, the antioxidant nutrients are the vitamins C and E and the carotenoids (particularly β-carotene). The definition is a convenient one that it may not be strictly valid because it assumes that the function in disease prevention of these nutrients is that of an antioxidant. This may be true in some instances, but it is necessary to make the reservation that other functions of these nutrients may be involved in their preventive role.

The idea that intervention with antioxidants may have a role to play in disease prevention is a new one. Three kinds of evidence have led to this possibility receiving serious consideration: (1) an understanding at the basic science level of the detail of the processes that may underly human disease causation, and the prevention of these factors by antioxidants; (2) the considerable body of evidence that now exists which links low dietary intake of the antioxidant nutrients with the observation of higher subsequent incidence of disease; and (3) evidence which is much more limited, that intervention by supplementation of human subjects with antioxidant nutrients may lead to lowered incidence of disease. In prospective epidemiological trials with human population groups, evidence accumulates extremely slowly, because the outcome of an intervention can only be assessed many years later in terms of disease prevention. At the present time, there are many trials in progress, or nearing completion, and conclusive evidence must await the final results of all these studies. Supplementation with the antioxidant nutrients is a practice that is undertaken voluntarily by large numbers of people throughout the world. Food quality and lifestyle, which may have altered recently, may restrict intake of these nutrients, and because of publicity about the evidence from epidemiological studies that is at present available which appears to indicate that supplements of these nutrients may lower the risk of degenerative disease in some circumstances, people around the world are opting to take supplements on a regular basis. In view of the great international interest in this topic, both among the general population and by governments, which may have major consequences for public health medicine world-wide and which has received a good deal of attention in the media, it is essential for regulatory bodies to ensure that supplements of antioxidants taken by persons in the general population are completely safe and free from side-effects. The present discussion attempts to evaluate the available evidence about the safety of vitamin E, vitamin C, and β-carotene when taken by human subjects as dietary supplements.

As a broad generalization, it is possible to say the vitamin C and E are remarkably nontoxic and that ingestion of quite large amounts daily has not been shown to have any serious toxicological consequences. β-Carotene has also been placed in the same category, and since it has been used as a colorant and a drug for many years, it has been subjected to detailed toxicological evaluation and has been found to have a very low toxicity. The publication of results of a study in Finland[1] which appears to show an increased incidence of lung cancer in heavy smokers given β-carotene supplements gave rise to anxiety as to the safety of such supplements in this population subgroup. This anxiety has been exacerbated by "results," which are said to be similar, of the CARET study[2,3] in the U.S. which were discussed early in 1996 at a press conference in Washington, D.C., the responsible agent being the National Cancer Institute of the U.S. No properly validated publication of these "results" has appeared, and it is therefore difficult to make any reasonable comment. These matters will be further considered in the appropriate section.

II. β-CAROTENE

The safety of β-carotene has been reviewed by Bendich (1988)[4] and by the present author;[5] further useful information on the absorption and metabolism of this nutrient are given in the recent review of Wang (1994).[6] β-Carotene has been used extensively as a colorant in the food and cosmetic industries and as a drug and nutrient; it has therefore been essential to conduct extensive reliable toxicity studies of this substance using an accepted range of techniques which have been agreed internationally as providing the best possible information as to the human toxicity of substances. When this was done,[7,8] the Ames test revealed no mutagenicity, a finding which was confirmed by studies using the mouse bone-marrow micronucleus test. Embryotoxicity was not found in rats and rabbits, and in a multiple-generation study in rats given up to 1 g/kg/day orally, reproductive function was normal, and there was no interference with embryonic morphology that was detectable by usual methods. A study conducted over a 2-year period in dogs revealed no tumorigenicity or chronic toxicity of any kind and in a mouse carcinogenicity study β-carotene was entirely without any discernible tumorigenic effect. In several organs of dogs and mice given high doses of β-carotene, vacuolated cells were seen but this was considered to be due to the formation of fat storage cells; this phenomenon was not dose-related and, in the absence of evidence to the contrary, it was thought to be harmless.

Detailed toxicity trials of the kind cited above were thus conducted some years ago and led to β-carotene being placed in the U.S. FDA category of Foods Generally Recognized as Safe (GRAS), both for use as a colorant in the food, drug, and cosmetic industries, and as a dietary supplement and nutrient.[9] In addition to these uses, β-carotene has been used for nearly 30 years to treat patients with genetically inherited photosensitivities; it has been reported in this context that "the ingestion of large amounts of pure β-carotene has not produced toxic side-effects."[10] Individuals taking supplements may experience some hypercarotenemia when amounts in excess of 30 mg/day are taken for extended periods, but the yellowing of the skin has been found to disappear quickly and spontaneously after discontinuing the treatment. Skin yellowing may also be seen when large amounts of carrots or products containing finely grated carrots or carrot juice are consumed by some individual subjects; this has also not been regarded as detrimental. Hypercarotenemia is an entirely benign condition, and no adverse effects have ever been reported. The largely anecdotal reports of leukopenia, reproductive disorders, increased prostatic cancer incidence, retinopathy, and allergic reactions in people taking large amounts of β-carotene have not been linked reliably to β-carotene toxicity in larger scale studies and may therefore be disregarded. None of these reports has been substantiated either in controlled clinical trials and it can therefore be concluded that no such side-effects of β-carotene ingestion need be of concern.

A short-term Phase I toxicity trial of supplemental β-carotene was carried out in a small number of human volunteers, and a progressive statistically significant decrease in serum vitamin E concentration was reported during supplementation for 9 months with 15, 30, 45, and 60 mg/day β-carotene.[11] The conclusion was reached that further studies were needed to determine how long-term β-carotene dosage might influence tissue distribution of dietary α-tocopherol. It was further suggested that careful monitoring of this and other potentially harmful nutrient interactions should become part of all long-term intervention studies, which is a view that cannot be endorsed too strongly. The question of interaction between β-carotene and α-tocopherol at the nutritional or biochemical level is one that needs careful consideration. This question had not been thought to be one that might give rise to difficulty, because earlier studies had not demonstrated any such interaction. In a study by McLarty (1992),[12] 50 mg/day β-carotene and 25,000 IU of retinol every other day were administered to 758 asbestos workers; plasma α-tocopherol levels were found to be stable after treatment for as long as 1 and 2 years. In a small study by Willett (1983),[13] 14 laboratory workers, aged 23 to 57, were supplemented with 25 mg/day β-carotene for 26 weeks. No variation in their plasma α-tocopherol level was reported. A study among 222 Finnish smokers aged 30 to 69[14] showed that 20 mg/day of β-carotene given as a supplement for 2 months caused no effect on the serum concentration of α-tocopherol. Nierenberg (1994),[15] in a randomized study of 241 participants in the Polyp Prevention Study, demonstrated no effect on serum α-tocopherol level when supplements of 25 mg/day of β-carotene, or of placebo, were given. This question has been addressed in a comprehensive substudy within the CARET study.[16] Participants, 2319 in number, given 30 mg/day β-carotene and 25,000 IU of retinol/day for up to 6 years were found to show no evidence of lowered vitamin E levels; there was, in fact, a small but statistically significant increase in the vitamin E level in the subjects who were given the β-carotene supplement. Similar results were obtained[15] when 505 subjects were given 25 mg/day β-carotene for 9 months and in a study of older women given a 90 mg β-carotene supplement for 3 weeks.[17] Although there is no satisfactory explanation available for the results of Xu (1992),[11] the balance of probability is that there is unlikely to be any interaction between β-carotene and α-tocopherol that would seriously alter the nutritional availability of vitamin E to human subjects. It is therefore possible to conclude that supplementation of normal individuals in the population with small supplements of β-carotene can be undertaken safely. The controversy with respect to a possible carotene-tocopherol interaction does however point up the importance of ensuring that all disease prevention trials involving human subjects should closely monitor serum concentrations of micronutrients, so that these can be correlated with the incidence of the disease under investigation.

Before leaving the subject of β-carotene safety, the question raised by the cancer intervention trials mentioned above must be addressed. The safety of the ingestion of moderate doses of β-carotene by heavy smokers who are at high risk of developing lung cancer has been raised by the ATBC Cancer Prevention Study in Finland.[1] This was a randomized double-blind placebo-controlled primary prevention trial in 29,133 Finnish male subjects, aged between 50 to 69 years; the criterion for entry into the study was that the subjects were habitual heavy smokers who had smoked on average 20 cigarettes/day for an average of 36 years, and none of the subjects had any clinical signs of lung cancer, or other degenerative diseases, at entry to the study. The objective was to determine the effect on subsequent lung cancer incidence of daily supplements of either 50 mg α-tocopherol, 20 mg β-carotene, both nutrients together, or a placebo. Among 876 new cases of lung cancer that occurred during the trial, there was no reduction in incidence of disease as judged by valid clinical parameters in subjects given α-tocopherol. There was however a statistically significant 18% higher incidence of lung cancer in those subjects given β-carotene (402 subjects with placebo vs. 474 subjects with β-carotene).

The design of the CARET study is given in a paper by Omenn et al. (1991).[2] The study was stopped in January 1996 by agreement between the U.S. National Cancer Institute and the responsible researchers, and the reasons communicated to the press in a conference called on the 18th of January. No proper report has yet appeared* of the results of this study, and it is not therefore possible to comment objectively about it. However, in view of the widespread concern that is currently being expressed as to the likely adverse effect of β-carotene in heavy smokers, it is necessary to attempt to address the question with the limited data that are available. The subjects were 14,254 current and former smokers with a long history of smoking and 4060 asbestos-exposed individuals (a total of 18,314 participants). The subjects were men and women aged 50 to 69 and smoking history required that they had smoked at least one pack of 20 cigarettes per day for at least 20 years (called 20 pack years); the average smoking history was 50 pack years of smoking. The asbestos workers were aged 45 to 69 years, and the criterion was extensive occupational exposure to asbestos beginning at least 15 years earlier, and they had to be either current smokers, or to have quit smoking recently. One half of the participants in both groups were given 30 mg of β-carotene and 25,000 IU of retinyl palmitate per day, and the other half received a placebo. After an average of 4 years of receiving these supplements, 28% more cases of lung cancer were diagnosed in the group taking the supplements than in those taking the placebo, and 17% more deaths occurred in the participants taking the supplements. The study was accordingly terminated early on ethical grounds.

Both the studies described above were conducted among free-living subjects whose chief characteristic was that they were likely to have a high risk of developing lung cancer during the course of the study. With an extensive background of epidemiological studies that indicated a negative correlation between intake or plasma level of β-carotene and lung cancer morbidity, the studies were expected to demonstrate a beneficial effect of supplementation with β-carotene. Clearly, the reverse is what was found. A possible explanation of these studies lies in an understanding of the cancer process; initiation of carcinogenesis first involves mutation of DNA structure which is usually repaired without noticeable detrimental effect to the subject concerned. Promotion and progression of cancer is a process that is thought to take many years and only when a mutation becomes established do the cells concerned become transformed and does true cancer develop. The subjects in the two β-carotene intervention studies could be expected to have moved some distance along the carcinogenic road before the intervention was applied, and it must therefore be considered that the intervention with β-carotene may have caused an exacerbation of a late, or very late, stage of the carcinogenic process. It is highly likely that antioxidants and β-carotene, if they do indeed lower the incidence of cancer, may do so by intervention at an early stage of the process of cancer causation, and that thus, with hindsight, it might be expected to be unlikely that intervention at a later stage would have a beneficial effect.

The public health implications with respect to β-carotene safety are considerable. Although as has been demonstrated above β-carotene has been shown to have a very low toxicity when judged by conventional toxicological methodology, the finding in subjects of high cancer risk of an apparent exacerbatory effect on cancer must be taken very seriously. The health benefits of consuming fruit and vegetable foods in

---

* Details of this study have recently appeared in Omenn et al. (1996) *New Engl. J. Med.* 334, 1150–1155. This report does not alter the conclusions reached here.

terms of cancer prevention are established and accepted,[18] and it is clear that many of these foods contain high levels of carotenoids, and that lung cancer in particular benefits from a high level of intake of such foods. Clearly, there is no suggestion of an adverse effect of consuming such foods even though extreme attention to such a practice might lead to levels of β-carotene intake approaching those used as supplements in the studies described above. The balance of probability is that β-carotene supplementation at levels up to 10 to 12 mg per day is entirely safe; until further work clarifies the situation in heavy smokers with respect to taking supplements, these should be avoided by these individuals. β-Carotene should remain a major candidate for the *prevention* of disease *de novo,* and the ATBC study "illustrates the pitfalls of relying on clinical trials to answer questions about the benefits of nutrients in disease prevention" (G. Block, 1994, personal communication).

III. VITAMIN C

There have been three reviews within the past 14 years that address the question of the tolerance and safety of ingestion by human subjects of large amounts of vitamin C.[5,19,20] Despite this, an exhaustive literature review by the present author has failed to reveal the existence of a placebo-controlled double-blind human study of this important question. Overload of ascorbic acid is unlikely to occur in humans even at very high levels of dietary intake;[20] this is because physiological mechanisms control ascorbic acid absorption, tissue concentrations, metabolic pathways in which ascorbate participates, and elimination of the vitamin by the kidney. Size of dose and the percentage absorbed are in an inverse relationship in humans and saturation kinetics with a K_m of 5.44 mM were demonstrated by a study using intestinal perfusion of vitamin C which was able to control these parameters precisely.[21] In the guinea pig, tissue levels of ascorbate increased very little[22] when massive doses of vitamin C were given; the small increase that was detected, which was not statistically significant, was thought to be due to ascorbate that was trapped in the extracellular fluid. There is without a doubt a consistent body pool size of ascorbate in humans of about 20 mg/kg body weight which is maintained by homeostatic mechanisms irrespective of intake; this mechanism has been shown to continue to operate even at very high levels of intake.[23]

The existing body of knowledge about the toxicology of vitamin C in animals was reviewed in detail by Hanck (1982),[19] who concluded from a very large body of extensive evidence that the acute, subacute, chronic, and subchronic toxicity of the vitamin is extremely low. Indeed Hanck (1982) concluded that vitamin C is very well tolerated by animals over a wide range of intake, with very few reported side-effects, none of which have been shown to be consistent and may therefore be disregarded. Possible adverse health effects in human subjects have been published occasionally, but exhaustive study of each by the present author and by others has failed to substantiate the reported toxic effect. However, despite the absence of such validation, in public health terms it is important to consider each with care so that a reasoned argument may be advanced about each claim that has been made. Thus, the formation of urinary oxalate stones in subjects ingesting large amounts of vitamin C over a long period was alleged and was for a time a cause of anxiety; this has, however, proved to be without foundation. Human subjects have been shown not to metabolize ascorbate to carbon dioxide, in contrast to the guinea pig which uses this metabolic pathway; the guinea pig is not therefore a useful model in this instance. Human excretion is mainly as unchanged ascorbate although this is accompanied by the urinary excretion of a range of metabolites, among which is oxalate; the important point is that intake of ascorbate at levels in excess of the level which is required to maintain plasma levels at about 10 mg/L is accompanied by excretion of the excess ascorbate unchanged.[23] Excretion of oxalate derived from ascorbate accounts for a constant amount of approximately 35 to 40% of the total daily excretion of oxalate, but ingestion of large amounts of vitamin C does not result in any more than a very small increase in the excretion of oxalate. The work of Schmidt (1981)[24] shows that there is no dose-response relationship at all between administered vitamin C and excreted oxalate and that the relatively constant daily excretion of oxalate is unaffected by increasing the intake of ascorbate over a very wide range. It can be stated unequivocally with the hindsight of a number of years that the explanation of the difference between more recent results and those of earlier workers is that in the early experiments the alkalinity of urine samples, that arises on standing, caused some conversion of ascorbate to oxalate, and that therefore the conversion *in vivo* of ascorbate to oxalate is minimal.[25] Similar anxieties were expressed some years ago with regard to urate excretion; it was suggested that ascorbate might therefore indirectly exacerbate the effect of urate on gout. There are two human studies that demonstrate that in healthy subjects ascorbate ingestion has no effect on the excretion of urate.[24,26] Furthermore, when high nonphysiological plasma levels of ascorbate were induced by continuous intravenous infusion of ascorbate in gouty, as compared to normal subjects,[27] there was little effect on the clearance of urate. This has been accepted as indicating that it is highly improbable that high dietary intake of ascorbate has any effect on the urinary excretion of urate in subjects with gout, and indeed the anecdotal experience of subjects with gout is that a high intake of ascorbate causes no discernable exacerbation of their condition.

It was reported by Herbert (1974)[28] that low plasma levels of vitamin B_{12} occurred in subjects who were taking large doses of ascorbic acid. This was, however, shown to be explained by analytical error. Low levels of plasma vitamin B_{12} can be reported in error if no cyanide is added to the assay to liberate protein-bound cobalamins and to stabilize the cobalamins so released;[29,30] this was the case in the work of Herbert (1974). It can therefore be concluded with confidence that high levels of intake of ascorbate in human subjects has no effect on plasma vitamin B_{12} levels. High ascorbic acid intake has also been shown to have no effect on iron absorption in healthy iron replete subjects which repudiates suggestions that iron overload could be a consequence of high ascorbate intake.[31] The regulation of body iron stores has been shown unequivocally not to be affected by ascorbate intake, which might be thought to cause increased availability of iron from the diet because of a chemical interaction between ascorbate and iron in the gastrointestinal tract. Even in patients with hemochromatosis, there is almost no effect of vitamin C. Cochrane (1965) and Rhead (1971)[32,33] reported what they interpreted as rebound scurvy in a small number of subjects following withdrawal of high vitamin C supplements. These studies were uncontrolled and have not been substantiated by more detailed studies designed to investigate this possibility. Studies in guinea pigs showed no evidence for these claims even when the study was designed to demonstrate a rebound effect. There was no increased catabolism of ascorbate during high vitamin C dosage, nor was there any such increase when the vitamin C dosage was abruptly withdrawn.[34,35] The human data available remain less clear cut and even somewhat contradictory, and there is a need for a definitive resolution of this question. However, evidence available at present leads one to conclude that the phenomenon, if it exists at all, does not constitute a significant problem, which could impinge on the public health arena.

There are many reports in the literature that indicate that ascorbic acid added to cells *in vitro* in culture increases the rate of mutagenesis (see, for example, Reference 20 for a review). Several detailed reports exist of increased DNA strand breakage, increased DNA repair, and a range of chromosome aberrations in cells cultured in media that include added ascorbate. However, these effects were only demonstrated in cultures that contained added Cu^{2+} or Fe^{3+} ions as part of the culture medium. When, however, steps were taken to ensure very low levels of these metals in the culture medium, no detrimental effect on DNA was observed. This is an important observation which requires frequent restatement because the public health implications of an alleged mutagenic effect of ascorbate are very serious. It can be concluded that in any such system *in vitro* the apparent mutagenic effect of ascorbate is most likely to be due to an ascorbate/metal ion-driven generation of oxygen-derived free radicals which cause the DNA damage. There is ample evidence that oxygen-derived free radicals are generated under such circumstances and that they have a mutagenic effect if this is not subject to any control.[36] There is no evidence of ascorbate-induced mutagenicity *in vivo,* so it is highly improbable that any effect that depends on metal ion-driven generation of free radicals caused by ascorbate has any significance. Efficient free radical-scavenging systems protect DNA *in vivo* from such effects, and intracellular concentrations of ascorbate, and metals which are efficiently sequestered on binding proteins, are so low as to be unlikely to be harmful.[37]

The conclusion from an exhaustive survey of the literature is that oral intake of high, or even very high, levels of vitamin C are safe and entirely free from side-effects. No consistently proven adverse effect of ascorbate on human health has ever been recorded.

IV. VITAMIN E

There have been three reliable reviews about the toxicological safety of oral intake of vitamin E in human subjects.[5,38,39] It therefore is not necessary to rehearse here again all the detail which is available but only to refer to the salient points in these reviews where full details can be found. The tables given here are taken from Diplock (1995)[5] and the original references that refer to each of the points quoted are given in that review. Study of conventional aspects of the toxicity of vitamin E in animals was undertaken by many workers over a long period of time, and Table 2.1 gives details of several of the subacute and subchronic toxicity studies that have been carried out.[40-45] There is no evidence of any detrimental effect attributable to vitamin E, and similar conclusions are possible with respect to the teratogenicity and reproductive toxicity of vitamin E in animals at even large levels of intake of

TABLE 2.1
Studies on Subacute and Subchronic Toxicity of Vitamin E

Species	Route	Dose	Duration	Result
Rat	Oral	130 mg/kg/day	2 mo	No abnormalities
Rat	Oral	100 mg/day	4 mo	Small increase in P metabolism only
Rat	Oral	10 mg/day	4 mo	No abnormalities
Rat	Feed	500 mg/kg diet	1 mo	Small effect on liver triglycerides
Rat	Feed	875, 1750 mg/kg	3 mo	No abnormalities
Rat	Feed	0.002, 0.2% in diet	3 mo	No abnormalities
Rat	Gavage	125,500 mg/kg	3 mo	No abnormalities
		2000 mg/kg	3 mo	Extended prothrombin time

TABLE 2.2
Studies on Teratogenesis and Reproductive Toxicity of Vitamin E

Species	Route	Dose	Duration	Result
Rat	In feed	0.002, 0.2, and 2.0%	Days 6 to 16 of pregnancy	No difference between treatment and placebo groups.
Rat	In feed	0.002, 0.2, and 2.0%	F_1 generation: mated on days 112 and 175 of dosage. F_0 generation: treated until day 268.	No effects on reproductive toxicity or teratogenicity. Clinical and haematological parameters normal.
Mouse	Gavage	591 IU/mouse	Days 7 to 11 of pregnancy	One malformation among 91 mice.

the vitamin. A summary of some of the available studies is given in Table 2.2, which is based on References 44 and 46.

The possibility that vitamin E might have anticlastogenic effects has been studied extensively and its potential mutagenicity was tested in several different ways. Thus, in cultures of Salmonella, there was a significant decrease in the presence of vitamin E in the formation of point mutations induced by malondialdehyde and beta-propionolactone.[47] Using a standard sex-linked recessive lethal test in Drosophila, vitamin E was without effect on the mutation rate in irradiated male animals. However, after mating with females raised on a diet containing vitamin E, there was a significant lowering of the rate of sex-linked recessive lethal mutations in subsequent generations.[48] The mutagenicity of vitamin E was also tested *in vitro* in human lymphocytes. No induction of chromosomal damage was found nor was an increase in sister chromatid exchange rates.[49] Vitamin E has thus been conclusively demonstrated to have no mutagenic properties, but it indeed appears to have some effect in reversing the mutagenic effects of other compounds. Early literature suggested that impure factions containing vitamin E had tumor-promoting capability. There is a very large body of evidence that refutes this claim in studies where pure compounds were used; the explanation of the earlier papers is that the extracts used probably contained other impurities that were themselves carcinogenic. Table 2.3 shows a summary of some of the available evidence[50,51] and demonstrates that, even at very

TABLE 2.3
Studies on Chronic Toxicity and Carcinogenicity of Vitamin E

Species	Route	Dose	Duration	Result
Rat	In feed	500, 1000, 2000 mg/kg/day	24 mo	No significant effects on a range of clinical chemical parameters. Slight increase in liver weight and in liver enzymes in serum. Hemhorrage (anti-vitamin K effect). *Decrease* in mammary tumors.
Rat	In feed	25, 250, 2500, 10,000 and 25,000 IU/kg	8 to 16 mo	No abnormalities at low doses. Increase in serum alkaline phosphatase and relative heart and spleen weight at high doses. No change in prothrombin time. No carcinogenicity.

high levels of inclusion in the feed, vitamin E has not been shown to have any carcinogenic activity.

There are very large numbers of reports in the literature that deal with, or purport to deal with, the toxicity in human subjects of vitamin E. Among these many reports, there are different levels of reliability that can be attributed to them. Published reports include those that describe single observations carried out on one subject, and studies that are planned and which may or may not include placebo groups, but which may include bias because they lack blinding. There are fewer, highly reliable studies which have been planned with all necessary rigor: these include sufficient numbers of subjects to enable proper statistical evaluation of the results, they use placebo groups, and they use careful double-blinding of the *modus operandi,* so as to ensure that the results obtained are valid and reliable. Fortunately sufficient such studies have been undertaken to enable an authoritative view of the human toxicity, or lack of toxicity, of vitamin E. It is strange, however, to observe that the most frequently cited observations in the literature are those that appear to have the least scientific rigor and validity. There are nevertheless a few studies which, despite the fact that they do not have adequate controls, are of some interest and three of these[52-54] are cited in Table 2.4. No consistent adverse effects of vitamin E emerge from these uncontrolled studies cited by Kappus and Diplock (1992).[39] However, the study of Corrigan (1982)[54] highlights the possibility that vitamin E supplementation may aggravate the vitamin K deficiency that results from Warfarin anticoagulant therapy and this point is discussed further later.

With regard to controlled double-blinded studies of vitamin E toxicity in humans, there are several reports which show conclusively that vitamin E has very low toxicity in human subjects with no consistent adverse effects being reported. Table 2.5 gives details of a number of such studies.[55-61] Some adverse effects were observed on prothrombin time, or on other factors associated with blood clotting. Kappus and Diplock (1992)[39] reviewed this question carefully and noted that in several studies no effect was observed on blood clotting whereas in other studies there was a marked effect of vitamin E on some aspect of blood-clotting mechanistics. It was concluded, following a study of all the reports available, that vitamin E

TABLE 2.4
Studies with Oral Vitamin E in Human Subjects Without Strict Controls

Subjects	Dose/substance	Duration	Result
28 adults	100 to 800 IU/day: "tocopherol"	4 months to 21 years (mean 2.9 y)	No evidence of toxicity judged by clinical chemical blood parameters (blood coagulation, liver enzymes and thyroid hormones, etc.).
10 adults	800 mg/day *All rac-*α-tocopheryl acetate	4 weeks	No adverse effects judged by clinical chemical parameters.
12 Warfarin-treated cardiology patients	100 to 400 IU *All rac-*α-tocopherol	4 weeks	Warfarin effect (vitamin K antagonism) was aggravated.

TABLE 2.5
Double-Blind Controlled Studies with Oral Vitamin E in Human Subjects

Subjects	Dosage	Duration	Results
75 cardiac patients	200 mg/day *all rac-*α-tocopheryl nicotinate	4 to 6 weeks	No differences between groups
202 volunteers	600 IU/day *all rac-*α-tocopheryl acetate	4 weeks	Serum T_3 and T_4 lower; triglycerides lower and cholesterol raised in women (no effect was statistically significant). No other effects.
30 volunteers	800 IU/day "vitamin E"	16 weeks	No differences between groups
19 volunteers	600 mg/day RRR-α-tocopherol	12 weeks	No objective or subjective adverse effects. (Clinical chemical parameters, liver kidney and thyroid function, serum lipids, prothrombin time, urinary parameters, all normal.)
52 angina pectoris patients	1600 IU per day RRR-α-tocopheryl succinate	6 months	No objective or subjective adverse effects. (Clinical chemical blood parameters, prothrombin time, urinary parameters normal.)
25 diabetics	2000 IU/day *All rac-*α-tocopheryl acetate	6 weeks	No subjective or objective adverse effects. (Blood parameters, e.g., cholesterol, T_3, T_4, blood coagulation, all normal.)
36 angina pectoris patients	3200 IU/day RRR-α-tocopheryl succinate	9 weeks	No subjective or objective adverse effects except some gastrointestinal disturbance.

at a high level of intake may affect the coagulation parameters if a low level of vitamin K is also present. The conclusion was thus that an underlying vitamin K deficiency level which is just tolerable, and which may be without symptoms, may be exacerbated following administration of vitamin E so that symptoms now become apparent. It is therefore clear that vitamin E cannot be recommended for administration under these conditions, which may have been caused by intestinal malabsorption in the subject concerned or by anticoagulant therapy that may have been administered. Alternatively administration of vitamin E must be accompanied by concomitant administration of vitamin K. It is important to recognize that vitamin E does not by itself cause coagulation abnormalities in persons who have no coagulation abnormalities, and that in such individuals who are the majority of the population, vitamin E supplementation is entirely free from adverse effects.

There is a wide range of levels of administration that have been recommended for human vitamin E intake. This range, which has arisen because those making recommendations have different goals, extends from the small amount that is considered necessary to prevent deficiency, through somewhat larger amounts that may be thought necessary to prevent degenerative disease, to the very large amounts that, it has been claimed with very limited verification, have a range of "therapeutic" effects. In public health terms, therefore, it must be appreciated that much larger levels of intake than those currently shown to have health benefit may be taken voluntarily by members of the public, and it is important that they should be safeguarded as well as those taking more modest levels of intake of the vitamin.

The following conclusions were reached[5,39] with respect to the safety of oral intake of vitamin E by human subjects.

1. The toxicity of vitamin E is very low.
2. Animal studies show vitamin E is not mutagenic, carcinogenic, or teratogenic.
3. Reported increases in serum lipids in human subjects following high oral dosage are inconsistent and of little significance.
4. In double-blind human studies, oral dosage resulted in few side-effects, even at a dosage as high as 3.2 g per day.
5. Dosage up to 1000 mg per day is considered to be entirely safe and without side-effects.
6. Oral intake of high levels of vitamin E can exacerbate the blood coagulation defect of vitamin K deficiency caused by malabsorption or anticoagulant therapy, and high vitamin E intake is contra-indicated in these subjects.

Some anxiety has been expressed[62] as to the safety of long-term ingestion of amounts of vitamin E in doses of 100 mg per day which were found[63,64] to confer significant protection against the risk of coronary artery disease. Higher doses than this (up to about 500 mg of vitamin E daily) have also recently been shown to confer benefit in subjects with angiographically proven cardiovascular disease.[65] While it is not possible at present to state categorically that oral ingestion of these amounts, during 5, 10, or 20 years, of vitamin E is entirely safe, because no one has been able to test the toxicity of the vitamin over such long periods, application of the premise universally in a prospective manner would result in the removal from the pharmacopoeia of most drugs currently on the market because their toxicity has not been evaluated at high dosage in human subjects over long periods of time. The ultimate test of any drug or other therapeutic agent must be in the human clinical situation, following careful toxicological evaluation in a range of animals, followed by close detailed study with clinical supervision in human subjects. These criteria have all been applied with considerable rigor to vitamin E, and common sense tells us that not only will long-term supplementation prove to be free from harmful side-effects but that this may also convey considerable health benefit.

REFERENCES

1. ATBC. The effect of vitamin E and beta carotene on the incidence of lung cancer and other cancers in male smokers. *New Engl. J. Med.* 1994, 330, 1029.
2. Omenn, G.S., Goodman, G., Grizzle, J., Thornquist, M., Rosenstock, L., Barnhart, S., et al. CARET, the beta-carotene and retinol efficacy trial to prevent lung cancer in asbestos-exposed workers and in smokers. *Anticancer Drugs* 1991, 2(1), 79.
3. Omenn, G.S., Goodman, G.E., Thornquist, M.D., Rosenstock, L., Barnhart, S., Gylys-Colwell, I., et al. The Carotene and Retinol Efficacy Trial (CARET) to prevent lung cancer in high-risk populations: pilot study with asbestos-exposed workers. *Cancer Epidemiology, Biomarkers & Prevention* 1993, 2(4), 381.
4. Bendich, A., The safety of beta-carotene. *Nutrit. Cancer* 1988, 11, 207.
5. Diplock, A.T., Safety of antioxidant vitamins and β-carotene. *Am. J. Clin. Nutr.* 1995, 62 (Suppl), 1510S.
6. Wang, X.D., Review: absorption and metabolism of beta-carotene. *J. Amer. Coll. Nutr.* 1994, 13, 314.
7. Bagdon, R.E., Zbinden, G., and Studer, A., Chronic toxicity studies of beta-carotene. *Toxicol. Appl. Pharmacol.* 1960, 2, 225.
8. Heywood, R., Palmer, A.K., Gregson, R.L., and Hummler, H., The toxicity of beta-carotene. *Toxicology* 1985, 36, 91.
9. Office LSR. Evaluation of the health aspects of carotene (β-carotene) as a food ingredient. *FASEB Bethesda MD, U.S.A.* 1979; Contract Number (FDA) 223-75-2004.
10. Matthews-Roth, M.M., Beta-carotene therapy for erythropoetic protoporphyria and other photo-sensitivity diseases. *Biochemie.* 1986, 68, 875.
11. Xu, M.J., Plezia, P.M., Alberts, D.S., Emerson, S.S., Peng, Y.M., Sayers, S.M., et al. Reduction in plasma or skin alpha-tocopherol concentration with long-term oral administration of beta-carotene in humans and mice. *J. Natl. Cancer Inst.* 1992, 84(20), 1559.
12. McLarty, J.W., An intervention trial in high-risk asbestos-exposed persons. In: Newell, G.R. and Hongs, W.K., Editors. *The Biology and Prevention of Aerodigestive Tract Cancer.* New York: Plenum Press Inc., 1992, 141.
13. Willett, W.C., Stampfer, M.J., Underwood, B.A., Taylor, J.O., and Hennekens, C.H., Vitamins A, E and carotene: effect of supplementation on their plasma levels. *Amer. J. Clin. Nutr.* 1983; 38, 559.
14. Albanes, D., Virtamo, J., Rautalahti, M., Haukka, J., Palmgren, J., Gref, C.G., et al. Serum β-carotene before and after β-carotene supplementation. *Eur. Clin. Nutr.* 1992, 46, 15.
15. Nierenberg, D.W., Stukel, T.A., Mott, L.A., and Greenberg, E.R., Steady-state serum concentration of alpha tocopherol not altered by supplementation with oral beta carotene. The Polyp Prevention Study 1 Group. *J. Natl. Cancer Inst.* 1994, 86(2), 117.
16. Goodman, G.E., Metch, B.J., and Omenn, G.S., The effect of long-term beta carotene and vitamin A administration on serum concentrations of alpha-tocopherol. *Cancer Epidemiol. Biomarkers Prevent.* 1994, 3, 429.
17. Ribaya-Mercado, J.D., Ordovas, J.M., and Russell, R.M., Effect of beta-carotene supplementation on the concentrations and distribution of carotenoids, vitamin E, vitamin A and cholesterol in plasma lipoprotein and non-lipoprotein fractions in healthy older women. *J. Amer. Coll. Nutr.* 1995, 14, 614.
18. Block, G., Patterson, B., and Subar, A., Fruit vegetables and cancer prevention: a review of the epidemiological evidence. *Nutr. Cancer* 1992, 18, 1.

19. Hanck, A., Tolerance and effects of high doses of ascorbic acid. Dosis facit venenum. *Int. J. Vitam. Nutr. Res. Suppl.* 1982, 23, 221.
20. Rivers, J.M., Safety of high-level vitamin C ingestion. *Int. J. Vitam. Nutr. Res. Suppl.* 1989, 30, 95.
21. Nelson, E.W., Lane, H., Fabri, P.J., and Scott, B., Demonstration of saturation kinetics in the intestinal absorption of vitamin C in man and the guinea pig. *J. Clin. Pharmacol.* 1978, 18, 325.
22. Sorensen, D.I., Devine, M.M., and Rivers, J.M., Catabolism and tissue levels of ascorbic acid following long-term massive doses in the guinea pig. *J. Nutr.* 1974, 104, 1041.
23. Kallner, A., Hartmann, D., and Hornig, D., Steady-state turnover and body pool of ascorbic acid in man. *Am. J. Clin. Nutr.* 1979, 32, 530.
24. Schmidt, K.H., Hagmaier, V., Hornig, D.H., Vuilleumier, J.P., and Rutishauser, G., Urinary oxalate excretion after large intakes of ascorbic acid in man. *Amer. J. Clin. Nutr.* 1981, 34, 305.
25. Wandzilak, T.R., D'Andre, S.D., Davis, P.A., and Williams, H.E., Effect of high dose vitamin C on urinary oxalate levels. *J. Urol.* 1994, 151(4), 834.
26. Mitch, W.E., Johnson, M.W., Kirshenbaum, J.M., and Lopez, R.E., Effect of large oral doses of ascorbic acid on uric acid excretion by normal subjects. *Clin. Pharmacol. Therp.* 1981, 29, 318.
27. Berger, L., Gerson, C.D., and Yu, T.F., The effect of ascorbic acid on uric acid excretion with a commentary on the renal handling of ascorbic acid. *Amer. J. Med.* 1977, 62, 71.
28. Herbert, V. and Hacob, E., Destruction of vitamin B_{12} by ascorbic acid. *J. Amer. Med. Assoc.* 1974, 230, 241.
29. Newmark, H.L., Scheiner, J., Markus, M., and Prabhudesai, M., Stability of vitamin B_{12} in the presence of ascorbic acid. *Amer. J. Clin. Nutr.* 1976, 29, 645.
30. Markus, M., Prabhudesai, M., and Wassef, S., Stability of vitamin B_{12} in the presence of ascorbic acid in food and serum: restoration by cyanide of apparent loss. *Am. J. Clin. Nutr.* 1980, 33.
31. Cook, J.D., Watson, S.S., Simpson, K.H., Lipschitz, D.A., and Skikne, B.S., The effect of high ascorbic acid supplementation on body iron stores. *Blood* 1984, 64, 721.
32. Cochrane, H.A., Overnutrition in prenatal life: a problem? *Canad. Med. Assoc. J.* 1965, 93, 893.
33. Rhead, W.A. and Schrauzer, G.N., Risks of long-term ascorbic acid overdosage. *Nutr. Rev.* 1971, 29, 262.
34. Norkus, E.P. and Rosso, P., Changes in the ascorbic acid metabolism of the offspring following high maternal intake of this vitamin in the pregnant guinea pig. *Ann. New York Acad. Sci.* 1975, 258, 401.
35. Norkus, E.P. and Rosso, P., Effects of maternal intake of ascorbic acid on the postnatal metabolism of this vitamin in the guinea pig. *J. Nutr.* 1981, 111, 624.
36. Dizdaroglou, M., Chemistry of free radical damage to DNA and nucleoproteins. In: Halliwell, B., Aruoma, O.I., Editors. *DNA and Free Radicals.* New York and London: Ellis Horwood, 1993, 19.
37. Halliwell, B. and Aruoma, O.I., *DNA and Free Radicals.* 1st ed. New York, London: Ellis Horwood, 1993.
38. Bendich, A. and Machlin, L.J., Safety of oral intake of vitamin E. *Amer. J. Clin. Nutr.* 1988, 48, 642.
39. Kappus, H. and Diplock, A.T., Tolerance and safety of vitamin E: a toxicological position report. *Free Rad. Biol. Med.* 1992, 13(1), 55.
40. Demole, V., Pharmakologisches über vitamin E. *Int. Z. Vitaminforsch.* 1939, 8, 338.
41. Weissberger, L.H. and Harris, P.L., Effect of tocopherols on phosphorus metabolism. *J. Biol. Chem.* 1943, 151, 543.
42. Levander, O.A., Morris, V.C., Higgs, D.J., and Varma, R.N., Nutritional relationships among vitamin E, selenium, antioxidants and ethyl alcohol in the rat. *J. Nutr.* 1973, 103, 536.
43. Dysma, H.A. and Park, J., Excess dietary vitamin E in rats. *Fed. Am. Soc. Exp. Biol.* 1975, 34, 912.
44. Krasavage, W.J. and Terhaar, C.J., D-alpha-tocopheryl-polyethyleneglycol 1000 succinate. Acute toxicity, subchronic feeding, reproduction and teratologic studies in the rat. *J. Sci. Agrc.* 1977, 25, 273.
45. Abdo, K.M., Rao, G., and Montgomery, C.A., Thirteen week toxicity study of D-alpha-tocopheryl acetate (vitamin E) in Fischer 344 rats. *Fd. Chem. Toxicol.* 1986, 24, 1043.
46. Hook, E.B., Healey, K.M., Niles, A.M., and Shalko, R.C., Vitamin E: teratogen or anti-teratogen? *Lancet* 1974, 809.

47. Shamberger, R.J., Corlett, C.L., Beaman, K.D., and Kasten, B.L., Antioxidants reduce the mutagenic effect of malonaldehyde and beta-propiolactone. Part IX, Antioxidants and cancer. *Mut. Res.* 1979, 66, 349.
48. Beckmann, C., Roy, R.M., and Sproule, A., Modification of radiation-induced sex-linked recessive lethal mutation frequency by tocopherol. *Mut. Res.* 1982, 105, 73.
49. Gebhart, E., Wagner, H., Grziwok, K., and Behnsen, M., The actions of anticlastogens in human lymphocyte cultures and their modification by rat liver S9 mix. Chap. II, Studies with vitamins C and E. *Mut. Res.* 1985, 149, 83.
50. Weldon, G.H., Bhatt, A., Keller, P., and Hummler, H., dl-α-Tocopheryl acetate (vitamin E): a long-term toxicity and carcinogenicity study in rats. *Int. J. Vit. Nutr. Res.* 1983, 53, 287.
51. Yang, N.Y. and Desai, I.D., Effect of high levels of dietary vitamin E on hematological indices and biochemical parameters in rats. *J. Nutr.* 1977, 107, 1410.
52. Farrell, P.M. and Bieri, J.G., Megavitamin E supplementation in man. *Am. J. Clin. Nutr.* 1975, 28, 1381.
53. Ernst, E. and Matrai, A., Einfluss von alpha-tocopherol (Vitamin E) auf die fliesseigenschaft des blutes. *Therapiewoche* 1985, 35, 5701.
54. Corrigan, J.J., The effect of vitamin E on Warfarin-induced vitamin K deficiency. *Ann. N.Y. Acad. Sci.* 1982, 393, 361.
55. Inagaki, Y., Kinoshita, M.O., Nakamura, Y., and Masuda, Y.A., Double-blind controlled study of the efficacy of DL-α-tocopherylnicotinate in patients with vascular disease. In: DeDuve, C. and Hayashi, O., Editors. *Tocopherol, Oxygen and Biomembranes.* Amsterdam, New York: Elsevier-North Holland Biomedical Press, 1978, 338.
56. Tsai, A.C., Kelly, J.J., Peng, B., and Cook, N., Study on the effect of megavitamin supplementation in man. *Am. J. Clin. Nutr.* 1978, 31, 831.
57. Stampfer, M.J., Willet, W., Castelli, W.P., Taylor, J.O., Fine, J., and Hennekens, V.H., Effect of vitamin E on lipids. *Am. J. Clin. Nutr.* 1983, 79, 714.
58. Kitagawa, M. and Mino, M., Effects of elevated D-α-(RRR)-tocopherol dosage in man. *J. Nutr. Sci. Vitaminol.* 1989, 35, 133.
59. Gillian, R.E., Mondell, B., and Warbasse, J.R., Quantitative evaluation of vitamin E in the treatment of angina pectoris. *Am. Heart J.* 1977, 93, 444.
60. Bierenbaum, M.L., Noonan, F.J., Machlin, L.J., Machlin, S., Stier, A., Watson, P.B., et al. The effect of supplemental vitamin E on serum parameters in diabetics, postcoronary and normal subjects. *Nutr. Res. Internat.* 1985, 31, 1171.
61. Anderson, T.W. and Reid, D.B., A double-blind trial of vitamin E in angina pectoris. *Am. J. Clin. Nutr.* 1974, 27, 1174.
62. Steinberg, D., Antioxidant vitamins and coronary heart disease [editorial; comment]. *N. Engl. J. Med.* 1993, 328(20), 1487.
63. Stampfer, M.J., Hennekens, C.H., Manson, J.E., Colditz, G.A., Rosner, B., and Willett, W.C., Vitamin E consumption and the risk of coronary disease in women. *N. Engl. J. Med.* 1993, 328(20), 1444.
64. Rimm, E.B., Stampfer, M.J., Ascherio, A., Giovannucci, E., Colditz, G.A., and Willett, W.C., Vitamin E consumption and the risk of coronary heart disease in men. *N. Engl. J. Med.* 1993, 328(20), 1450.
65. Stephens, N.G., Parsons, A., Schofield, P.M., Kelly, F., Cheeseman, K., and Mitchinson, M.J., Randomised controlled trial of vitamin E in patients with coronary disease: Cambridge Heart Antioxidant Study (CHAOS). *Lancet* 1996, 347, 781.

Chapter 3

ANTIOXIDANTS AND IMMUNE FUNCTION

Paula F. Inserra, Sussan K. Ardestani, and Ronald Ross Watson

Contents

I. Free Radicals, Antioxidants, and Immune Function 19
   A. Introduction 19
   B. Antioxidants: Mechanism of Action 21
      1. Antioxidant Enzymes 21
      2. Antioxidant Compounds 22
   C. Immune Function and Free Radical Reactions 22
      1. Effect of Free Radicals on Immune Cells 22
      2. Free Radicals and T-Cell Activation 22
      3. Free Radicals and Cytokine Production 23
      4. Summary 25
   D. Antioxidant Nutrients and Immune Function 26
      1. Effect of Antioxidants on Nonspecific Immune Responses 26
      2. Effect of Antioxidants on Specific Immune Responses 26
   E. Summary 26

Acknowledgments 27

References 27

I. FREE RADICALS, ANTIOXIDANTS, AND IMMUNE FUNCTION

A. INTRODUCTION

Free radicals, reactive oxygen species (ROS), are produced during normal cellular metabolism by oxidation. It is the primary means by which humans and other animals derive energy. Oxidant catalysts provide the stable electrons that are necessary for oxidation. The most common biological oxidant catalysts are copper and iron, with iron being most abundant and most readily available. As electrons are transferred from oxidant catalysts to oxygen, a variety of new oxygen species are formed, each characterized by an unpaired set of electrons in their outer orbital. Therefore, one free radical can begin a destructive process of removing electrons from stable compounds and forming many ROS, transforming stable compounds into a variety of free radicals (Table 3.1). Other sources of free radicals are also

TABLE 3.1
Free Radicals Produced by the Reduction
of Dioxygen and by Ionizing Radiation,
Reactive Metals, Enzymes, and Other
Endogenous and Environmental Initiators

.O^{2-}	Superoxide
HO_2-	Superoxide conjugate acid
$1O_2$	Singlet oxygen
.OH	Hydroxyl radical
R.	Organic free radical
ROO	Peroxy free radical

common: inflammation, strenuous exercise, detoxification, exposure to certain chemicals, radiation, ultraviolet light, alcohol, cigarette smoke, air pollutants, excess free calcium, excess stored or unbound iron, and high fat diets.

ROS are toxic via their effects on cellular components such as denaturing proteins, membrane lipids, and DNA. The latter is a major initiator of cancer. Damage caused by ROS tend to accumulate over time and is a major reason facilitating cancer development in the elderly.

Free radicals can be detrimental by reacting with, and sometimes destroying, critical cellular components including the polyunsaturated fatty acids (PUFA) that comprise lipoprotein particles and plasma membranes. ROS attack the unsaturated bonds of fatty acids in lipid membranes, altering membrane structure and function.[1] The products of lipid peroxidation are diffusible and since lipoproteins travel throughout the body, the ensuing damage can spread far beyond the site of original attack. Therefore, in order to reach the point of oxidative stress a significant amount of oxidant exposure must occur. The basic prerequisite for lipid peroxidation, as well as other types of oxidative damage, is inadequate free radical scavengers. Free radicals that react with polyunsaturated long carbon chain lipids results in the formation of chemotactic products, aldehydric nonanoic acids, and various other aldehydes.[2] Aldehydes can bind with biological amines such as proteins, nucleic acids, and amino lipids, altering their structure and functions.[2] Free radical damage results in a loss of membrane fluidity, receptor alignment, potential cell lysis, damage to sulfur containing enzymes and other proteins, resulting in inactivation, cross-linking, and denaturation. Damage to carbohydrates can alter cellular receptor functions including those associated with cytokine activities and prostaglandin formation. Free radicals can also induce brain disorders,[3] atherosclerosis,[4] and colon cancer.[4]

Since ROS are produced abundantly by a variety of pathways, humans and other animals have evolved defense mechanisms against these free radicals. Antioxidants are small molecules that act as scavengers of ROS and prevent them from causing further cellular damage. In addition to antioxidants, free radicals can also be inactivated by enzymes. Aging results in a decrease in the amount of antioxidant enzymes. Such decreases in antioxidant enzymes contribute to the increased risk for developing cancer and the increased incidence of immune dysfunction seen with aging. In addition to the decline in antioxidant enzymes, the accumulation of free radical damage also contributes to these increased risk factors.

However, when free radicals are not excessive, they can play a positive role in human health and development. For example, the fetus uses oxidants to stimulate cellular differentiation. Free radicals can contribute to, and alter, gene expression.[5] Free radicals also play a pivotal role in the activation of natural detoxification systems such as cytochrome P450.[6] They are also produced by neutrophils and macrophages in an effort to kill invading microorganisms.[6] With chronic or high microorganism infection, the antigen burden in white blood cells can produce excessive amounts of free radicals increasing the antioxidant requirement.

B. ANTIOXIDANTS MECHANISM OF ACTION
1. Antioxidant Enzymes

Antioxidant enzymes have the capacity to lower the free radical burden. Free radical reactions can be broken down into three stages: initiation, propagation, and termination. Antioxidants enzymes can affect the generation of free radicals during all of these stages. The initiation phase of free radical reactions can be inhibited by two metalloenzymes: superoxide dismutase and catalase. They work by inactivating precursor molecules of free radicals, preventing the formation of ROS. Superoxide dismutase is a Mn-containing metalloenzyme in mitochondria and a Cu/Zn-containing metalloenzyme in the cytoplasm. Catalase is a Fe-containing metalloenzyme in peroxisomes. It catalyzes the decomposition of hydrogen peroxide, which is produced as a result of superoxide dismutase. Both enzymes, however, catalyze the reaction seen in Table 3.2. In addition, glutathione peroxidase which contains selenium also works as an antioxidant. Glutathione peroxidase is important for the decomposition of hydrogen peroxides and lipid peroxides and thereby works by interfering with the propagation phase of free radical generation. Although Mn, Cu, Zn, and Se are necessary components, they are only considered antioxidants when incorporated into their respective enzymes.[7]

TABLE 3.2
Antioxidant Enzymes

Enzyme	Mineral	Reaction
Superoxide dismutase (SOD)	CuZn Mn Fe (bacterial)	$2O_2^- + 2H^+ \rightarrow O_2 + H_2O_2$
Glutathione peroxidase (GSHPx)	Se (4)	$H_2O_2 + 2GSH \rightarrow GSSG + 2H_2O$ $ROOH + 2GSH \rightarrow GSSG + ROH + H_2O$
Phospholipid hydroperoxide glutathione peroxidase (PLGSHPx)	Se (1)	$H_2O_2 + 2GSH \rightarrow GSSG + H_2O$ $ROOH + 2GSH \rightarrow GSSG + ROH + H_2O$ $PLOOH + 2GSH \rightarrow GSSG + PLOH + H_2O$
Catalase (CT)	Fe	$H_2O_2 \rightarrow H_2O + O_2$
Glutathione-S-transferase (GS-T)	None	$ROOH + 2GSH \rightarrow GSSG + ROH + H_2O$

2. Antioxidant Compounds

Three compounds act only by directly interfering with propagation of free radical generation: vitamin E, vitamin C, and β-carotene. In addition to the direct action of these nutrients, riboflavin, a B vitamin, is a constituent of the enzyme glutathione reductase. Glutathione reductase is important for the regeneration of antioxidant defenses.[8]

C. IMMUNE FUNCTION AND FREE RADICAL REACTIONS
1. Effect of Free Radicals on Immune Cells

Free radicals can be detrimental to lymphocytes. High levels of dietary polyunsaturated fatty acid (PUFA) are immunosuppressants.[9] The unsaturated double bonds found in PUFAs are prime targets for free radical damage and initiation of chain reactions resulting in lipid peroxide formation. Lipid peroxides and aldehydes can alter cellular, including immunocellular, functions and even result in lysis of oxidized cell membranes. Lipoproteins in the plasma can also be oxidized and become lymphotoxic.[10] Lipid peroxidation also causes a decrease in membrane fluidity. Loss of membrane fluidity in lymphocytes has been directly related to a decreased ability of lymphocytes to respond to immunological challenges.[11-13]

Antigen presenting cells (APCs) generate an oxidative burst in response to many stimuli, which targets intracellular proteins. Intracellular proteins could either be normal cellular proteins, which are not needed, or they could be of viral origin. APCs contain proteolytic complexes, proteasomes, that selectively recognize and degrade oxidatively modified proteins. Oxidative modification exposes hydrophobic core residues which are acted on by proteasomes[14,15] to generate peptides of nine amino acids in length. Normal rates of protein oxidation within cells "mark" proteins for proteolysis by proteasomes. Peptides of nine amino acids in length travel to the endoplasmic reticulum where they associate with Major Histocompatibility Complex (MHC Class I) molecules and β$_2$-macroglobulin. Such complexes traverse the golgi apparatus and get presented on MHC class I cell surface molecules. Once these proteins are properly presented on class I MHC, CD8$^+$ T-cells can distinguish between self and nonself antigens[16] and selectively destroy only those cells which are infected. In this scenario, oxidation and generation of free radicals is an essential component for the proper functioning of cell-mediated immunity.

2. Free Radicals and T-Cell Activation

Free radicals are necessary compounds for maintaining optimal immune function. The proliferation of T-lymphocytes is a pivotal event in cell-mediated immunity and it too requires the action of free radicals. Foreign antigens are partially degraded by antigen-presenting cells and presented on their surface in association with MHC Class II to CD4$^+$ T-cells. This initiates a complex series of events with production of cytokines, particularly interleukin-1 (IL-1) by accessory cells and IL-2 by CD4$^+$ T-cells. Cytokines are small, locally acting molecules which stimulate various events including proliferation of CD4$^+$ T-lymphocytes. These T-cells also express cell surface receptors for IL-2 and the iron transport molecule, transferrin.

Hydroxyl radical scavengers such as dimethyl sulfoxide, thiouren, dimethyl urea, and mannitol inhibit mitogenic responses of human peripheral blood lymphocytes to phorbol myristate acetate (PMA), ConA, and phytohaemagglutinin (PHA) mitogens.[16] These findings suggest that hydroxyl radicals might be involved in mediating the signal(s), perhaps those from cytokines, that trigger T-cell activation and proliferation. Further evidence to support this theory is that antioxidants such as butylated hydroxy anisole (BHA), desferrioxamine (DES), and desferrithiocin (DFT) inhibit the antigen-driven proliferation in a dose-dependent manner. These compounds, however, do not inhibit the production of IL-1 by accessory cells or that of IL-2 by T-cells, but they do inhibit cell surface expression of IL-2 receptors. An exception to this rule is that the amino thiol cystamine can inhibit IL-2 production by human peripheral blood lymphocytes stimulated with mitogen. DES, DFT, BHA, and ferriganide all inhibit DNA synthesis induced by PHA or PMA/ionomycine.[17] It has therefore been proposed that free radicals are involved in the activation of T-lymphocytes.[18] Iron is also necessary for T-cell activation as iron in the +2 state can convert O_2 to a free radical which then activates T-cells. Iron chelators exert antiproliferative effects through interactions with intracellular iron pools. These chelators might influence cellular activities by binding iron and preventing its involvement as a catalyst for hydroperoxides or by inhibiting ribonucleotidesynthesis. Furthermore, Terada showed that small traces of iron are necessary for the production of the cell-cycle regulatory protein kinase, P34[cdc2][19].

B-lymphocytes possess a functional NADPH oxidase, which also works by producing free radicals. The proliferation of B-cells is also inhibited by antioxidants,[17] while T-lymphocytes do not have NADPH oxidase,[20] other leukocytes provide the "help" necessary for T-lymphocytes to produce ROS.[21]

Cystamine amino thiol compounds block the binding of AP-1 and NF-KB to DNA. These two proto-oncogenes are necessary for T-cell proliferation. Also, cysteamine inhibits intracellular DCFH oxidation, IL-2 mRNA, IL-2, and DNA synthesis. A speculative interpretation of these results is that mitogens induce intracellular formation of ROS in T-cells, leading to oxidation of AP-1 and/or NF-KB and thus might need free radicals for their transport into the nucleus. Binding of transcription factors to DNA only occurs under reducing conditions. The redox factor, Ref-1, in the nucleus, is capable of reducing oxidized transcription factors. Among the genes regulated by AP-1 is the gene encoding for IL-2 production. IL-2 production is essential for T-cell passage through G1 into DNA synthesis.

Lipoxygenase (LO) inhibitor blockade increases intracellular Ca^{2+} in response to binding of the T-cell receptor (TCR) to MHC and CD3 accessory cell surface molecules. This results in the inhibition of inositol-triphosphate synthesis which impedes signal transduction and ultimately cell activation. However, LO inhibitors do not effect the activation of Na^+ and H^+ antiport by PMA. These compounds can increase pH in stimulated cells and activate protein kinase C (PKC) which will amplify signal transduction pathways.[22] LO inhibitors decrease IL-2 production in Jurkat cells and do not inhibit IL-2 production in PMA-treated Jurkat cells.[22]

3. Free Radicals and Cytokine Production

Since free radicals are extremely reactive, they can modify various biochemical substances. Hydrogen peroxide elevates cytoplasmic free Ca^{2+} levels and activates PKC, facilitating signal transduction.[23] Additionally, hydrogen peroxide can cause reversible inhibition of DNA synthesis in murine osteoblastic cells when added during the late G1 phase. This function of hydrogen peroxide is also seen with TGF-β1. TGF-β1 and hydrogen peroxide both increase expression of the HIC-5 gene which encodes a novel Zn-finger protein (molecular weight 5 KDa). It also increases phosphorylation of 30 KDa heat shock protein. Thus, hydrogen peroxide can be a second messenger when activated by TGF-β1.[24] Low concentrations (10 nm to 1 mM) of superoxide anions and hydrogen peroxide can stimulate growth or growth responses. Intracellular pH increases within 10 seconds, activating PKC. Production of superoxide anions and hydrogen peroxide involves the activity of a plasma membrane NADPH-oxidase. Cytokines are required for the generation of free radicals.[25] TNF-α specifically induces extensive mitochondrial superoxide generation.[26] In contrast to TNF-α, a variety of human tumor cells, neuroblastoma, melanoma, and colon, pancreatic, ovarian, and breast carcinoma release large amounts of hydrogen peroxide without any specific growth stimulus.[27] The growth responses that involve the release of superoxide or hydrogen peroxide may be mediated through the oxidative inactivation of serum proteinase inhibitors. This would allow serum proteinase to remodel the cell surface, or glycocalyx, thereby facilitating or modulating the action of normal growth factors.[28] Oncogenes or transformed cells respond significantly better to growth promoting effects in the presence of low levels of superoxide or hydrogen peroxide. This may be due to the fact that reduced levels of antioxidant enzymes contribute to a cellular redox state. These free radicals facilitate the growth of neoplastic cells as part of a constitutively active autocrine system, or from adjacent inflammatory cells.[28]

At low concentrations, active oxygen is an important mediator of cellular response and growth. Exogenous addition of active oxygen to resting cells stimulates DNA synthesis and the induction of proto-oncogenes, c-fos and c-myc.[29] The presence of oxygen radicals increases the production and reception of IL-1. Oxygen radicals can increase IL-1 production by monocytes and the proliferation of lymphocytes in PHA-induced blast transformation reactions stimulated by recombinant IL-2.[30] There are two major mechanisms of lymphocyte stimulation by oxygen radicals, activation of PKC and lipoxygenase. The effect of lipoxygenase activation is supported by the strong inhibitory effect of NDGA (a lipoxygenase inhibitor and antioxidant).[31]

Antioxidants, diamide and ascorbic acid, have inhibitory effects on protein tyrosine phosphatase in murine fibroblast cells transfected with human EGF-receptor. In view of its effects on cellular growth, oxidative stress plays a role in growth factor-mediated signal transduction.[32] IL-1β stimulates IL-6 secretion in a dose and time-dependent manner. The antioxidants pyrolidine dithiocarbamate, N-acetyl-cysteine, two thiol-reacting molecules, trolox, and hydrosoluble analogue of vitamin E, completely inhibit IL-6 secretion in a dose-dependant manner. However, a mixture of verapamil (a calcium channel blocker), neomycin sulfate (a phospholipase C cascade inhibitor), and 2'5'-dideoxyadenosine (an adenylate cyclase inhibitor), did not affect IL-6 induction by IL-1.[33]

The nuclear transcription factor, NF-KB, is constitutively present in the cytoplasm as an inactive complex. NF-KB is involved in the transmission of signals from the cytoplasm to the nucleus by binding to the 5′-GGGACTTTCC-3′ sequence in the K enhancer. NF-KB can activate genes involved in immune, inflammatory, or acute phase responses. IL-1, TNF, PMA and other activating factors can activate NF-KB. Activated NF-KB translocates the nucleus where it recognizes a specific DNA sequence,[34] the gene coding for IL-6.[35] *N*-acetylcysteine (NAC), an antioxidant, inhibits, and diamid, an oxidant, stimulates NF-KB activation.[36] The mechanism of action of NAC is that it increases intracellular glutathione and decreases reduced glutathione. NAC also blocks TNF-α induced NF-KB activation,[37] while hydrogen peroxide leads to NF-KB activation.[38] These changes should produce an immunological environment that contains higher levels of cytokines produced by T-helper 2 cells, TNF and IL-6. In murine and human AIDS, leukemia, and other cancers, high levels of IL-6 are associated with suppressed cellular immune defenses.[39,40]

The role of cytokines in ROS production is still unclear. It has been shown[41] that isolated rat islet cells exposed to a combination of cytokines had diminished insulin release, increased ROS production, and islet necrosis. The *in vitro* toxic effect of cytokines on islet cells is mediated by ROS release. However, *in vivo* effects of cytokines in the production of ROS and induction of oxidative damage are not well understood. In rodents, macrophages produce ROS following stimulation with other compounds. This process does not occur spontaneously. *In vivo* production of cytokines significantly enhanced macrophage response to infectious agents.[42] Biologically, cytokines such as TNF-α and IL-1 are highly conserved and are capable of causing extreme toxicity and even death at certain doses. Blockade of IL-1 by the use of its specific receptor antagonists and blockade of TNF by the use of TNF antibodies preserved the effects of endotoxin, i.e., bacterial lipoprotein polysaccharide (LPS) cell surface molecule. This implies that each cytokine is partially responsible for lethal endotoxin effects. Thus, both administration of cytokines and strategies to block their effects can be beneficial to the host.

Organisms need to evolve mechanisms to control or regulate cytokine responses. One mechanism of cytokine protection against cellular toxicity is generation of protective enzymes that limit the effects of ROS.[43]

4. Summary

Although free radicals at high levels can decrease immune function, at physiologic concentrations they are vital for antigen presentation and cell proliferation. Cytokines like TNF-α are necessary for the generation of free radicals and at low concentration, free radicals act as second messengers to mediate cellular growth. Free radicals can also increase TNF-α, IL-6, and IL-1 production. IL-6 production stimulated by free radicals can occur via two mechanisms, either by increasing IL-1 or by activating NF-KB. IL-1 and TNF-α can be extremely toxic and even induce death at certain doses. IL-6 inhibits T-helper 1 cells and secretion of IL-2 is needed for normal cellular immunity. The body has therefore evolved defense mechanisms to detoxify free radicals. Instead of investigating ways to minimize the production of free radicals, perhaps studies should focus on how to regulate their production more effectively.

D. ANTIOXIDANT NUTRIENTS AND IMMUNE FUNCTION
1. Effect of Antioxidants on Nonspecific Immune Responses

Antioxidants can increase immune responses by controlling the amount of free radicals generated in a cell. Neutrophils kill extracellular pathogens by generation of oxidative bursts, which are toxic to the invading organism. Neutrophils are not destroyed because they take up vitamin E[44] before the oxidative burst. Following activation, neutrophil vitamin C concentration is lower.[45,46] This suggests that vitamin C works with vitamin E to decrease the free radical burden within the neutrophil.[47] Vitamin C and vitamin E supplementation has also been found to normalize the reduced chemotactic and bactericidal activities of neutrophils in individuals with inherited phagocytosis disorders,[48] as well as in newborns.[49] Vitamin E deficient rats have impaired neutrophil and macrophage chemotaxis, reduced ingestion of complement coated beads, and decreased protection from auto-oxidative damage.[50] Chronic immune-mediated inflammation such as that found in experimentally induced granulomas has been decreased in animals given superoxide dismutase, catalase, or vitamin E.[51] The synovial fluid in the joints of rheumatoid arthritis patients contains high levels of ROS with infiltrating neutrophils and T-lymphocytes in the infected joints. Local lipid peroxidation has been correlated with the degree of inflammation in animal models of arthritis. Administration of antioxidants such as superoxide dismutase and catalase directly into arthritic joints decreases inflammation.[52] Ascorbic acid levels are low in patients with rheumatoid arthritis, despite normal ascorbic acid absorption.[53] In this sense, both a balanced generation of free radicals as well as an adequate level of antioxidant nutrients are essential to destroy invading organisms while preserving immune cells.

2. Effect of Antioxidants on Specific Immune Responses

In laboratory animals, T- and B-cell proliferation is correlated with dietary and serum vitamin E levels.[54] Vitamin E deficiency affects T-lymphocytes to a greater degree than B-lymphocytes. T-lymphocyte function is reduced to a greater degree than that of B-lymphocytes, macrophages, and stem cells with age.[55,56] T-lymphocyte cell membranes in young mice are more fluid than B-cell membranes. However, as mice age, T-cells lose their fluidity, whereas B-cells retain theirs. This occurs because T-cell lipids are more susceptible to peroxidation than B-cell lipids.[57] The ability of T-lymphocytes to form rosettes is significantly inhibited following exposure to oxygen radicals, whereas B-lymphocyte rosette formation is not affected.[58] As aging progresses, the level and activity of antioxidant enzymes decreases which results in impaired T-lymphocytes. Dietary β-carotene and carotenoids of similar chemical structure (but lacking pro vitamin A activity) enhance cytotoxic T-cell activity and lower tumor levels in animal models.[55]

E. SUMMARY

Inflammation results in the production of excessive amounts of free radicals. Vitamin E, C, and glutathione are necessary for increasing the immune response, controlling inflammation, and reducing tissue damage.

ACKNOWLEDGMENTS

Supported by grants from Wallace Genetic Foundation, Inc., which has funded research in the area of this review.

REFERENCES

1. Sun, Y., Free radicals, antioxidant enzymes and carcinogenesis, *Free. Cited. Med.,* 8, 1879, 1990.
2. Kamimura, S., et al., Increased 4-hydroxynonenal levels in experimental alcoholic liver disease: association of lipid peroxidation with liver fibrogenesis, *Hepatology,* 16, 448, 1992.
3. Volicer, L., et al., Involvement of free radicals in dementia of Alzheimer type: a hypothesis, *Neurobiol. Aging,* 43(2), 63, 1990.
4. Yagi, K., Lipid peroxides in human diseases, *Chem. Phys. Lipids,* 45, 337, 1987.
5. Franson, R. C., et al., Mechanisms of cytoprotective and anti-inflammatory activity of PGB1 oligomers: PGBx has potent anti-phospholipase A2 and anti-oxidant activity, *Prostaglandin Leukot. Essent. Fatty Acid,* 43(2), 63, 1991.
6. Bast, A., et al., Oxidants and antioxidants: state of the art, *Am. J. Med.,* 91(3c), 2s, 1991.
7. Willett, W. C., et al., Dietary fat and risk if breast cancer, *N. Engl. J. Med.,* 316, 22, 1987.
8. Machlin, L. J., et al., Free radical tissue damage: protection role of antioxidant nutrients, *FASEB J.,* 1, 441, 1987.
9. Gurr, M. I., The role of lipids in the regulation of the immune system, *Prog. Lipid Res.,* 22, 257, 1983.
10. Cathcart, M. K., et al., Monocytes and neutrophils oxidize low density lipoprotein making cytotoxic, *J. Leukocyte Biol.,* 38, 341, 1985.
11. Fountain, M. W., et al., Effects of enrichment of phosphatidylcholine liposomes with cholesterol or alpha-tocopherol on the responses of lymphocytes to phytohemagglutinin, *Mol. Immunol.,* 19, 59, 1982.
12. Cinder, B., et al., Dietary fat alters the fatty acid composition of lymphocyte membranes and the rate at which suppressor capacity is lost, *Immunol. Lett.,* 6, 331, 1983.
13. Wedner, H. J., Biochemical events associated with lymphocyte activation, *Surv. Immunol. Res.,* 3, 295, 1984.
14. Davies, K. J. A. and Goldberg, A. L., Protein damage by oxygen radicals are rapidly degraded in extracts of red blood cells, *J. Biol. Chem.,* 262, 8227, 1987.
15. Pacific, R. E. and Davies, K. J. A., Protein degradation as an index of oxidative stress, *Meth. Enzymol.,* 186, 485, 1990.
16. Ivovogrodosky, A., et al., Hydroxyl radical scavengers inhibit lymphocyte mitogenesis, *Proc. Natl. Acad. Sci. U.S.A.,* 79, 1171, 1982.
17. Hunt, N. H., et al., Interference with oxidative processes inhibits proliferation of human peripheral blood lymphocytes and murine β-lymphocytes, *Int. J. Immunopharmacol.,* 13, 1019, 1991.
18. Chaudhri, C., et al., Effect of antioxidants on primary alloantigen-induced T cell activation and proliferation, *J. Immunol.,* 137, 2646, 1986.
19. Terada, N., et al., Definition of the roles for iron and essential fatty acids in cell cycle progression of normal human T lymphocytes, *Exp. Cell Res.,* 204, 260, 1993.
20. Pick, E. and Gadbe, R. Certain lymphoid cells contain the membrane-associated component of the phagocyte-specific NADPH oxidase, *J. Immunol.,* 140, 1611, 1983.
21. Rabesandratana, H., et al., Implication of oxidative phenomena in T cell activation, *Int. J. Immunopharmacol.,* 14, 895, 1992.
22. Gerber, M. and Domand, J., Increased oxidative metabolism in PMA-activated lymphocytes: a flow cytometric study, *Oxidative Stress Cell Activation and Viral Infection,* Pasquier, C., Olivier, R.Y., Auclair, C., and Parker, L., Eds., Birkhauser Press, 1993, 253.

23. Yamada, T., Hydrogen peroxide generation in whole rat pancreatic islets: synergistic regulation by cytoplasmic free calcium and protein kinase C, *Biochem. Biophys. Res. Commun.*, 155, 569, 1988.

24. Nose, K., et al., Involvement of hydrogen peroxide in the action of TGF-B1, in *Oxidation Stress, Cell Activation and Viral Infection*, Pasquier, C. Ed., Birkhauser Press, 1993, 21.

25. Meier, B., et al., Identification of a superoxide generating NADPH oxidase system in human fibroblsts, *Biochem. J.*, 275, 241, 1991.

26. Heennet, T., et al., Tumor necrosis factor-α induces superoxide generation in mitochondria of 929 cells, *Biochem. J.*, 289, 587, 1993.

27. Szatrowski, T. P. and Nathan, C. F., Production of large amounts of hydrogen peroxide by human tumor cells, *Cancer Res.*, 51, 794, 1991.

28. Burdon, R. H., Cellular generated active oxygen species as signals in the activation of tumor cell growth, *Oxidative Stress, Cell Activation and Viral Infection,* Pasquier, C., Olivier, R.Y., Auclair, C., and Parker, L., Eds., Birkhauser Press, 1993, 43.

29. Crawford, D., et al., Oxidant stress induces the proto-oncogenes c-fos and c-myc in mouse epidermal cells, *Oncogeny*, 3, 27, 1988.

30. Afanas'ev, I. B. and Korkina, L. G., Effect of oxygen radicals on the IL-1 production by monocytes and IL-2 receptor expression in lymphocytes during primary and secondary immunodeficiency, *Oxidative Stress, Cell Activation and Viral Infection,* Pasquier, C., Olivier, R.Y., Auclair, C., and Parker, L., Eds., Birkhauser Press, 1993, 53.

31. Dornand, J. and Gerber, M., Inhibition of murine T-cell response by antioxidants: the targets of lipoxygenase pathway inhibitors, *Immunology*, 68, 384, 1989.

32. Stein, A., Oxidative stress and growth factor mediated signal transduction, *Oxidative Stress, Cell Activation and Viral Infection,* Pasquier, C., Olivier, R. Y., Auclair, C., and Parker, L., Eds., Birkhauser Press, 1993, 35.

33. Raes, M., et al., Effects of antioxidants on IL-6 secretion induced by IL-1 in human cultured lung fibroblasts, *Oxidative Stress, Cell Activation and Viral Infection,* Pasquier, C., Olivier, R. Y., Auclair, C., and Parker, L., Eds., Birkhauser Press, 1993, 77.

34. Grimm, S. and Baeuerle, P. A., The inducible transcription factor NF-KB:structure-function relationship of its protein subunits, *Biochem. J.*, 290, 297, 1993.

35. Zhang, Y., et al., Interleukin-6 induction by tumor necrosis factor and interleukin-1 in human fibroblasts involves activation of a nuclear factor binding to a KB-like sequence. *Mol. Cell. Biol.*, 10, 3818, 1990.

36. Roederer, M., et al., Cytokine-stimulated human immunodeficiency virus replication is inhibited by N-acetyl-L-cysteine, *Proc. Natl. Acad. Sci. U.S.A.*, 87, 4884, 1990.

37. Mihm. S., et al., Inhibition of HIV-1 replication and NF-KB activity by cysteine and cysteine derivatives, *AIDS,* 5, 497, 1991.

38. Schreck, R., et al., Reactive oxygen intermediates as apparently widely used messengers in the activation of the NF-KB transcription factor and HIV-1, *EMBO J.,* 10, 2247, 1991.

39. Wang, Y., Huang, D., Liang, B., and Watson, R. R., Nutritional status and immune responses in mice with murine AIDS are normalized by vitamin E supplementation. *J. Nutr.,* 124, 2024, 1994.

40. Wang, Y., Huang, D., Wood, S., and Watson, R. R., Modulation of immune function and cytokine production by various levels of vitamin E supplementation during murine AIDS, *Immunopharmacology,* 29, 225, 1995.

41. Robinovitch, A., et al., Cytotoxic effects of cytokines on rat islets: evidence for involvement of free radicals and lipid peroxidation, *Diabetologia*, 35, 409, 1992.

42. Wolf, J. E. and Mossol, S. E., *In vivo* activation of macrophage oxidative burst activity by cytokines and amphotericin B, *Infect. Immun.*, 58, 1296, 1990.

43. Visner, G. A., et al., Regulation of manganese superoxide dismutase by lipopolysaccharide, IL-1 and TNF, *J. Biol. Chem.*, 265, 2856, 1990.

44. Moser, U. and Weber, F., Uptake of ascorbic acid by human granulocytes, *Int. J. Vit. Nutr. Res.,* 54, 47, 1984.

45. Hemila, H., et al., Activated polymorphonuclear leucocyte consume vitamin C, *Febs. Lett.*, 178, 25, 1985.

46. Oberritter, H., et al., Effect of functional stimulation on ascorbate content in phagocytes under physiological and pathological conditions, *Int. Archs. Allergy Appl. Immun.*, 81, 46, 1986.

47. Anderson, R., et al., Ascorbate and cysteine-mediated selective neutralization of extracellular oxidants during N-formyl peptide activation of human phagocytes, *Agents and Actions*, 20(1/2), 77, 1987.

48. Weening, R. S., et al., Effect of ascorbate on abnormal neutrophil, platelet and lymphocyte function in a patient with Chediak-Higashi syndrome, *Blood*, 57, 856, 1981.

49. Vohra, K., et al., Correction of defective chemotaxis of neonatal neutrophilis with ascorbic acid, *Pediatr. Res.*, 17, 340, 1983.

50. Harris, R. E., et al., Consequences of vitamin E deficiency on the phagocyte and oxidative function of the rat polymorphonuclear leukocyte, *Blood*, 55, 338, 1980.

51. Chensue, S. W., et al., Role of oxygen reactive species in schistosoma mansoni egg-induced granulomatous inflammation, *Biochem. Biophys. Res. Commun.*, 122, 184, 1984.

52. Sies, H., *Oxidative Stress*, Academic Press, London, 1984.

53. Lunec, J., et al., Oxidative damage and its relevance to inflammatory joint disease in *Cellular Antioxidant Defense Mechanisms*, Ching Kuang Chow, Ed., CRC Press Inc., 1988, Boca Raton, Florida.

54. Bendich, A., et al., Dietary vitamin E requirement for optimum immune responses in the rat, *J. Nutr.*, 116(4), 675, 1986.

55. Bendich, A., et al., A role for carotenoids in immune function, *Clinical Nutrition*, 7(3), 113, 1988.

56. Makinodamt, T., Cellular basis of immunological aging, *Biological Mechanisms of Aging*, Shimke, R. T., Eds., USDA, NIH, 1981.

57. Hendricks, L. C., et al., Susceptibility to lipid peroxidation and accumulation of fluorescent products with age is greater in T-cells than B-cells, *Free Radical Biology and Medicine*,

58. Crever, M. R., et al., The effect of oxidant stress on human lymphocytotoxicity, *Blood*, 56, 284, 1980.

Chapter 4

ANTIOXIDANTS AND AIDS

Zhen Zhang, Paula F. Inserra, and Ronald Ross Watson

Contents

I. Introduction..32

II. Oxidative Stress and HIV Infection 32

III. Antioxidants and AIDS 33
    A. Glutathione and *N*-Acetylcysteine 33
    B. Vitamin E (Tocopherol)..34
    C. α-Lipoic Acid 34
    D. Vitamin C (Ascorbic Acid) 34
    E. Carotenoids...35
    F. Other Vitamins...35
    G. Zinc..35
    H. Selenium...36
    I. Copper 36
    J. Antioxidant Enzymes 36
    K. Diethyldithiocarbamate (DDTC)..37
    L. Desferrioxamine (DFX) 37
    M. Plant-Derived Metabolites with Synergistic Antioxidant Activity 37
        1. Phenolic Compounds (Hydroxyl Derivatives of Aromatic
           Hydrocarbons) 37
           a. Ubiquinone 37
           b. Flavonoids 38
           c. Coumarins (Benzopyrones)...38
        2. Nitrogen Containing Compounds: Di- and Polyamines....................38
        3. Enzyme Systems and Polypeptides...38
        4. Vitamins...38

IV. Conclusion 38

References..39

I. INTRODUCTION

Acquired immunodeficiency syndrome (AIDS) is a result of infection with human immunodeficiency virus (HIV-1 or HIV-2) which eventually destroys a subset CD4[+] helper T-lymphocyte. This results in enhanced susceptibility to opportunistic infection and neoplasms.[1] Oxidative stress plays a major role in the progression of HIV infection to AIDS and has been suggested to contribute to the decline of CD4[+] lymphocytes.[2] The existence of oxidative stress in HIV infection and AIDS is exemplified by the excess production of reactive oxygen species (ROS) and a general loss of antioxidant defenses in HIV-infected patients.[3] Therefore, the reduction of oxidative stress by antioxidant treatment may be a desirable therapy during the asymptotic HIV infection as well as advanced AIDS.[4]

II. OXIDATIVE STRESS AND HIV INFECTION

Oxidative stress is a pathologic phenomenon resulting from an imbalance between the system producing ROS and the antioxidant defense systems which function synergistically to prevent or destroy ROS.[5] An increased production of ROS is caused by infecting agents in neutrophils and macrophages,[6] as well as from abnormal production of TNF-α in HIV-infected patients.[7,8] Increased secretion of TNF-α results from direct stimulation by free radicals and the antigens of opportunistic bacteria only in AIDS when severe immunedysfunction permits persistent infection. In the asymptomatic stage, activation of the TNF gene occurs by the viral replication machinery.[5] TNF may play an important role in causing a further increase in the levels of oxidants by providing an "amplification loop" that feeds back to excite further production of ROS from macrophages and neutrophils.[9] It may also react with T-cells to enhance expression of autocrine cell activators, such as IL-2, and receptors, thereby promoting activation of T-cell respiratory activity for greater intracellular ROS.[10,11] The excessive production of oxygen free radicals causes the oxidation of circulating or membrane lipids, proteins, and DNA and functions as a potent inducer of viral activation, DNA damage, and immunosuppression.[12]

Apoptosis, programmed cell death of CD4[+] lymphocytes, is of fundamental importance in progression towards AIDS.[3] The cascade of events that results from oxidative stress can initiate apoptosis, a possible pathway of immune cell loss in patients with HIV infection.[3] It includes oxidation of cellular membranes, alteration in metabolic pathways, disruption of electron transport systems, depletion of cellular ATP production, loss of CA[2+] homeostasis, endonuclease activation, and DNA/chromatin fragmentation. The DNA damage caused by oxidative stress may be related to HIV-associated malignancies and disease progression.[13] Downstream events secondary to these effects may also play a role in activation of the latent virus and subsequent viral replication.[3] Oxidative stress is a known activator of HIV replication *in vitro* through the activation of a nuclear factor κB (NF-κB). NF-κB in turn stimulates HIV gene expression by acting on the promoter region of the viral long terminal repeat (LTR), a critical region for transcription in the integrated virus.[13] TNF-α is an important activator of HIV by generating ROS which activates NF-κB.[14]

III. ANTIOXIDANTS AND AIDS

The suggestion that oxidative stress is a feature of HIV infection and AIDS is also supported by multiple nutritional deficiencies and increased metabolism of antioxidants in HIV-infected patients.[3] This results from malabsorption of nutrients, hypermetabolism, and drug-nutrient interactions.[15] The antioxidant status of lymphocytes is important for their functioning, which is closely linked to their redox potential, particularly to their cysteine and glutathione levels.[5] In a weakened antioxidant system, DNA repair capacity of the cells may be altered and lymphocytes may be killed or impaired.[16-18] Since ROS is involved in the signal transduction mechanisms for HIV activation, a possible therapeutic use of antioxidants in preventing HIV activation has been suggested.[19-23]

A. GLUTATHIONE AND N-ACETYLCYSTEINE

Glutathione (GSH), a thiol derived from cysteine, is important in scavenging reactive oxygen intermediates released by activated neutrophils and monocytes.[24] It regulates many lymphocyte functions, including their proliferative response to mitogens, responsiveness of cytotoxic T-cells to IL-2, and cytotoxicity of lymphokine-activated killer cells.[25-29] Depletion of GSH inhibits proliferation of T-lymphocytes, particularly those from HIV-infected patients.[30] Another important effect of GSH is its ability to inhibit HIV replication when stimulated by TNF or phorbol myristate acetate (PMA) in infected macrophages and lymphoid cells.[31]

HIV-infected patients have greatly decreased levels of GSH in their plasma and peripheral blood lymphocytes.[32,33] The decreased levels of GSH is highly correlated with depressed numbers of CD4+ cells.[24] GSH is a good candidate for clinical investigation, as flow cytometry can measure glutathione levels in T-cell subsets and has been used to show GSH changes in such subsets following HIV infection.[18] Since GSH and vitamin E spare each other, vitamin E appears to prevent the drop in GSH levels and thus TNF-α-induced HIV replication.[34]

N-Acetylcysteine (NAC) has both a direct and indirect antioxidant role. It is a cysteine precursor which is converted intracellularly into GSH and can also act directly as an antioxidant.[4] By increasing cellular GSH levels and decreasing TNF-α, it can also inhibit TNF-α-induced HIV replication and prevent TNF-α-induced apoptosis of T-lymphocytes and other cells in HIV-infected people.[35,36] NAC has been reported to increase antibody-dependent cell mediated cytotoxicity of neutrophils.[35] Early clinical trials have shown that NAC prevents the decline in CD4+ cells in GSH-deficient individuals.[37] Unfortunately, oral and intravenous GSH are not effective at enhancing cellular GSH stores.[38] Although aerosolized GSH does increase cellular stores, the most effective means for raising cellular GSH levels is oral or intravenous administration of the GSH precursor NAC.[34,38] Therefore, treating patients with NAC may be a useful strategy in slowing the progression of the disease.

L-2-oxothiazolidine 4-carboxylate (OTC) is another pro-GSH drug that has been proposed for AIDS therapy. Although NAC and OTC blocked cytokine induction of HIV *in vitro,* NAC was far more effective than OTC.[4] In isolated peripheral blood mononuclear cells, NAC fully replenishes depleted intracellular GSH whereas OCT only minimally replenishes GSH.[4] Although NAC is markedly more effective at blocking HIV expression than OCT *in vitro,* both drugs could prove equally effective in the clinical setting.[4] A report studying rats noted that procysteine, also a pro-drug for glutathione, effectively reduced heart damage caused by ischemia by increasing levels of cellular GSH.[39] Whether procysteine will be effective in people with AIDS remains to be determined.

B. VITAMIN E (TOCOPHEROL)

Vitamin E, a fat soluble vitamin, is also a well known natural antioxidant. It attaches to free radicals and prevents the further generation of free radicals which ultimately prevents membranes lipid peroxidation.[40] Deficiencies in vitamin E lead to prooxidant status and have detrimental effects on the immune system.[15]

Plasma vitamin E levels were lower in HIV-infected patients than in controls.[41] Vitamin E derivatives such as vitamin E acetate, α-tocopheryl succinate, and 2,2,5,7,8-Pentamethyl-6-hydroxychromane (PMC) exhibited a concentration dependent inhibition of NF-κB activation by TNF-α.[1] Thus, vitamin E acetate, which is a natural, safe compound and PMC, which was demonstrated to be very effective in blocking NF-κB activation, should be considered for possible inclusion in combination therapies for AIDS.[1] The intake of supplementary vitamin E is significantly associated with slower progressions to AIDS in HIV seropositive men.[42] Vitamin E has also been shown to increase the CD4+/CD8+ lymphocyte ratio in AIDS patients by enhancing CD4+ cell counts.[43]

C. α-LIPOIC ACID

Recently, α-lipoic acid was found to exert antioxidant action *in vivo* and *in vitro.*[44] In addition, α-lipoic acid has been shown to inhibit HIV-1 replication in infected cells.[45,46] This may be due to the inhibition of NF-κB activation imposed by the antioxidant properties of dihydrolipoic acid (DHLA) generated from α-lipoate.[14] DHLA can cause a complete inhibition of NF-κB activation induced by TNF-α by scavenging free radicals and recycling vitamin E.[14] The inhibitory action of α-lipoic acid was found to be very potent as only 4 mM was needed for a complete inhibition, whereas 20 mM was required for NAC,[45] which indicates that α-lipoic acid may be effective in AIDS therapeutics.

D. VITAMIN C (ASCORBIC ACID)

Vitamin C has a role in modeling the immune system, possibly by affecting natural killer cell, macrophage, and T-cell activities.[47] Unfortunately, most of these studies were done on mice, and mice can synthesize vitamin C internally. In humans, vitamin C properties seem to make it a potential anticancer treatment.[47] Vitamin C also appears to have direct effects on HIV, thus enhancing its importance in treating people with AIDS. *In vitro* vitamin C inhibits the replication of HIV by more than 90% at levels of no toxicity of vitamin C.[48,49] Vitamin C is apparently more efficient than GSH or NAC in reducing HIV-1 replication in chronically infected T-lymphocytes[49] The effects of vitamin C on HIV can also be increased by the addition of NAC.[67]

Large amounts of vitamin C are consummated by HIV-infected patients.[50] No clinical benefit is associated with ingestion of vitamin C, in spite of the report that vitamin C can improve the clinical situation of patients suffering from different viral disease and their CD4[+] cell count with massive doses of vitamin C.[5] The survey of the nutritional status of HIV seropositive patients[51] showed a nonsignificant decrease in serum vitamin C and no significant difference in the prevalence of a low status, even with an increase in vitamin C intakes (10 times the RDA) due to the supplementation (7p, 10).

E. CAROTENOIDS

There is a severe deficit in plasma carotenoid including β-carotene levels in HIV-infected patients.[5] The degree of reduction in carotene levels is secondary to its depletion, given its ability to act as an antioxidant and scavenge the excess active oxygen.[52]

F. OTHER VITAMINS

In a study of micronutrients in HIV-infected patients, there was a decrease in vitamin A and vitamin B2 (riboflavin) levels.[51] Vitamin B2 deficiency results in a decreased activity of glutathione reductase, which regenerates oxidized GSH to reduced GSH, enabling it to rejuvenate its antioxidant functions. Mean serum levels of vitamin B1 (thiamin), vitamin B6 (pyridoxal), folate, and vitamin B12 were unchanged by HIV infection, whereas the prevalence of deficiencies in vitamin A and B6, vitamin B12 and E were significantly increased.[5]

G. ZINC

Zinc has a very interesting role in HIV infection. Zinc not only functions as an antioxidant, but it also has a more direct effect on the immune system. Zinc increases the secretion of IL-2 and the activity of thymulin, and it prevents apoptosis.[5] Zinc penetrates cells, enabling regulatory proteins to bind DNA, which results in expression of the IL-2 gene.[53] The addition of zinc to a serum-free culture medium increases the proliferation of T-lymphocytes and the synthesis of IL-2 in response to stimulation.[54] In the presence of zinc, thymulin assumes an active cyclic form enabling zinc to be recognized by high affinity receptors on T-lymphocytes. This results in the differentiation of T-lymphocytes by the induction of antigen B and in response to concanavalin.[56] It is very important to note that Zn^{2+} inhibits the endogenous endonuclease activated by Ca^{2+} which is responsible for the apoptosis of CD4[+] cells induced by TNF.[54] Additionally, zinc acts as an antiviral agent by inhibiting the reverse transcriptase.[5]

HIV-infected patients whose status remained stable for 2 years had normal plasma zinc levels,[56] whereas zinc levels of those who progressed towards AIDS were lower. Thymulin, which is also considered as a good marker of zinc status, was found to be extremely low in the blood of patients with AIDS.[57]

Faced with this decreased zinc status,[58] the effect of zinc supplementation was investigated in these patients. The most worrisome risk was that of an upsurge of viral activity due to the existence of several zinc-finger proteins in the structure of HIV-1.[59,60] It has been reported that the supplementation of zinc in AIDS patients can increase the CD4[+]/CD8[+] lymphocyte ratio;[61] however, very few studies can confirm these results.

H. SELENIUM

Selenium is a cofactor of glutathione peroxidase (GPx). Due to its antiviral effects and its importance for all immunological functions, the administration of selenium is suggested as a supportive therapy in early as well as in advanced stages of HIV infection.[62] A characteristic of the protective effects of selenium against viral pathogens is that its benefits occur at supplemental levels above physiological requirements. This suggests that it may not be associated solely with its function in GPx.[62] Selenium inhibits reverse transcriptase activity in RNA-virus-infected animals; therefore, supplemental selenium could also prevent the replication of HIV and retard the development of AIDS in newly HIV-infected subjects. Selenium is required for lymphocyte proliferation, macrophage-initiated tumor cytodestruction, and natural killer cell activity.[63]

Subnormal serum or plasma selenium levels and erythrocyte GPx activities have been observed in patients with AIDS and AIDS-related complex (ARC).[64] Selenium levels and GPx activity were correlated to the total number of lymphocytes in HIV-infected patients.[64,65]

Selenium supplementation in HIV-infected patients causes symptomatic improvements, especially in appetite and intestinal functions,[66] and possibly slows the course of the disease. During the period of supplementation, CD4$^+$ cell numbers still tended to decline; however, this decline was often only slight, or not observed at all. CD8$^+$ cells counts tended to decrease more often than to increase, causing the CD4$^+$/CD8$^+$ lymphocyte ratio to increase.[66]

I. COPPER

It is extremely difficult to study the copper status in patients with inflammations. Cytokines, IL-1 and TNF, cause serum copper to undergo a clear-cut increase, due to the increase in ceruloplasmin, an "acute phase protein," even in copper-deficient subjects.[67]

Serum copper increased in AIDS patients after a decrease in the asymptomatic stage. Low serum zinc levels with high copper levels are predictive of progression towards AIDS, independent of the basal level of CD4$^+$ cell counts.[51,58,68]

The measurement of copper-zinc superoxide dismutase (Cu-Zn SOD) in red cells is a more reliable marker of the zinc status with no variation in the enzyme, regardless of the stage of the disease.[67]

J. ANTIOXIDANT ENZYMES

The study of antioxidant enzyme activities, in addition to the changes in GPx described above, has shown a progressive and considerable increase in serum catalase,[69] while red cell SOD remains normal.[67]

Serum catalase activity increased progressively with advancing HIV infection (i.e., AIDS > symptomatic infection > asymptomatic infection > controls).[69] This correlates with increases in serum hydrogen peroxide (H$_2$O$_2$) scavenging ability and may reflect or compensate for systemic GSH and other antioxidant deficiencies in HIV-infected individuals.[69]

Manganese-containing superoxide dismutase (Mn-SOD) is the key enzyme in cellular protection from apoptosis induced by TNF,[70] via expression of the gene for

Mn-SOD and for metallothioneins.[5] A decreased population of Mn-SOD was seen while mRNA of this enzyme was overproduced in HIV-infected patients.[71] This results from the inhibition of translation of SOD mRNA caused by the binding of HIV tat protein to an RNA hairpin.[5] The sequence on which tat binds presents a sequence homology with a part of viral RNA, which is the biological target of tat, permitting the regulation of viral expression. The anomaly of Mn-SOD production is accompanied by signs of oxidizing stress in cells.[5]

K. DIETHYLDITHIOCARBAMATE (DDTC)

DDTC has a GPx-like activity. It is the only antioxidant drug that has been extensively studied in clinical trials, although it has not shown any *in vitro* antiviral activity.[72,73] In animals, DDTC increased GSH levels in a variety of tissues.[13] A significant reduction in these rates of new opportunistic infections was reported in AIDS patients receiving DDTC as compared to placebo.[73] However, a subsequent study apparently failed to demonstrate the similar benefit in a cohort study of HIV-infected asymptomatic patients.[13]

L. DESFERRIOXAMINE (DFX)

DFX is an iron chelator with strong antioxidant properties. DFX can inhibit *in vitro* HIV-1 replication in the H-9 T-lymphocyte cell line. The rationale for this work is to explain the low rate of symptomatic HIV-1 infection in multiple transfused thalassaemic patients who have been intensively chelated with DFX.[74]

M. PLANT-DERIVED METABOLITES WITH SYNERGISTIC ANTIOXIDANT ACTIVITY

Plants experience death due to oxidative stress which closely parallels the process of apoptosis in human, particularly as related to the destructive phenomena seen in HIV infection and AIDS. Primary and secondary metabolites found in plants act as synergistic antioxidants and can protect plants from oxidation-induced cell death. Some of these same metabolites can inhibit cell killing by HIV.[3] These metabolites are exemplified by phenolic compounds, nitrogen containing compounds, enzyme systems and polypeptides, and vitamins. Therefore, use of these antioxidants in patients with HIV/AIDS are proposed as a mechanism by which viral replication and cell killing in HIV infection can be inhibited.[3]

1. Phenolic Compounds (Hydroxyl Derivatives of Aromatic Hydrocarbons)
a. *Ubiquinone*

Ubiquinone (coenzyme Q_{10}, CoQ_{10}) is known for its activity as a redox component of transmembrane electron transport in mitochondria. In its reduced form, ubiquinol is an active antioxidant. Ubiquinol scavenges products from the peroxidation of membrane lipids even after the peroxidation process has been initiated. Lipid peroxidation will not occur, in fact, until all ubiquinol is consumed, which spares vitamin E in the process.[75]

Patients with AIDS had significantly lower blood CoQ_{10} levels than healthy controls, while patients with ARC and asymptomatic HIV-seropositive infection had decreased blood levels of CoQ_{10}, but not to the extent of those of AIDS patients.[76]

Supplementation with CoQ_{10} retarded the progression from ARC to AIDS and have a positive effect on the T4/T8 lymphocyte ratio.[66] However, CoQ_{10} may actually increase the level of free radicals thereby increasing oxidative stress.[66]

b. Flavonoids

Flavonoids (plant phenolic pigment products, particularly the catechins and quercitin) scavenge peroxyl and hydroxyl free radical.[77] They are protective against lipid peroxidation, probably by donating H^+ atoms to peroxyl radicals and terminating the chain radical reaction.[78] They can also control the release of reactive oxygen products from macrophages and neutrophils by regulation enzymes such as NADPH oxidase.[79] Quercitin, in particular, can inhibit the PKC-induced phosphorylation of I-κB that can liberate NF-κB to play a role in activation viral replication.[21,80]

c. Coumarins (Benzopyrones)

Coumarins are effective against oxidative stress by acting in a similar manner to flavonoids.[81]

2. Nitrogen Containing Compounds: Di- and Polyamines (e.g., Spermine, Putrescine, Cadaverine)

Nitrogen containing compounds effectively inhibit lipid peroxidation and impede the release of superoxide radicals form senescing membranes. They exert their stabilizing affects by binding with negative charges of both nucleic acids and phospholipids.[82] They inhibit protease and RNAase activity which is observed as a consequence of oxidative stress in plants.[82] Similar actions of polyamines in humans have been shown to help maintain intracellular Ca^{2+} homeostasis.[3]

Polyamines decline during oxidative stress, particularly when their necessary precursor, arginine, is either deficient or diverted; arginine is consumed during nitric oxide production in HIV infection.[3]

3. Enzyme Systems and Polypeptides

Dismutase, catalases, and peroxidases all exist in plants and their enhancement can increase resistance to oxidative stress.[83] The reduced form of GSH (a tri-peptide), so integral to the discussion of oxidative stress in HIV infection, is a scavenger of peroxides in plants and arrest senescence.[84]

4. Vitamins

Vitamin C and E and the various carotenoids are ubiquitous in plants. As in humans, they do not suffice as protection from superoxidative stress. This is confirmed by the multiplicity of the antioxidant systems that are necessary to synergize with vitamins and provide adequate protection.[85,86]

IV. CONCLUSION

Oxidizing stress is not merely an epiphenomenon, but is at the heart of the pathogenesis of HIV disease. This has incited researchers to test the effect of antioxidants in cell models, showing the high efficacy of certain micronutrients, but also of some other antioxidants. It is indispensable to combine the return of a deficient antioxidant nutritional status to normal (zinc, selenium, carotene, vitamins C and E) with the supply of high doses of synthetic antioxidant generating glutathione as *N*-acetylcysteines.

Generally, supplementation with antioxidants appears to offer some hope in slowing the progression of HIV infection. Currently, there is considerable debate over the use of antioxidant therapies in many illnesses, although more and more mainstream practitioners are considering the potential benefits of such therapies.[87] While the substances discussed here are largely free of toxic effects, caution still must be taken, and the development of adverse effects should be carefully monitored. It is also important for practitioners to stress to their patients the importance of a basic balanced diet as the essential groundwork underlying any additional supplementation or drug treatment. The research into antioxidants is still at an early stage of development, but future studies will likely resolve which of these substances can be used effectively in treating HIV infection.[67]

REFERENCES

1. Yuichiro, J. S., Bharat, B. A., and Lester, P., Inhibition of NF-κB activation by vitamin E derivatives, *Biochem. Biophys. Res. Commun.,* 193, 277, 1993.
2. Buttke, T. M. and Sandstron, P. A., Oxidative stress as a mediator of apoptosis. *Immunol. Today,* 15, 7, 1994.
3. Greenspan, H. C. and Arouma, O., Could oxidative stress initiate programmed cell death in HIV infection? A role for plant derived metabolites having synergistic antioxidant activity, *Chem. Biol. Interact.,* 91, 187, 1994.
4. Raju, A. P., Herzenberg, A. L., Herzenberg, A. L., and Roederer, C., Glutathione precursor and antioxidant activities of N-acetylcysteine and oxothiazolidine carboxylate compared in *in vitro* studies of HIV replication, *AIDS Res. Hum. Retrovi.,* 10, 961, 1994.
5. Favier, A., Sappey, C., Leclerc, P., Faure, P., and Micoud, M., Antioxidant status and lipid peroxidation in patients infected with HIV, *Chem. Biol. Interact.,* 91, 165, 1994.
6. Bruan, D. P., Kessler, H., Falk, L., Paul, D., Harris, J. E., Blauw, B., and Landay, A., Monocyte functional studies in asymptomatic human immunodeficiency disease virus (HIV) infected individuals, *J. Clin. Immunol.,* 8, 486, 1988.
7. Folks, T., Justement, J., Kinter, A., Dinarello, C., and Fauci, A., Cytokine induced expression of HIV-1 in a chronically infected promonocyte cell line, *Science,* 238, 800, 1987.
8. Poli, G., Kinter, A., Justement, J., Kehrl, J., Bressler, P., Stanley, S., and Fauci, A., Tumor necrosis factor a function in an autocrine manner in the induction of human immunodeficiency virus expression, *Proc. Natl. Acad. Sci. U.S.A.,* 87, 782, 1990.
9. Greenspan, H. C. and Arouma, O., Oxidative stress and apoptosis in HIV infection: a role for plant-derived metabolites with synergistic antioxidant activity, *Immunol. Today,* 15, 209, 1994.
10. Greenspan, H. C., The role of reactive oxygen species, antioxidants and phytopharmaceuticals in human immunodeficiency virus activity, *Med. Hypotheses,* 40, 85, 1993.
11. Scott-algara, D., Vuillier, F., Marasescu, M., de Saint Martin, J., and Dighiero, G., Serum levels of IL-2, IL-1 alpha, TNF-αlpha, and soluble receptor of IL-2 in HIV-infected patients, *AIDS Res. Hum. Retrovir.,* 7, 381, 1991.
12. Floyd, R. A. and Schneider, J. E., Hydroxyl free radicals damage to DNA, in *Membrane Lipid Oxidation,* Vol. I, Vigo-pelfrey, C., Ed., CRC Press, Boca Raton, FL, 1990.

13. Salvain, B. and Mark, A. W., The role of oxidative stress in disease progression in individuals infected by the human immunodeficiency virus, *J. Leukocyte Biol.,* 52, 111, 1992.
14. Lester, P. and Yuichire, J. S., Vitamin E and alpha-lipoate: role in antioxidant recycling and activation of the NF-κB transcription factor, *Molec. Aspects Med.,* 14, 229, 1993.
15. Kelleher, J., Vitamin E and the immune response, *Proc. Nutr. Soc.,* 50, 245, 1991.
16. Droge, W., Eck, H. P., Peckar, U., and Caniel, V., Glutathione augments the activation of cytotoxic T lymphocytes *in vivo, Immunology,* 172, 151, 1986.
17. Gougerot-Poccidalo, M. A., Fay, M., Roche, Y., Chollet, M., and Martin, S., Mechanism by which oxidative injury inhibits the proliferative response for human lymphocytes to PHA. Effect of the thiol compound 2-mercaptoethanol, *Immunology,* 164, 281, 1989.
18. Roederer, M., Staal, F. J., Osada, H., and Herzenberg, L. A., CD4 and CD8 T cells with high intracellular glutathione levels are selectively lost as the HIV infection progresses, *Int. Immunol.,* 199, 933, 1990.
19. Staal, F. J. T., Roederer, M., and Herzenberg, L. A., Intracellular thiols regulate activation of nuclear factor kappa B and transcripation of human immunodeficiency virus, *Proc. Natl. Acad. Sci. U.S.A.,* 87, 9943, 1990.
20. Mihm, S., Ennen, J., Pessare, U., Kurth, R., and Droge, W., Inhibition of HIV-1 replication and NF-kappa B activity by cysteine and cysteine derivatives, *AIDS,* 5, 497, 1991.
21. Schreck, R., Meier, B., Mannel, D. N., Droge, W., and Vaeuerle, P. A., Dithiocarbamates as potent inhibitors of nuclear factor Kappa B activation in intact cells, *J. Exp. Med.,* 175, 1181, 1992.
22. Schreck, R., Rieber, P., and Baeuerle, P. A., Reactive oxygen intermediates as apparently widely used messengers in the activation of the NF-kappa B transcription factor and HIV-1, *EMBO. J.,* 10, 2247, 1991.
23. Schreck, R., Albermann, K., and Baeuerle, P. A., Nuclear factor kappa B: an oxidative stress-responsive transcription factor of eukaryotic cells, *Free Radic. Res. Commun.,* 17, 221, 1992.
24. Quey, B., Malinverni, R., and Lauterburg, B. H., Glutathione depletion in HIV-infected patients: role of cysteine deficiency and effect of oral N-acetyl-cysteine, *AIDS,* 5, 814, 1992.
25. Fidelus, R. K. and Tsan, M., Enhancement of intracellular glutathione promotes lymphocyte activation by mitogen, *Cell Immunol.,* 97, 155, 1986.
26. Fidelus, R. K., Ginouves, P., Lawrence, D., and Tsan, M., Modulation of intracellular glutathione concentrations alters lymphocyte activation and proliferation, *Exp. Cell Res.,* 170, 269, 1987.
27. Suthanthiran, M., Anderson, M. E., Sharma, V. K., and Meister, A., Glutathione regulates activation-dependent DNA synthesis in highly purified normal human T lymphocytes stimulated via the CD2 and CD3 antigens, *Proc. Natl. Acad. Sci. U.S.A.,* 87, 3343, 1990.
28. Liang, S. M., Lee, N., Finbloom, D. S., and Liang, C. M., Regulation by glutathione of interleukin-4 activity on cytotoxic T cells, *Immunol.,* 75, 435, 1992.
29. Droge, W., Eck, H. P., Gmunder, H., and Mihm, S., Modulation of lymphocyte functions and immune responses by cysteine and cysteine derivatives, *Am. J. Med.,* 91 (suppl), 140, 1991.
30. Levy, D. M., Wu, J., Salibian, M., and Black, P. H., The effect of changes in thiol subcompartments on T-cell colony formation and cell cycle progression: relevance of AIDS. *Cell Immunol.,* 140, 370, 1992.
31. Kalebic, T., Kinter, A., Poli, G., Anderson, M. E., Meister, A., and Fauci, A. S., Suppression of human immunodeficiency virus expression in chronically infected monocytic cells by glutathione, glutathione ester, and N-acetyl-cysteine, *Proc. Natl. Acad. Sci. U.S.A.,* 88, 986, 1991.
32. Papadopulos-Eleopulos, E., Turner, V. F., and Papadimitriou, J. M., Oxidative stress, HIV, and AIDS, *Res. Immunol.,* 143, 145, 1992.
33. Droge, W., Eck, H. P., and Mihm, S., HIV-induced cysteine deficiency and T-cell dysfunction — a rationale for treatment with N-acetylcysteine, *Immunol. Today,* 13, 211, 1992.
34. Gilden, D., Nutritional intervention in HIV disease, *BETA,* March: 3–11, 1994.
35. Rortert, L. R., Vanita, R. A., and Bonnie, J. A., N-Acetylcysteine enhances antibody-dependent cellular cytotoxicity in neutrophils and mononuclear cells from healthy adults and human immunodeficiency virus-infected patients, *J. Infect. Dis.,* 172, 1492, 1995.

36. Angela, K. T., Stephen, D., Seth, W. P., Sheila, C. D., Suryaram, G., Steven, M. F., Deborah, N., Leon, G. E., Howard, E. G., and Harris, A. G., Tumors necrosis factors alpha-induced apoptosis in human neuronal cells: protection by the antioxidant N-acetylcysteine and the genes *bcl-2* and *crm*A, *Mol. Cell. Biol.,* 15, 2359, 1995.
37. Kinscherf, R., Fishbach, T., and Mihm, S., Effect of glutathione depletion and oral N-acetyl-cysteine treatment of CD4+ and CD8+ cells, *FASEB J.,* 8, 448, 1994.
38. Salbemini, D. and Botting, R., Modulation of platelet function by free radicals and free-radical scavengers, *TIPS,* 14, 36, 1993.
39. Shug, A. L. and Madsen, D. C., Protection of the ischemic rat heart by procysteine and amino acids, *J. Nutr. Biochem.,* 5, 356, 1994.
40. Combs, G. F. Jr., *The Vitamins: Fundamental Aspects in Nutrition and Health,* Academic Press, San Diego, 1992.
41. Passi, S., Picardo, D. M., Morrone, A., and Ippolito, F., I valori ematici deficitari degli acidi grassi poliinsaturi dei fosfolipidi, della vitamin E e della glutathione peossidasi come possibili fattori di rischio nell' insorgenza e nello sviluppo della sindrome da immunodeficienza acquisita, *G. Ital. Dermatol. Venereol.,* 125, 125, 1990.
42. Abrams, B., Duncan, D., and Hertz-Picciotto, I., A prospective study of dietary intake and acquired immune deficiency syndrome in HIV-seropositive homosexual men, *J. AIDS,* 6, 949, 1993.
43. Myrvik, Q. N., Immunology and nutrition, in *Modern Nutrition in Health and Disease,* 8th ed., Shils, M. E., Olson, J. A., and Shike, M., Eds., Lea & Febiger, Philadelphia, 1994, 62362.
44. Peinado, J., Sies, H., and Akerboom, T. P., Hepatic lipoate uptake, *Arch. Biochem. Biophys.* 273, 389, 1989.
45. Yuichiro, J., Suzuki, B. B. A., and Lester, P., α-Lipoic acid is a potent inhibitor of NF-κB activation in human T cells, *Biochem. Biophys. Res. Commun.,* 189, 1709, 1992.
46. Baur, A., Harrer, T., Peukert, M., Jahn, G., Kalden, J. R., and Fleckenstien, B., Alpha-lipoic acid is an effective inhibitor of human immuno-deficiency virus replication, *Klin. Wochenschr.,* 69, 722, 1991.
47. Siegel, B. V., Vitamin C and the immune response in health and disease, in *Human Nutrition: A Comprehensive Treatise, Vol. 8: Nutrition and Immunology,* Plenum Press, New York, 1993, 167.
48. Harakeh, S., Jariwalla, R. J., and Pauling, L., Suppression of human immunodeficiency virus replication by ascorbate in chronically and acutely infected cells, *Proc. Natl. Acad. Sci. U.S.A.,* 87, 7245, 1990.
49. Harakeh, S. and Jariwalla, R. J., Comparative study of the anti-HIV activities of ascorbate and thiol-containing reducing agents in chronically HIV-infected cells, *Am. J. Clin. Nutr.,* 54, 1231s, 1991.
50. Cathart, R., Vitamin C in the treatment of acquired immune deficiency syndrome (AIDS), *Med. Hypotheses,* 14, 423, 1984.
51. Beach, R., Mantero-Antienza, E., and Shor-Posner, G., Specific nutrient abnormalities in asymptomatic HIV-1 infection, *AIDS,* 6, 701, 1992.
52. Bendich, A. and Olson, J. A., Biological actions of carotenoids, *FASEB J.,* 3, 1927, 1989.
53. Schwabe, J. and Rhodes, D., Beyond zinc fingers: a steroid hormone receptors have a novel structural motif for DNA recognition, *Tibs,* 16, 291, 1991.
54. Tanala, Y., Shiozawa, S., Morito, I., and Fujita, T., Role of zinc in interleukin 2 mediated T-cell activation, *Scand. J. Immunol.,* 31, 547, 1990.
55. Dardenne, M., Savino, W., Berrih, S., and Bach, J. F., A zinc dependent epitope in the molecule of thymulin athymic hormone, *Proc. Natl. Acad. Sci. U.S.A.,* 82, 7035, 1985.
56. Graham, N., Sorensen, D., Odaka, N., Brookmeyer, R., Chan, D., Willett, W., Morris, J., and Saah, A., Relationship of serum copper and zinc levels to HIV-1 seropositivity and progression to AIDS, *J. AIDS,* 4, 976, 1991.
57. Fabris, N., Mocchegiani, E., Galli, M., Irato, L., Lazzarin, A., and Moroni, M., AIDS, zinc deficiency and thymic hormone failure, *J. Am. Med. Assoc.,* 259, 839, 1988.
58. Sergio, W., Zinc salts that may be defective against the AIDS virus HIV, *Med. Hypotheses,* 26, 251, 1988.

59. Maekawa, T., Sakura, H., Sudo, T., and Ishii, S., Putative metal finger structure of the human immuno-deficiency virus type 1 enhancer binding protein HIV-EP1, *J. Biol. Chem.,* 64, 14591, 1989.

60. South, T., Kim, B., Hare, D., and Summers, M., Zinc fingers and molecular recognition, structure and nucleic acid binding studies of an HIV zinc finger-like domain, *Biochem. Pharmacol.,* 40, 123, 1990.

61. Zazzo, J. F., Rouveix, B., Rajagopolan, P., Leracher, M., and Girard, P. M., Effect of zinc on immune status of zinc depleted ARC patients, *Clin. Nutr.,* 8, 259, 1989.

62. Schrauzer, G. N. and Sacher, J., Selenium in the maintenance and therapy of HIV-infected patients, *Chem. Biol. Inter.,* 91, 199, 1994.

63. Kiremidjian-Schumacher, L. and Stotzky, G., Selenium and immune responses, *Environ. Res.,* 42, 277, 1987.

64. Dwodkin, B. M., Rosenthal, W. S., Wormser, G. P., Weiss, L., Numez, M., Coline, C., and Herp, A., Abnormalities of blood selenium and glutathione peroxidase in patients with acquired immunodeficiency syndrome and AIDS-related complex, *Biol. Trace Elemen. Res.,* 20, 86, 1988.

65. Dworkin, B., Rosenthal, W., Wormser, G., and Weiss, L., Selenium deficiency in the acquired immuno-deficiency syndrome, *J. Parenteral. Enteral. Nutr.,* 10, 405, 1986.

66. Adam, E. S., Antioxidant supplementation in HIV/AIDS, *Nurse Practit.,* 20, 8, 1995.

67. Walter, R., Oster, M., Lee, T., Flynn, N., and Keen, C., Zinc status in human immunodeficiency virus infection, *Life Sci.,* 47, 1579, 1990.

68. Beck, K., Scramel, P., Hedl, A., Jaeger, H., and Kaboth, W., Serum trace element levels in HIV-infected subjects, *Biol. Trace Elem. Res.,* 25, 89, 1990.

69. Leff, J., Oppegard, M., Curiel, T., Brown, K., Schooley, R., and Repine, J., Progressive increases in serum catalase activity in advancing human immunodeficiency virus infection, *Free Rad. Biol. Med.,* 13, 143, 1992.

70. Wong, G. H., Elwell, J., Oberley, L., and Goeddel, D., Manganous superoxide dismutase is essential for cellular resistance to cytotoxicity of tumor necrosis factor, *Cell,* 58, 923, 1989.

71. Flores, S. C., Marecki, J. C., Harper, Kp., Bose, S. K., Nelson, S. K., and McCoed, J. M., Tat protein of human immunodeficiency virus type 1 represses expression of manganese superoxide dismutase in Hela Cells, *Proc. Natl. Acad. Sci. U.S.A.,* 90, 7632, 1993.

72. Reisinger, E. C., Kern, P., Ernst, M., Bock, P., Flad, H. D., and Dietrich, M., Inhibition of HIV progression by dithiocarb, *Lancet,* 335, 679, 1990.

73. Hersh, E. M., Brewton, G., Abrams, D., Bartlett, J., Galpin, J., Parkash, G., Gorter, R., Gottlieb, M., Jonikas, J. J., Landesman, S., Levine, A., Marcel, A., Petersin, E. A., Whiteside, M., Zahradnik, J., Negron, C., Boutitie, F., Caraux, J., Dupuy, J.-M., and Salmi, L. R., Dithiocarb sodium (diethyldithiocarbmate) therapy in patients with symptomatic HIV infection and AIDS. A randomized double blind, placebo-controlled multicenter study, *J. Am. Med. Assoc.,* 265, 1538, 1991.

74. Baruchel, S., Gao, Q., and Wainberg, M. A., Desferrioxamine and HIV, *Lancet,* 337, 1356, 1991.

75. Feid, B., Kim, M. C., and Ames, B. N., Ubiquinol-10 is an effective lipid-soluble antioxidant at physiological concentrations, *Proc. Natl. Acad. Sci. U.S.A.,* 87, 4879, 1990.

76. Langsjoen, P. H., Folkers, K., and Richardson, P., Treatment of patients with human immunodeficiency virus infection with coenzyme Q_{10}, in *Biomedical and Clinical Aspects of Coenzyme Q,* Vol. 6, Folkers, K., Litatarru, G. ., and Yamagami, T., Eds., Elsevier, Amsterdam, 1991, 40916.

77. Afanas'ev, I. B. and Dorozhko, A. I., Chelating and free radical scavenging mechanisms of inhibitory action of rutin and quercitin in lipid peroxidation, *Biochem. Pharmacol.,* 38, 1763, 1989.

78. Laughton, M. J., Evans, P. J., Moroney, M. A., Hoult, J. R. S., and Halliwell, F., Inhibition of mammalian 5-lipoxygenase and cyclo-oxygenase by flavonoids and phenolic dietary additives, *Biochem. Pharmacol.,* 42, 1673, 1993.

79. Torel, J., Cillard, J., and Dillard, P., Antioxidant activity of flavonoids and reactivity with peroxy radical, *Phytochemistry,* 25, 383, 1986.

80. Greenspan, H. C., The role of reactive oxygen species, antioxidants and phytopharmaceuticals in human immunodeficiency virus activity, *Med. Hypotheses,* 40, 85, 1993.

81. Paya, M., Halliwell, B., and Hoult, J. R. W., Interactions of a series of coumarins with reactive oxygen species, *Biochem. Pharmacol.,* 44, 205, 1992.

82. Drolet, G., Dumbroff, E. B., Legge, R. L., and Thompson, J. E., Radical scavenging properties of polyamines, *Phytochemistry,* 25, 367, 1986.
83. Bowler, C. and Slooten, L., Manganese superoxide dismutase can reduce cellular damage mediated by oxygen radicals in transgenic plants, *EMBO J.,* 10, 1732, 1991.
84. Alscher, R. G., Biosynthesis and antioxidant function of glutathione in plants, *Physiol. Plant,* 77, 457, 1989.
85. Garewal, H. S., Ampel, N. M., Watson, R. R., Prabhala, R. H., and Dols, C. L., A preliminary trial of beta-carotene in subjects infected with the human immunodeficiency virus, *J. Nutr.,* E22, 728, 1992.
86. Watson, R. R., Prabhala, R. H., Plezia, P. M., and Alberts, D. S., Effect of beta-carotene on lymphocyte subpopulations in elderly humans; evidence for a dose-response relationship, *Am. J. Clin. Nutr.,* 53, 90, 1991.
87. Voelker, R., Recommendations for antioxidants: how much evidence is enough? *J. Am. Med. Assoc.,* 271, 1148, 1994.

Chapter 5

ANTIOXIDANTS AND CANCER: THE EPIDEMIOLOGIC EVIDENCE

Jerry W. McLarty

Contents

I. Introduction...45
   A. Background..45
   B. Kinds of Epidemiologic Studies 46
   C. Methods 46

II. Results...47
   A. Recent Reviews 48
   B. Retrospective Dietary Studies 48
   C. Prospective Dietary Studies 50
   D. Retrospective Serum Studies...50
   E. Prospective Serum Studies 52

III. Conclusions...54

References..56

I. INTRODUCTION

A. BACKGROUND

The idea that diet may have something to do with cancer risk has been around for decades. At first, the emphasis was upon potential carcinogens in the diet that could be eliminated. However, population-based studies conducted in the 1960s[1] and early 1970s[2,3] shifted the focus toward a radical new idea: that perhaps certain diets could even protect against cancer. Now, after hundreds of studies have been conducted in populations around the world, in both sexes and many ethnic/racial groups and with many different kinds of cancer, it is clear that populations whose diets are rich in certain micronutrients have lower cancer risks than populations with diets deficient in these micronutrients. There is also evidence that antioxidants such as β-carotene, ascorbic acid (vitamin C), α-tocopherol (vitamin E), and selenium are significantly associated with reduced cancer risks. This chapter summarizes and discusses the considerable epidemiologic evidence for an association between antioxidants and cancer risk. The focus will be on the number of studies conducted for each antioxidant/nutrient and the results, by tumor site.

0-8493-8509-1/97/$0.00+$.50
© 1997 by CRC Press LLC

45

B. KINDS OF EPIDEMIOLOGIC STUDIES

The evidence for possible antioxidant cancer preventive roles includes dietary studies, studies of serum concentrations of antioxidants, experimental laboratory and animal studies, and human clinical trials. Only the human dietary and serum studies will be discussed in this chapter. There are several common study designs for both dietary and serum studies: retrospective studies, prospective studies, and other designs such as case-cohort or ecological studies. By far the most commonly reported type of study has been the retrospective dietary case-control study, in which diets of persons with cancer (cases) are compared with the diets of similar persons, often matched by age, race, sex, and other characteristics, who do not yet have cancer (controls). The obvious criticism for this kind of study is that the disease, e.g., cancer, may affect diet, so any differences found may be the result of cancer and not related to the cause of cancer. Also, persons with cancer may have a different dietary recall than persons without cancer, resulting in a reporting bias. Efforts to avoid this criticism have included interviewing spouses and other significant persons about the dietary habits of the cases or trying to estimate dietary habits some months or years before the diagnosis of cancer. Stronger evidence often comes from prospective studies in which the diets of persons (often as part of an identified cohort, such as an occupational group, a community, etc.) are documented, and then after some years have past, the baseline diets of those who developed cancer are compared to those who did not get cancer. There are two common variants of prospective studies: nested case-control studies, for which controls are selected from the same cohort as the cases, and case-cohort studies for which data from all persons in the cohort without cancer are compared to the cases' data. Even prospective dietary studies can be criticized on the grounds that diet could be associated with reduced cancer risk but may only be a surrogate for other lifestyle/environmental factors that are causing the observed reduced risk. Furthermore, dietary studies are not specific enough. For example, fruits and vegetables contain hundreds of chemical compounds, any one of which may be the protective agent. Studies which have measured specific micronutrients in plasma, serum, or other human tissue (such as nail clippings) have been used in an attempt to address the specificity issue. As with dietary studies, serum studies can be either retrospective or prospective. Another less commonly used study design is an ecologic study, which compares grouped data such as population cancer rates and population lifestyle characteristics (such as per capita food consumption).

C. METHODS

A computer search of the National Library of Medicine's MEDLINE®* biomedical database was conducted for all years since 1966. Publications related to diet and cancer, vitamins and cancer, or antioxidants and cancer were selected for study. The list of publications selected for this review represents a thorough, but not exhaustive collection. The large number of studies precludes a complete listing, so some selection criteria were imposed. Studies related to therapy, animal experiments, or mechanistic laboratory experiments were excluded. Ecologic studies and reports of lesser studied sites were excluded. Additionally, studies related solely

---

* Registered Trademark of the National Library of Medicine

to preneoplasia or premalignant conditions were excluded. The cancer sites included were lung, colorectal, head and neck, breast, prostate, and gastric (esophagus and stomach). Finally, studies specific to dietary or serum antioxidants β-carotene, vitamin C, vitamin E, or selenium were selected. Studies that reported retinol (vitamin A) also were included, since many early studies did not discriminate between preformed vitamin A (not an antioxidant) and β-carotene. Indeed, vegetable sources of vitamin A are the carotenoids. Vitamin A may have mechanisms of cancer prevention not related to antioxidants. A number of promising studies of other nonantioxidant nutrients, such as folic acid, were not included.

II. RESULTS

As can be seen from Figure 5.1, the body of literature on antioxidants and cancer has been growing exponentially. Although most of the early studies were dietary studies, Wahi,[4] as early as 1962, investigated the relationship of serum vitamin A and carcinoma of the oral cavity. Other, more epidemiologic, studies followed within the next few years. The large-scale studies in Scandinavia,[3] Hawaii,[2] and elsewhere[5-7] in the 1970s added weight to the hypothesis that certain dietary components might be inversely related to cancer risk. By the early 1980s, the evidence was strong enough that several large-scale intervention studies using specific nutrients were initiated.[8] Since that time, many studies have added support to the protective hypothesis by investigating more nutrients, other cancer sites, and other populations. Although the large clinical trial results have, for the most part, been negative,[9-11] the evidence of an inverse relationship of antioxidants (or something related to them in the diet) is overwhelming. The tables that follow will summarize and categorize this evidence in terms of study outcome.

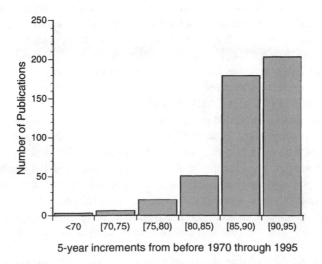

Figure 5.1. The number of antioxidant and cancer, diet and cancer, or vitamins and cancer-related publications per 5-year increments, since before 1970. On the horizontal axis, left brackets, i.e., "[", mean "greater than or equal to," and right parentheses, i.e., ")", mean "less than."

TABLE 5.1
Recent Reviews of Antioxidants and Cancer

Antioxidant/nutrient	Author, year	Site(s)	Reference
Vitamin A	Comstock, 1992	Multiple	27
	Willett, 1994	Lung, breast	28
	Fontham, 1990	Lung	29
β-Carotene	Flagg, 1995	Multiple	30
	Mayne, 1990	Multiple	31
	Fontham, 1990	Lung	29
	Willett, 1994	Lung, breast	28
Vitamin C	Block, 1992	Multiple	13
	Cohen, 1995	Gastrointestinal	32
	Flagg, 1995	Multiple	30
Vitamin E	Comstock, 1992	Multiple	27
	Knekt, 1991	Multiple	33
Selenium	Fontham, 1990	Lung	29
	Comstock, 1992	Multiple	27
Fruits and vegetables	Block, 1992	Multiple	12
	Fontham, 1990	Lung	29

A. RECENT REVIEWS

Numerous reviews and summaries have been published concerning the evidence, or lack thereof, for a protective antioxidant and cancer association. Table 5.1 shows several recent reviews (since 1990), categorized by micronutrient. One of the most comprehensive dietary reviews is by Block,[12] which summarizes the possible fruit and vegetable protective effects for a number of sites. Another review by Block[13] relates the evidence for vitamin C efficacy against cancer of the lung, cervix, colon, rectum, pancreas, and breast. There have been few recent reviews on vitamin E and on selenium, and the evidence presented is equivocal or negative, especially for selenium. Other reviews, such as by Garewal,[13-15] have been organized more by the tumor site rather than the specific antioxidant/nutrients. Most of the studies covered by the reviews listed in Table 5.1 are also included in this chapter.

B. RETROSPECTIVE DIETARY STUDIES

By far the most common type of study conducted has been the retrospective (case-control) dietary study. Table 5.2* summarizes the results of 145 retrospective dietary studies. The entries in the table are the number of studies reported by site, nutrient, and results. For example, out of 21 β-carotene and lung cancer studies, 15 found a significant inverse association, 4 found an equivocal association (e.g., inconsistent results, such as a significant association for one sex but not the other, or an inverse association that did not reach statistical significance), and 4 found no association. Note that the row and column totals are not consistent: some studies

* **Reading Tables 5.2–5.5:** The references at the bottom of the tables correspond to the number of studies for each site, nutrient, and outcome. For example, in Table 5.2 there are four studies listed concerning vitamin C and breast cancer: three (References 112, 118, and 122) are positive, none are equivocal, and one (Reference 10) is negative.

TABLE 5.2
Results of 145 Retrospective Dietary Studies

Nutrient[a]/outcome[b]

Cancer site	A +	A ±	A –	β-c +	β-c ±	β-c –	C +	C ±	C –	E +	E ±	E –	Se +	Se ±	Se –	F&V +	F&V ±	F&V –	Studies per site
Lung	8	5	8	15	4	2	4	2	4	2	0	1	0	0	0	10	3	1	34
Colorectal	2	0	2	7	0	0	7	2	1	1	1	1	0	0	0	13	1	2	25
Head and neck	3	0	2	8	2	2	6	1	2	2	1	2	0	0	0	9	1	0	20
Breast	0	1	6	3	4	3	3	0	1	2	1	2	0	0	1	1	0	2	17
Prostate	3	5	2	4	2	4	1	1	5	0	0	1	0	0	1	4	0	1	17
Gastric[c]	2	1	5	7	3	1	8	4	0	1	0	2	0	0	0	25	1	1	34
Number of studies per nutrient	55			71			52			20			2			73			

[a] A, vitamin A; β-c, β-carotene; C, vitamin C; E, vitamin E; Se, selenium; F&V, fruits and/or vegetables.
[b] Table entries are number of studies per site per nutrient per outcome:
   + significant protective association between nutrient and disease
   ± equivocal results, i.e., significant in some subgroups and not others, or nonsignificant protective association found
   – no association found between nutrient and outcome or, rarely, an increase in disease associated with the nutrient
[c] Gastric, esophagus and/or stomach.

References (+/±/–):

1. Lung-A: 34-41/38, 42-45/26, 46-52
2. Lung-β-c: 26, 37-41, 46-50, 52-55/38, 42, 45, 56/43, 51
3. Lung-C: 38, 43, 57, 58/46, 48/36, 42, 49, 56
4. Lung-E: 50, 55//56
5. Lung-Se: //
6. Lung-F&V: 46, 49, 50, 59-65/44, 53, 66/51
7. Colorectal-A: 67, 68//69, 70
8. Colorectal-β-c: 69, 71-76//
9. Colorectal-C: 69-71, 75-78/79, 80/81
10. Colorectal-E: 75/69/71
11. Colorectal-Se: //
12. Colorectal-F&V: 5, 74-78, 82-88/89/90, 91
13. Head and neck-A: 25, 92, 93//94, 95
14. Head and neck-β-c: 25, 93, 94, 96-100/89, 101/95, 102
15. Head and neck-C: 25, 92, 95, 97, 99, 101/89/96, 102
16. Head and neck-E: 25, 103/101/96, 10
17. Head and neck-Se: //
18. Head and neck-F&V: 97, 101, 102, 104-109/89/
19. Breast-A:/110/111-116
20. Breast-β-c: 116-118/111, 112, 119, 120/113, 115, 121
21. Breast-C: 112, 118, 122//110
22. Breast-E: 112, 123/119/115, 124
23. Breast-Se: //121
24. Breast-F&V: 125//110, 121
25. Prostate-A: 126-128/129-133/134, 135
26. Prostate-β-c: 128, 136-138/130, 132/129, 131, 133, 139
27. Prostate-C: 136/135/131, 133, 134, 138, 140
28. Prostate-E: //131
29. Prostate-Se: //133
30. Prostate-F&V: 129, 138, 139, 141//142
31. Gastric-A: 143, 144/145/146-150
32. Gastric-β-c: 147, 150-155/143, 145, 156/146
33. Gastric-C: 144, 146, 149-153, 157/145, 156, 158, 159/
34. Gastric-E: 151//153, 158
35. Gastric-Se: //
36. Gastric-F&V: 2, 7, 84, 106, 144, 146, 147, 150, 151, 155, 157, 158, 160-172/145/91

investigated more than one antioxidant, i.e., contributed to more than one column in Table 5.2, and some studies investigated more than one site, i.e., contributed to more than one row. References for each cell of the table are given at the bottom in the order of the results. Table 5.2 confirms the well-established conclusion that certain fruits and vegetables are associated with a decreased risk of lung cancer; in fact, 13 out of 14 studies reported a significant (10 studies) or equivocal (3 studies) inverse relationship; only one dietary study did not find an association. Surprisingly, only about 61% of the lung cancer-vitamin A retrospective dietary studies reported an inverse association. However, for all of the antioxidants except selenium, some studies reported a significant or other inverse association with lung cancer. The vitamin A evidence seems to be most consistent for prostate cancer: 80% of the studies reported an inverse association. β-Carotene results were quite consistent for lung cancer (19 out of 21 studies), colorectal cancer (all 7 studies), head and neck cancer (10 out of 12 studies) and gastric cancer (10 out of 11 studies). Vitamin C results were most encouraging for colorectal cancer (9 out of 10 studies) and gastric cancer (all 12 studies). Although protective vitamin E associations were reported for all of the cancer sites listed in Table 5.1; except prostate cancer, the number of studies was small and almost as many negative results were reported. There were 2 retrospective dietary selenium studies, but neither found significant inverse associations with cancer. Diets high in fruits and vegetables were inversely associated with cancer risk for all six cancer sites, but most consistently for head and neck, lung, colorectal, and gastric cancer. Only one out of three breast cancer studies reported a significant inverse association with fruits and vegetables. The results suggest that there may be a unique, tissue-specific response to each of the antioxidants.

C. PROSPECTIVE DIETARY STUDIES

Fewer prospective studies have been completed than retrospective studies, but perhaps their results should be given more weight because they were designed to eliminate the reporting bias of patients and surrogates and to minimize the possibility that the disease could cause the dietary differences found. Table 5.3 summarizes the results of 23 prospective dietary studies. For the most part, the prospective studies reflect the findings of the retrospective studies. The proportion of positive studies (i.e., showing a protective association) was even lower for the prospective dietary vitamin A-lung cancer studies — only three out of eight studies. The lung cancer β-carotene and lung cancer fruits and vegetables links were still highly consistent among the prospective studies. Although there were only two prospective vitamin C and gastric cancer studies reported, each showed an inverse correlation. The vitamin E results were about the same as for retrospective studies, but neither of the two breast cancer studies found an association. Selenium had a potential benefit in lung, prostate, and gastric cancer, but the number of studies was low. The fruits and vegetables-lung cancer findings were consistent: all 5 studies found an effect.

D. RETROSPECTIVE SERUM STUDIES

Table 5.4 shows the results of 27 retrospective serum studies. These studies typically measured antioxidant levels at time of diagnosis in cancer cases and compared them to control patient levels or cohort or population levels. Lung cancer results were consistent with the dietary studies: vitamin A and β-carotene had a protective association in all studies and one prospective vitamin E study also found

TABLE 5.3
Results of 23 Prospective Dietary Studies

| | Nutrient[a]/outcome[b] | | | | | | | | | | | | | | | | | |
Cancer site	A +	A ±	A –	β-c +	β-c ±	β-c –	C +	C ±	C –	E +	E ±	E –	Se +	Se ±	Se –	F&V +	F&V ±	F&V –	Studies per site
Lung	1	2	5	4	3	1	2	2	1	1	1	1	1	0	1	4	1	0	14
Colorectal	1	0	2	1	0	3	2	0	2	1	0	1	0	0	0	0	0	0	5
Head and neck	0	0	0	0	0	0	0	0	0	0	0	0	0	0	0	0	0	0	0
Breast	2	1	0	0	1	0	0	1	1	0	0	2	0	0	0	1	0	0	3
Prostate	0	1	0	0	1	0	0	0	0	0	0	0	1	0	0	0	0	1	2
Gastric[c]	1	0	0	1	0	1	2	0	0	1	0	0	2	0	0	1	0	0	5
Number of studies per nutrient	14			14			11			8			3			8			

[a] A, vitamin A; β-c, β-carotene; C, vitamin C; E, vitamin E; Se, selenium; F&V, fruits and/or vegetables.
[b] Table entries are number of studies per site per nutrient per outcome:
   + significant protective association between nutrient and disease
   ± equivocal results, i.e., significant in some subgroups and not others, or nonsignificant protective association found
   – no association found between nutrient and outcome or, rarely, an increase in disease associated with the nutrient
[c] Gastric, esophagus and/or stomach.

References (+/±/–):

1. Lung-A: 173/174, 175/176-180
2. Lung-β-c: 176, 178, 181, 182/180, 183, 184/185
3. Lung-C: 180, 181/174, 175/185
4. Lung-E: 181/175/176
5. Lung-Se: 186//180
6. Lung-F&V: 174, 179, 181, 187/184/
7. Colorectal-A: 175//188, 189
8. Colorectal-β-c: 175//185, 188, 189
9. Colorectal-C: 189, 190//185, 188
10. Colorectal-E: 188//189
11. Colorectal-Se: //
12. Colorectal-F&V: //
13. Head and neck-A: //
14. Head and neck-β-c: //
15. Head and neck-C: //
16. Head and neck-E: //
17. Head and neck-Se: //
18. Head and neck-F&V: //
19. Breast-A: 191, 192/193/
20. Breast-β-c: /193/
21. Breast-C: /193/192/
22. Breast-E: //192, 193
23. Breast-Se: //
24. Breast-F&V: 193//
25. Prostate-A: /194/
26. Prostate-β-c: /194/
27. Prostate-C: //
28. Prostate-E: //
29. Prostate-Se: 191//
30. Prostate-F&V: //194
31. Gastric-A: 191//
32. Gastric-β-c: 195//185
33. Gastric-C: 185, 195//
34. Gastric-E: 196//
35. Gastric-Se: 186, 191//
36. Gastric-F&V: 197//

a protective association. Both vitamin C studies of breast cancer found a positive effect, and the single gastric cancer study was consistent with the dietary findings of a beneficial relationship. Positive vitamin E effects were also found for prostate, breast, and gastric cancer, although the number of studies was small and negative findings were more prevalent. Selenium studies were mostly negative, but three out of seven selenium and breast cancer studies found a beneficial relationship.

TABLE 5.4
Results of 27 Retrospective Serum Studies

Cancer site	A +	A ±	A −	β-c +	β-c ±	β-c −	C +	C ±	C −	E +	E ±	E −	Se +	Se ±	Se −	Studies per site
Lung	2	2	0	2	0	0	0	0	0	1	0	0	0	0	0	5
Colorectal	0	0	1	0	0	1	0	0	1	0	0	1	0	0	2	2
Head and neck	4	1	0	2	1	0	0	0	0	0	0	0	0	0	0	5
Breast	2	0	3	1	1	3	2	0	0	3	0	2	3	0	4	11
Prostate	0	0	0	0	0	0	0	0	0	1	0	0	0	0	0	1
Gastric[c]	3	1	0	2	1	0	1	0	0	2	0	1	0	0	0	5
Number of studies per nutrient	18			12			4			11			9			

(Column group header: **Nutrient[a]/outcome[b]** spanning A, β-c, C, E, Se)

[a] A, vitamin A; β-c, β-carotene; C, vitamin C; E, vitamin E; Se, selenium.
[b] Table entries are number of studies per site per nutrient per outcome:
    + significant protective association between nutrient and disease
    ± equivocal results, i.e., significant in some subgroups and not others, or nonsignificant protective association found
    − no association found between nutrient and outcome or, rarely, an increase in disease associated with the nutrient
[c] Gastric, esophagus and/or stomach.

References (+/±/−):

1. Lung-A: 198, 199/44, 200/
2. Lung-β-c: 44, 201//
3. Lung-C: //
4. Lung-E: 199//
5. Lung-Se: //
6. Colorectal-A: //202
7. Colorectal-β-c: //202
8. Colorectal-C: //202
9. Colorectal-E: //202
10. Colorectal-Se: //202, 203
11. Head and neck-A: 4, 97, 204, 205/206/
12. Head and neck-β-c: 97, 205/206/
13. Head and neck-C: //
14. Head and neck-E: //
15. Head and neck-Se: //
16. Breast-A: 113, 207//114, 123, 208
17. Breast-β-c: 114/207/113, 123, 208
18. Breast-C: 209//
19. Breast-E: 207, 210, 211//123, 208
20. Breast-Se: 207, 209, 211/208, 212-214
21. Prostate-A: //
22. Prostate-β-c: //
23. Prostate-C: //
24. Prostate-E: 124//
25. Prostate-Se: //
26. Gastric-A: 201, 215, 216/206/
27. Gastric-β-c: 201, 216/206/
28. Gastric-C: 201//
29. Gastric-E: 201/216
30. Gastric-Se: //

E. PROSPECTIVE SERUM STUDIES

Table 5.5 summarizes the results of 18 prospective serum studies, arguably the most specific of all epidemiologic antioxidant studies, and perhaps the ones to which most weight should be attached. Typically, for these studies serum for a large number of people was saved, and after some years had elapsed, the blood antioxidant levels of cancer cases were compared with serum levels for control subjects. The inverse β-carotene and lung cancer association was strikingly consistent: all seven studies

TABLE 5.5
Results of 18 Prospective Serum Studies

	Nutrient[a]/outcome[b]															
	A			**β-c**			**C**			**E**			**Se**			**Studies**
Cancer site	+	±	–	+	±	–	+	±	–	+	±	–	+	±	–	**per site**
Lung	1	2	1	7	0	0	0	0	0	3	0	1	0	0	1	11
Colorectal	0	1	1	0	0	3	0	0	0	0	1	3	0	1	1	5
Head and neck	0	0	0	1	0	0	0	0	0	1	1	1	0	0	1	2
Breast	0	0	2	0	1	1	0	0	0	1	0	2	0	0	0	3
Prostate	2	0	0	0	0	2	0	0	0	0	0	2	0	0	0	3
Gastric[c]	2	1	1	2	1	1	3	0	0	2	0	1	1	0	1	7
Number of studies per nutrient		12			11			3			12			4		

[a] A, vitamin A; β-c, β-carotene; C, vitamin C; E, vitamin E; Se, selenium.
[b] Table entries are number of studies per site per nutrient per outcome:
+ significant protective association between nutrient and disease
± equivocal results, i.e., significant in some subgroups and not others, or nonsignificant protective association found
– no association found between nutrient and outcome or, rarely, an increase in disease associated with the nutrient
[c] Gastric, esophagus and/or stomach.

References (+/±/–):

1. Lung-A: 217/218, 219/220
2. Lung-β-c: 219-225//
3. Lung-C: //
4. Lung-E: 221, 223, 226//220
5. Lung-Se: //227
6. Colorectal-A: /228/220
7. Colorectal-β-c: //220, 221, 228
8. Colorectal-C: //
9. Colorectal-E: /224/220, 221, 228
10. Colorectal-Se: /227/228
11. Head and neck-A: //
12. Head and neck-β-c: 229//
13. Head and neck-C: //
14. Head and neck-E: 229/224/221
15. Head and neck-Se: //229
16. Breast-A: //230, 231
17. Breast-β-c: /231/221
18. Breast-C: //
19. Breast-E: 231//221, 230
20. Breast-Se: //
21. Prostate-A: 232, 233//
22. Prostate-β-c: //194, 221
23. Prostate-C: //
24. Prostate-E: //194, 221
25. Prostate-Se: //
26. Gastric-A: 222, 225/224/220
27. Gastric-β-c: 219, 225/224/220
28. Gastric-C: 219, 222, 225//
29. Gastric-E: 225, 234//220
30. Gastric-Se: 234//227

found the inverse association. Again, the β-carotene, colorectal cancer link was not found. All three of the vitamin C and prostate cancer studies were consistently positive, i.e., they showed a protective relationship. The vitamin E results were mixed, as with the retrospective studies. Unlike the retrospective studies, the prospective serum studies found an inverse selenium association with colorectal cancer and gastric cancer, but twice as many studies reported no effect.

III. CONCLUSIONS

It has been shown that there is considerable evidence suggesting the benefits of ingestion of at least some of the antioxidants. It is clear that diets rich in fruits and vegetables are associated with protection from lung cancer, gastric cancer, and colorectal cancer. The lung cancer evidence is especially strong and consistent: a total of more than 23,000 lung cancer cases were identified and compared to an even larger number of controls in the 168 dietary studies reported and more than 3000 cases were studied in the 45 serum reports. This is a staggering number of cancer cases and represents populations of millions from which the cases were identified. In addition to fruits and vegetables, diets high in β-carotene were consistently associated with reduced lung cancer risk: 35 of the 38 lung cancer β-carotene studies report this association. Only gastric cancer (esophagus or stomach) had the same consistently lower risk with vitamin C: all 18 of the studies reported a lowered risk. Almost 5000 cases of gastric cancer were included in the 18 vitamin C studies. Of the 20 β-carotene gastric cancer studies (also with more than 5,000 cases), 17 also found a protective association. Results for the other sites and antioxidants are less consistent. Protective associations were reported for all sites with all antioxidants except one: no head and neck-selenium effect was reported, although only one study had looked at this. A subjective ranking of the evidence for a protective cancer association is that fruits and vegetables are first, followed by β-carotene, vitamins C and A (in no clear order), vitamin E, and lastly, selenium. In terms of cancers that may be protected against, the evidence suggests a ranking of lung cancer, then gastric cancer, colorectal, and head and neck cancer, then prostate and breast cancer. There are several studies, not included in this review, suggesting that pancreatic cancer[16] and cancer of the cervix[17] may also be inversely associated with antioxidants. Another conclusion seems clear: the effects of an antioxidant may be tissue/site specific. If this is so, then studies which include all cancers or multiple sites may have reduced power to detect an inverse association with antioxidants.

The major weakness of the review, as presented, is that there has been no consideration of quality of the study or strength of the relationships between antioxidants and cancer: only numbers of publications have been presented. It is likely that a single, large, well-conducted study may be stronger evidence (whether negative or positive) than many studies with marginal statistical power. Also, a finding of a highly significant risk ratio far from 1.0 is likely to be stronger evidence of an effect than a marginally significant risk ratio close to 1.0. However, such considerations are beyond the scope of this review. Another problem, unique to all literature reviews, is the possibility of publication bias: negative studies may not get published as easily, or as often, as positive studies. However, it is not likely that this is a problem with antioxidants and cancer; by now, the field is mature enough that all kinds of studies have been reported) (in many countries, with many population groups) and negative studies abound. The field is controversial enough (and important enough) that any study, positive or negative, is of interest. Vitamin A, one of the first purported protective agents, has had many later negative findings. Other evidence of lack of a publication bias is the fact that multiple sites and multiple nutrients are often reported within the same study, with some of them being negative and some positive. Such studies could not have a selection bias toward positive or negative findings, since both are found within the same publications.

As shown by the large number of studies, there has been considerable interest in the topic of antioxidants and cancer. The possibility of preventing cancer by simple dietary means is attractive, especially since for some cancers, like lung cancer, there has been little progress in treatment for decades. The totality of evidence, epidemiological and experimental, has been sufficient to justify conducting large, expensive intervention trials using one or more antioxidants as potential preventive agents.[8] Unfortunately, most of the large-scale intervention trials that have been concluded did not find protective benefits,[9-11,18,19] and have even suggested that β-carotene may increase cancer risk in certain populations.[9,18] The reasons for the failure of the randomized clinical trials are not clear, and the puzzle of how to resolve these negative findings with the considerable epidemiologic evidence remains an important research issue. The evidence for a protective effect of antioxidants fit many of the philosophical criteria for causality. For example, the case-control studies, especially the prospective studies, show that diets or serum levels are low before the patients are diagnosed with cancer, e.g., a temporal relationship has been established. Many of the cited studies found not only a significant association, but a significant dose-response relationship as well. There is also biologic plausibility, i.e., there are sound biochemical and physiological mechanisms by which antioxidants could protect against cancer. Even the tissue specificity of some antioxidants lends plausibility: not every agent is associated with a reduced cancer risk for every cancer. Although not covered by this review, there are a number of studies that have found significant inverse relationships between antioxidants and preneoplastic conditions:[11,20] the same agents related to the ultimate cancer risk are also related to their precursor lesions, adding to the biologic, and temporal, plausibility. Ecological studies, not covered in this review, have found population differences in risks associated with the same dietary differences found in the case-control studies, adding strength to the causality hypothesis. Similarly, migration studies have found that subsequent generations of children and grandchildren have the same cancer risks as the host populations to which they migrated, ruling out a solely genetic reason for the population differences.

The major problem with dietary evidence is that the agents being studied may be significantly associated with something else in the diet (or the lifestyle) that is responsible for the protective effect. It is also possible that no single agent is by itself protective and that several or many dietary components together may be necessary. If this is the case, it may be impossible to sort them out with epidemiologic studies alone. Perhaps the intervention trials of the future will be conducted with foods such as fruits and vegetables, rather than with isolated micronutrients. However, not all randomized clinical trials with single agents have been failures: studies of synthetic retinoids have shown promise against head and neck cancer[21] and cervical cancer.[22] β-Carotene has been shown to reverse the prevalence and incidence of leukoplakia,[23] and vitamin E has shown promise in oral lesions.[24] Also, there have been a few studies, not reviewed, that looked at individual vitamin supplements and subsequent cancer risk, with mixed results.[25,26]

In conclusion, it is abundantly clear that people who consume certain fruits and vegetables have a lower risk of some cancers. It is less clear, but still likely, that diets rich in these fruits and vegetables may be protective. People whose blood levels of certain antioxidants are high are at lower risk of subsequent cancer, at least for some cancers. It is not yet known whether supplementation with antioxidants will reduce cancer risk. However, the epidemiologic evidence is so consistently suggestive, and the cancer problem so terrible, that we must try to find out.

REFERENCES

1. Magnus, K., Pedersen, E., Mork, T., Hougen, A. and Bjelke, E., Lung cancer in Finland and Norway: an epidemiological study, *Acta Pathol. Microbiol. Scand., Suppl* 199:1+, 1969.
2. Haenszel, W., Kurihara, M., Segi, M. and Lee, R. K. C., Stomach cancer among Japanese in Hawaii, *JNCI,* 49, 969, 1972.
3. Bjelke, E., Epidemiologic studies of cancer of the stomach, colon, and rectum; with special emphasis on the role of diet, *Scand. J. Gastroenterol. Suppl.,* 31, 1, 1974.
4. Wahi, P. N., Bodkhe, R. R., Arora, S. and Srivastava, M. C., Serum vitamin A studies in leukoplakia and carcinoma of the oral cavity, *Indian J. Path. Bact.,* 5, 10, 1962.
5. Graham, S., Dayal, H., Swanson, M., Mittelman, A. and Wilkinson, G., Diet in the epidemiology of cancer of the colon and rectum, *J. Natl. Cancer Inst.,* 61, 709, 1978.
6. Hirayama, T., Epidemiology of prostate cancer with special reference to the role of diet, *Natl. Cancer Inst. Monogr.,* 149, 1979.
7. Cook-Mozaffari, P. J., Azordegan, F., Day, N. E., Ressicaud, A., Sabai, C. and Aramesh, B., Oesophageal cancer studies in the Caspian Littoral of Iran: results of a case-control study, *Br. J. Cancer,* 39, 293, 1979.
8. Greenwald, P., Chemoprevention research at the U.S. National Cancer Institute, *Mil. Med.,* 159, 505, 1994.
9. The effect of vitamin E and beta carotene on the incidence of lung cancer and other cancers in male smokers. The Alpha-Tocopherol, Beta Carotene Cancer Prevention Study Group, *N. Engl. J. Med.,* 330, 1029, 1994.
10. Greenberg, E. R., Baron, J. A., Stukel, T. A., et al., A clinical trial of beta carotene to prevent basal-cell and squamous-cell cancers of the skin. The Skin Cancer Prevention Study Group, *N. Engl. J. Med.,* 323, 789, 1990.
11. McLarty, J. W., Holiday, D. B., Girard, W. M., Yanagihara, R. H., Kummet, T. D. and Greenberg, S. D., Beta-Carotene, vitamin A, and lung cancer chemoprevention: results of an intermediate endpoint study, *Am. J. Clin. Nutr.,* 62, 1431S, 1995.
12. Block, G., Patterson, B. and Subar, A., Fruit, vegetables, and cancer prevention: a review of the epidemiological evidence, *Nutr. Cancer,* 18, 1, 1992.
13. Block, G., Vitamin C status and cancer. Epidemiologic evidence of reduced risk, *Ann. N.Y. Acad. Sci.,* 669, 280, 1992.
14. Garewal, H., Chemoprevention of oral cancer: beta-carotene and vitamin E in leukoplakia, *Eur. J. Cancer Prev.,* 3, 101, 1994.
15. Garewal, H., Meyskens, F., Jr., Friedman, S., Alberts, D. and Ramsey, L., Oral cancer prevention: the case for carotenoids and anti-oxidant nutrients, *Prev. Med.,* 22, 701, 1993.
16. Baghurst, P. A., McMichael, A. J., Slavotinek, A. H., Baghurst, K. I., Boyle, P. and Walker, A. M., A case-control study of diet and cancer of the pancreas, *Am. J. Epidemiol.,* 134, 167, 1991.
17. Herrero, R., Potischman, N., Brinton, L. A., et al., A case-control study of nutrient status and invasive cervical cancer. I. Dietary indicators, *Am. J. Epidemiol.,* 134, 1335, 1991.

18. Omenn, G. S., Goodman, G. E., Thornquist, M. D., et al., Effects of a combination of beta carotene and vitamin A on lung cancer and cardiovascular disease, *N. Engl. J. Med.,* 334, 1150, 1996.
19. Hennekens, C. H., Buring, J. E., Manson, J. E., et al., Lack of effect of long-term supplementation with beta carotene on the incidence of malignant neoplasms and cardiovascular disease, *N. Engl. J. Med.,* 334, 1145, 1996.
20. Liu, T., Soong, S. J., Wilson, N. P., et al., A case control study of nutritional factors and cervical dysplasia, *Cancer Epidemiol. Biomarkers Prev.,* 2, 525, 1993.
21. Hong, W. K., Lippman, S. M., Itri, L. M., et al., Prevention of second primary tumors with isotretinoin in squamous-cell carcinoma of the head and neck, *N. Engl. J. Med.,* 323, 795, 1990.
22. Meyskens, F. L., Studies of retinoids in the prevention and treatment of cancer, *J. Am. Acad. Dermatol.,* 6, 824, 1982.
23. Stich, H. F., Mathew, B., Sankaranarayanan, R. and Nair, M. K., Remission of precancerous lesions in the oral cavity of tobacco chewers and maintenance of the protective effect of beta-carotene or vitamin A, *Am. J. Clin. Nutr.,* 53, 298S, 1991.
24. Benner, S. E., Wargovich, M. J., Lippman, S. M., et al., Reduction in oral mucosa micronuclei frequency following alpha-tocopherol treatment of oral leukoplakia, *Cancer Epidemiol. Biomarkers Prev.,* 3, 73, 1994.
25. Gridley, G., McLaughlin, J. K., Block, G., Blot, W. J., Gluch, M. and Fraumeni, J. F., Jr., Vitamin supplement use and reduced risk of oral and pharyngeal cancer, *Am. J. Epidemiol.,* 135, 1083, 1992.
26. Wu, A. H., Henderson, B. E., Pike, M. C. and Yu, M. C., Smoking and other risk factors for lung cancer in women, *J. Natl. Cancer Inst.,* 74, 747, 1985.
27. Comstock, G. W., Bush, T. L. and Helzlsouer, K., Serum retinol, beta-carotene, vitamin E, and selenium as related to subsequent cancer of specific sites, *Am. J. Epidemiol.,* 135, 115, 1992.
28. Willett, W. C., Micronutrients and cancer risk, *Am. J. Clin. Nutr.,* 59, 1162S, 1994.
29. Fontham, E. T., Protective dietary factors and lung cancer, *Int. J. Epidemiol.,* 19 Suppl 1, S32, 1990.
30. Flagg, E. W., Coates, R. J. and Greenberg, R. S., Epidemiologic studies of antioxidants and cancer in humans, *J. Am. Coll. Nutr.,* 14, 419, 1995.
31. Mayne, S. T., Beta-carotene and cancer prevention: what is the evidence?, *Conn. Med.,* 54, 547, 1990.
32. Cohen, M. and Bhagavan, H. N., Ascorbic acid and gastrointestinal cancer, *J. Am. Coll. Nutr.,* 14, 565, 1995.
33. Knekt, P., Role of vitamin E in the prophylaxis of cancer, *Ann. Med.,* 23, 3, 1991.
34. Bjelke, E., Dietary vitamin A and human lung cancer, *Int. J. Cancer,* 15, 561, 1975.
35. Bond, G. G., Thompson, F. E. and Cook, R. R., Dietary vitamin A and lung cancer: results of a case-control study among chemical workers, *Nutr. Cancer,* 9, 109, 1987.
36. Byers, T., Vena, J., Mettlin, C., Swanson, M. and Graham, S., Dietary vitamin A and lung cancer risk: an analysis by histologic subtypes, *Am. J. Epidemiol.,* 120, 769, 1984.
37. Dartigues, J. F., Dabis, F., Gros, N., et al., Dietary vitamin A, beta carotene and risk of epidermoid lung cancer in south-western France, *Eur. J. Epidemiol.,* 6, 261, 1990.
38. Fontham, E. T., Pickle, L. W., Haenszel, W., Correa, P., Lin, Y. P. and Falk, R. T., Dietary vitamins A and C and lung cancer risk in Louisiana, *Cancer,* 62, 2267, 1988.
39. Humble, C. G., Samet, J. M. and Skipper, B. E., Use of quantified and frequency indices of vitamin A intake in a case-control study of lung cancer, *Int. J. Epidemiol.,* 16, 341, 1987.
40. Kune, G. A., Kune, S., Watson, L. F., et al., Serum levels of beta-carotene, vitamin A, and zinc in male lung cancer cases and controls, *Nutr. Cancer,* 12, 169, 1989.
41. Kvale, G., Bjelke, E. and Gart, J. J., Dietary habits and lung cancer risk, *Int. J. Cancer,* 31, 397, 1983.
42. Hinds, M. W., Kolonel, L. N., Hankin, J. H. and Lee, J., Dietary vitamin A, carotene, vitamin C and risk of lung cancer in Hawaii, *Am. J. Epidemiol.,* 119, 227, 1984.
43. Koo, L. C., Dietary habits and lung cancer risk among Chinese females in Hong Kong who never smoked, *Nutr. Cancer,* 11, 155, 1988.
44. Pastorino, U., Pisani, P., Berrino, F., et al., Vitamin A and female lung cancer: a case-control study on plasma and diet, *Nutr. Cancer,* 10, 171, 1987.

45. Samet, J. M., Skipper, B. J., Humble, C. G. and Pathak, D. R., Lung cancer risk and vitamin A consumption in New Mexico, *Am. Rev. Respir. Dis.,* 131, 198, 1985.
46. Candelora, E. C., Stockwell, H. G., Armstrong, A. W. and Pinkham, P. A., Dietary intake and risk of lung cancer in women who never smoked, *Nutr. Cancer,* 17, 263, 1992.
47. Ho, S. C., Donnan, S. P., Martin, C. W. and Tsao, S. Y., Dietary vitamin A, beta-carotene and risk of epidermoid lung cancer among Chinese males, *Singapore Med. J.,* 29, 213, 1988.
48. Huang, C., Zhang, X., Qiao, Z., et al., A case-control study of dietary factors in patients with lung cancer, *Biomed. Environ. Sci.,* 5, 257, 1992.
49. Le Marchand, L., Yoshizawa, C. N., Kolonel, L. N., Hankin, J. H. and Goodman, M. T., Vegetable consumption and lung cancer risk: a population-based case-control study in Hawaii, *J. Natl. Cancer Inst.,* 81, 1158, 1989.
50. Mayne, S. T., Janerich, D. T., Greenwald, P., et al., Dietary beta carotene and lung cancer risk in U.S. nonsmokers, *J. Natl. Cancer Inst.,* 86, 33, 1994.
51. Pierce, R. J., Kune, G. A., Kune, S., et al., Dietary and alcohol intake, smoking pattern, occupational risk, and family history in lung cancer patients: results of a case-control study in males, *Nutr. Cancer,* 12, 237, 1989.
52. Ziegler, R. G., Mason, T. J., Stemhagen, A., et al., Dietary carotene and vitamin A and risk of lung cancer among white men in New Jersey, *J. Natl. Cancer Inst.,* 73, 1429, 1984.
53. Harris, R. W., Key, T. J., Silcocks, P. B., Bull, D. and Wald, N. J., A case-control study of dietary carotene in men with lung cancer and in men with other epithelial cancers, *Nutr. Cancer,* 15, 63, 1991.
54. Le Marchand, L., Hankin, J. H., Kolonel, L. N., Beecher, G. R., Wilkens, L. R. and Zhao, L. P., Intake of specific carotenoids and lung cancer risk [published erratum appears in Cancer Epidemiol Biomarkers Prev 1994 Sep;3(6):523], *Cancer Epidemiol. Biomarkers Prev.,* 2, 183, 1993.
55. LeGardeur, B. Y., Lopez, A. and Johnson, W. D., A case-control study of serum vitamins A, E, and C in lung cancer patients, *Nutr. Cancer,* 14, 133, 1990.
56. Byers, T. E., Graham, S., Haughey, B. P., Marshall, J. R. and Swanson, M. K., Diet and lung cancer risk: findings from the Western New York Diet Study, *Am. J. Epidemiol.,* 125, 351, 1987.
57. Jensen, H. and Madsen, J. L., Diet and cancer. Review of the literature, *Acta. Med. Scand.,* 223, 293, 1988.
58. Holst, P. A., Kromhout, D. and Brand, R., For debate: pet birds as an independent risk factor for lung cancer, *Br. Med. J.,* 297, 1319, 1988.
59. Dorgan, J. F., Ziegler, R. G., Schoenberg, J. B., et al., Race and sex differences in associations of vegetables, fruits, and carotenoids with lung cancer risk in New Jersey (United States), *Cancer Causes Control,* 4, 273, 1993.
60. Forman, M. R., Yao, S. X., Graubard, B. I., et al., The effect of dietary intake of fruits and vegetables on the odds ratio of lung cancer among Yunnan tin miners, *Int. J. Epidemiol.,* 21, 437, 1992.
61. Fraser, G. E., Beeson, W. L. and Phillips, R. L., Diet and lung cancer in California Seventh-day Adventists, *Am. J. Epidemiol.,* 133, 683, 1991.
62. Gao, C. M., Tajima, K., Kuroishi, T., Hirose, K. and Inoue, M., Protective effects of raw vegetables and fruit against lung cancer among smokers and ex-smokers: a case-control study in the Tokai area of Japan, *Jpn. J. Cancer Res.,* 84, 594, 1993.
63. Jain, M., Burch, J. D., Howe, G. R., Risch, H. A. and Miller, A. B., Dietary factors and risk of lung cancer: results from a case-control study, Toronto, 1981-1985, *Int. J. Cancer,* 45, 287, 1990.
64. MacLennan, R., Da Costa, J., Day, N. E., Law, C. H., Ng, Y. K. and Shanmugaratnam, K., Risk factors for lung cancer in Singapore Chinese, a population with high female incidence rates, *Int. J. Cancer,* 20, 854, 1977.
65. Pisani, P., Berrino, F., Macaluso, M., Pastorino, U., Crosignani, P. and Baldasseroni, A., Carrots, green vegetables and lung cancer: a case-control study, *Int. J. Epidemiol.,* 15, 463, 1986.
66. Freudenheim, J. L., Graham, S., Horvath, P. J., Marshall, J. R., Haughey, B. P. and Wilkinson, G., Risks associated with source of fiber and fiber components in cancer of the colon and rectum, *Cancer Res.,* 50, 3295, 1990.

67. Tomkin, G. H., Scott, L., Ogbuah, C. and OShaughnessy, M., Carcinoma of the colon — association with low dietary vitamin A in females: preliminary communication, *J. R. Soc. Med.,* 79, 462, 1986.

68. Tuyns, A. J., Haelterman, M. and Kaaks, R., Colorectal cancer and the intake of nutrients: oligosaccharides are a risk factor, fats are not. A case-control study in Belgium, *Nutr. Cancer,* 10, 181, 1987.

69. Ferraroni, M., La Vecchia, C., D'Avanzo, B., Negri, E., Franceschi, S. and Decarli, A., Selected micronutrient intake and the risk of colorectal cancer, *Br. J. Cancer,* 70, 1150, 1994.

70. Potter, J. D. and McMichael, A. J., Diet and cancer of the colon and rectum: a case-control study, *J. Natl. Cancer Inst.,* 76, 557, 1986.

71. Freudenheim, J. L., Graham, S., Marshall, J. R., Haughey, B. P. and Wilkinson, G., A case-control study of diet and rectal cancer in western New York, *Am. J. Epidemiol.,* 131, 612, 1990.

72. Lee, H. P., Gourley, L., Duffy, S. W., Esteve, J., Lee, J. and Day, N. E., Colorectal cancer and diet in an Asian population — a case-control study among Singapore Chinese, *Int. J. Cancer,* 43, 1007, 1989.

73. Slattery, M. L., Potter, J. D. and Sorenson, A. W., Age and risk factors for colon cancer (United States and Australia): are there implications for understanding differences in case-control and cohort studies?, *Cancer Causes Control,* 5, 557, 1994.

74. West, D. W., Slattery, M. L., Robison, L. M., et al., Dietary intake and colon cancer: sex- and anatomic site-specific associations, *Am. J. Epidemiol.,* 130, 883, 1989.

75. Yang, G., Gao, Y. and Ji, B., Comparison of risk factors between left and right-sided colon cancer, *Chung Kuo I Hsueh Ko Hsueh Yuan Hsueh Pao,* 16, 63, 1994.

76. Zaridze, D., Filipchenko, V., Kustov, V., Serdyuk, V. and Duffy, S., Diet and colorectal cancer: results of two case-control studies in Russia, *Eur. J. Cancer,* 29A, 112, 1992.

77. Kune, S., Kune, G. A. and Watson, L. F., Case-control study of dietary etiological factors: the Melbourne Colorectal Cancer Study, *Nutr. Cancer,* 9, 21, 1987.

78. Tuyns, A. J., A case-control study on colorectal cancer in Belgium. Preliminary results, *Soz Praventivmed,* 31, 81, 1986.

79. Howe, G. R., Miller, A. B., Jain, M. and Cook, G., Dietary factors in relation to the etiology of colorectal cancer, *Cancer Detect. Prev.,* 5, 331, 1982.

80. Macquart-Moulin, G., Riboli, E., Cornee, J., Charnay, B., Berthezene, P. and Day, N., Case-control study on colorectal cancer and diet in Marseilles, *Int. J. Cancer,* 38, 183, 1986.

81. Jain, M., Cook, G. M., Davis, F. G., Grace, M. G., Howe, G. R. and Miller, A. B., A case-control study of diet and colo-rectal cancer, *Int. J. Cancer,* 26, 757, 1980.

82. Haenszel, W., Locke, F. B. and Segi, M., A case-control study of large bowel cancer in Japan, *J. Natl. Cancer Inst.,* 64, 17, 1980.

83. Hu, J. F., Liu, Y. Y., Yu, Y. K., Zhao, T. Z., Liu, S. D. and Wang, Q. Q., Diet and cancer of the colon and rectum: a case-control study in China, *Int. J. Epidemiol.,* 20, 362, 1991.

84. La Vecchia, C., Negri, E., Decarli, A., et al., A case-control study of diet and colo-rectal cancer in northern Italy, *Int. J. Cancer,* 41, 492, 1988.

85. Manousos, O., Day, N. E., Trichopoulos, D., Gerovassilis, F., Tzonou, A. and Polychronopoulou, A., Diet and colorectal cancer: a case-control study in Greece, *Int. J. Cancer,* 32, 1, 1983.

86. Slattery, M. L., Sorenson, A. W., Mahoney, A. W., French, T. K., Kritchevsky, D. and Street, J. C., Diet and colon cancer: assessment of risk by fiber type and food source [published erratum appears in J Natl Cancer Inst 1989 Jul 5;81(13):1042], *J. Natl. Cancer Inst.,* 80, 1474, 1988.

87. Steinmetz, K. A., Kushi, L. H., Bostick, R. M., Folsom, A. R. and Potter, J. D., Vegetables, fruit, and colon cancer in the Iowa Women's Health Study, *Am. J. Epidemiol.,* 139, 1, 1994.

88. Young, T. B. and Wolf, D. A., Case-control study of proximal and distal colon cancer and diet in Wisconsin, *Int. J. Cancer,* 42, 167, 1988.

89. Day, G. L., Shore, R. E., Blot, W. J., et al., Dietary factors and second primary cancers: a follow-up of oral and pharyngeal cancer patients, *Nutr. Cancer,* 21, 223, 1994.

90. Miller, A. B., Howe, G. R., Jain, M., Craib, K. J. and Harrison, L., Food items and food groups as risk factors in a case-control study of diet and colo-rectal cancer, *Int. J. Cancer,* 32, 155, 1983.

91. Tajima, K. and Tominaga, S., Dietary habits and gastro-intestinal cancers: a comparative case-control study of stomach and large intestinal cancers in Nagoya, Japan, *Jpn. J. Cancer Res.*, 76, 705, 1985.

92. Graham, S., Mettlin, C., Marshall, J., Priore, R., Rzepka, T. and Shedd, D., Dietary factors in the epidemiology of cancer of the larynx, *Am. J. Epidemiol.*, 113, 675, 1981.

93. Marshall, J., Graham, S., Mettlin, C., Shedd, D. and Swanson, M., Diet in the epidemiology of oral cancer, *Nutr. Cancer*, 3, 145, 1982.

94. Mackerras, D., Buffler, P. A., Randall, D. E., Nichaman, M. Z., Pickle, L. W. and Mason, T. J., Carotene intake and the risk of laryngeal cancer in coastal Texas, *Am. J. Epidemiol.*, 128, 980, 1988.

95. Rossing, M. A., Vaughan, T. L. and McKnight, B., Diet and pharyngeal cancer, *Int. J. Cancer*, 44, 593, 1989.

96. Freudenheim, J. L., Graham, S., Byers, T. E., et al., Diet, smoking, and alcohol in cancer of the larynx: a case-control study, *Nutr. Cancer*, 17, 33, 1992.

97. Kune, G. A., Kune, S., Field, B., et al., Oral and pharyngeal cancer, diet, smoking, alcohol, and serum vitamin A and beta-carotene levels: a case-control study in men, *Nutr. Cancer*, 20, 61, 1993.

98. Negri, E., La Vecchia, C., Franceschi, S. and Tavani, A., Attributable risk for oral cancer in northern Italy, *Cancer Epidemiol. Biomarkers Prev.*, 2, 189, 1993.

99. Zheng, T., Boyle, P., Willett, W. C., et al., A case-control study of oral cancer in Beijing, People's Republic of China. Associations with nutrient intakes, foods and food groups, *Eur. J. Cancer B. Oral Oncol.*, 29B, 45, 1993.

100. Tavani, A., Negri, E., Franceschi, S., Barbone, F. and La Vecchia, C., Attributable risk for laryngeal cancer in northern Italy, *Cancer Epidemiol. Biomarkers Prev.*, 3, 121, 1994.

101. Gridley, G., McLaughlin, J. K., Block, G., et al., Diet and oral and pharyngeal cancer among blacks, *Nutr. Cancer*, 14, 219, 1990.

102. McLaughlin, J. K., Gridley, G., Block, G., et al., Dietary factors in oral and pharyngeal cancer, *J. Natl. Cancer Inst.*, 80, 1237, 1988.

103. Lee, H. P., Gourley, L., Duffy, S. W., Esteve, J., Lee, J. and Day, N. E., Preserved foods and nasopharyngeal carcinoma: a case-control study among Singapore Chinese, *Int. J. Cancer*, 59, 585, 1994.

104. Franceschi, S., Bidoli, E., Baron, A. E., et al., Nutrition and cancer of the oral cavity and pharynx in north-east Italy, *Int. J. Cancer*, 47, 20, 1991.

105. Franco, E. L., Kowalski, L. P., Oliveira, B. V., et al., Risk factors for oral cancer in Brazil: a case-control study, *Int. J. Cancer*, 43, 992, 1989.

106. Notani, P. N. and Jayant, K., Role of diet in upper aerodigestive tract cancers, *Nutr. Cancer*, 10, 103, 1987.

107. Oreggia, F., De Stefani, E., Correa, P. and Fierro, L., Risk factors for cancer of the tongue in Uruguay, *Cancer*, 67, 180, 1991.

108. Winn, D. M., Ziegler, R. G., Pickle, L. W., Gridley, G., Blot, W. J. and Hoover, R. N., Diet in the etiology of oral and pharyngeal cancer among women from the southern United States, *Cancer Res.*, 44, 1216, 1984.

109. Zheng, W., Blot, W. J., Shu, X. O., et al., Diet and other risk factors for laryngeal cancer in Shanghai, China, *Am. J. Epidemiol.*, 136, 178, 1992.

110. Graham, S., Marshall, J., Mettlin, C., Rzepka, T., Nemoto, T. and Byers, T., Diet in the epidemiology of breast cancer, *Am. J. Epidemiol.*, 116, 68, 1982.

111. Brisson, J., Verreault, R., Morrison, A. S., Tennina, S. and Meyer, F., Diet, mammographic features of breast tissue, and breast cancer risk, *Am. J. Epidemiol.*, 130, 14, 1989.

112. Graham, S., Hellmann, R., Marshall, J., et al., Nutritional epidemiology of postmenopausal breast cancer in western New York, *Am. J. Epidemiol.*, 134, 552, 1991.

113. Marubini, E., Decarli, A., Costa, A., et al., The relationship of dietary intake and serum levels of retinol and beta-carotene with breast cancer. Results of a case-control study, *Cancer*, 61, 173, 1988.

114. Potischman, N., McCulloch, C. E., Byers, T., et al., Breast cancer and dietary and plasma concentrations of carotenoids and vitamin A, *Am. J. Clin. Nutr.*, 52, 909, 1990.

115. Richardson, S., Gerber, M. and Cenee, S., The role of fat, animal protein and some vitamin consumption in breast cancer: a case control study in southern France, *Int. J. Cancer*, 48, 1, 1991.

116. Rohan, T. E., McMichael, A. J. and Baghurst, P. A., A population-based case-control study of diet and breast cancer in Australia, *Am. J. Epidemiol.,* 128, 478, 1988.

117. Lee, H. P., Gourley, L., Duffy, S. W., Esteve, J., Lee, J. and Day, N. E., Dietary effects on breast-cancer risk in Singapore, *Lancet,* 337, 1197, 1991.

118. Zaridze, D., Lifanova, Y., Maximovitch, D., Day, N. E. and Duffy, S. W., Diet, alcohol consumption and reproductive factors in a case-control study of breast cancer in Moscow, *Int. J. Cancer,* 48, 493, 1991.

119. Ambrosone, C. B., Marshall, J. R., Vena, J. E., et al., Interaction of family history of breast cancer and dietary antioxidants with breast cancer risk (New York, United States), *Cancer Causes Control,* 6, 407, 1995.

120. Cooper, J. A., Rohan, T. E., Cant, E. L., Horsfall, D. J. and Tilley, W. D., Risk factors for breast cancer by oestrogen receptor status: a population-based case-control study, *Br. J. Cancer,* 59, 119, 1989.

121. Van 't Veer, P., Kolb, C. M., Verhoef, P., et al., Dietary fiber, beta-carotene and breast cancer: results from a case-control study, *Int. J. Cancer,* 45, 825, 1990.

122. Landa, M. C., Frago, N. and Tres, A., Diet and the risk of breast cancer in Spain, *Eur. J. Cancer Prev.,* 3, 313, 1994.

123. London, S. J., Stein, E. A., Henderson, I. C., et al., Carotenoids, retinol, and vitamin E and risk of proliferative benign breast disease and breast cancer, *Cancer Causes Control,* 3, 503, 1992.

124. Gerber, M., Richardson, S., Cavallo, F., et al., The role of diet history and biologic assays in the study of "diet and breast cancer", *Tumori,* 76, 321, 1990.

125. La Vecchia, C., Decarli, A., Franceschi, S., Gentile, A., Negri, E. and Parazzini, F., Dietary factors and the risk of breast cancer, *Nutr. Cancer,* 10, 205, 1987.

126. Hayes, R. B., Bogdanovicz, J. F., Schroeder, F. H., et al., Serum retinol and prostate cancer, *Cancer,* 62, 2021, 1988.

127. Heshmat, M. Y., Kaul, L., Kovi, J., et al., Nutrition and prostate cancer: a case-control study, *Prostate,* 6, 7, 1985.

128. Ohno, Y., Yoshida, O., Oishi, K., Okada, K., Yamabe, H. and Schroeder, F. H., Dietary beta-carotene and cancer of the prostate: a case-control study in Kyoto, Japan, *Cancer Res.,* 48, 1331, 1988.

129. Giovannucci, E., Ascherio, A., Rimm, E. B., Stampfer, M. J., Colditz, G. A. and Willett, W. C., Intake of carotenoids and retinol in relation to risk of prostate cancer, *J. Natl. Cancer Inst.,* 87, 1767, 1995.

130. Kolonel, L. N., Hankin, J. H. and Yoshizawa, C. N., Vitamin A and prostate cancer in elderly men: enhancement of risk, *Cancer Res.,* 47, 2982, 1987.

131. Rohan, T. E., Howe, G. R., Burch, J. D. and Jain, M., Dietary factors and risk of prostate cancer: a case-control study in Ontario, Canada, *Cancer Causes Control,* 6, 145, 1995.

132. Ross, R. K., Shimizu, H., Paganini-Hill, A., Honda, G. and Henderson, B. E., Case-control studies of prostate cancer in blacks and whites in southern California, *J. Natl. Cancer Inst.,* 78, 869, 1987.

133. West, D. W., Slattery, M. L., Robison, L. M., French, T. K. and Mahoney, A. W., Adult dietary intake and prostate cancer risk in Utah: a case-control study with special emphasis on aggressive tumors, *Cancer Causes Control,* 2, 85, 1991.

134. Bravo, M. P., Castellanos, E. and del Rey Calero, J., Dietary factors and prostatic cancer, *Urol. Int.,* 46, 163, 1991.

135. Kaul, L., Heshmat, M. Y., Kovi, J., et al., The role of diet in prostate cancer, *Nutr. Cancer,* 9, 123, 1987.

136. Kolonel, L. N., Yoshizawa, C. N. and Hankin, J. H., Diet and prostatic cancer: a case-control study in Hawaii, *Am. J. Epidemiol.,* 127, 999, 1988.

137. Mettlin, C., Selenskas, S., Natarajan, N. and Huben, R., Beta-carotene and animal fats and their relationship to prostate cancer risk. A case-control study, *Cancer,* 64, 605, 1989.

138. Oishi, K., Okada, K., Yoshida, O., et al., A case-control study of prostatic cancer with reference to dietary habits, *Prostate,* 12, 179, 1988.

139. Le Marchand, L., Hankin, J. H., Kolonel, L. N. and Wilkens, L. R., Vegetable and fruit consumption in relation to prostate cancer risk in Hawaii: a reevaluation of the effect of dietary beta-carotene, *Am. J. Epidemiol.,* 133, 215, 1991.

140. Graham, S., Haughey, B., Marshall, J., et al., Diet in the epidemiology of carcinoma of the prostate gland, *J. Natl. Cancer Inst.*, 70, 687, 1983.

141. Mishina, T., Watanabe, H., Araki, H. and Nakao, M., Epidemiological study of prostatic cancer by matched-pair analysis, *Prostate*, 6, 423, 1985.

142. Talamini, R., La Vecchia, C., Decarli, A., Negri, E. and Franceschi, S., Nutrition, social factors and prostatic cancer in a Northern Italian population, *Br. J. Cancer*, 53, 817, 1986.

143. Graham, S., Haughey, B., Marshall, J., et al., Diet in the epidemiology of gastric cancer, *Nutr. Cancer*, 13, 19, 1990.

144. Mettlin, C., Graham, S., Priore, R., Marshall, J. and Swanson, M., Diet and cancer of the esophagus, *Nutr. Cancer*, 2, 143, 1981.

145. Ziegler, R. G., Morris, L. E., Blot, W. J., Pottern, L. M., Hoover, R. and Fraumeni, J., Jr., Esophageal cancer among black men in Washington, D.C. II. Role of nutrition, *J. Natl. Cancer Inst.*, 67, 1199, 1981.

146. Brown, L. M., Blot, W. J., Schuman, S. H., et al., Environmental factors and high risk of esophageal cancer among men in coastal South Carolina, *J. Natl. Cancer Inst.*, 80, 1620, 1988.

147. Decarli, A., Liati, P., Negri, E., Franceschi, S. and La, V. C., Vitamin A and other dietary factors in the etiology of esophageal cancer, *Nutr. Cancer*, 10, 29, 1987.

148. Graham, S., Marshall, J., Haughey, B., et al., Nutritional epidemiology of cancer of the esophagus, *Am. J. Epidemiol.*, 131, 454, 1990.

149. Ramon, J. M., Serra-Majem, L., Cerdo, C. and Oromi, J., Nutrient intake and gastric cancer risk: a case-control study in Spain, *Int. J. Epidemiol.*, 22, 983, 1993.

150. You, W. C., Blot, W. J., Chang, Y. S., et al., Diet and high risk of stomach cancer in Shandong, China, *Cancer Res.*, 48, 3518, 1988.

151. Gao, Y. T., McLaughlin, J. K., Gridley, G., et al., Risk factors for esophageal cancer in Shanghai, China. II. Role of diet and nutrients, *Int. J. Cancer*, 58, 197, 1994.

152. Gonzalez, C. A., Riboli, E., Badosa, J., et al., Nutritional factors and gastric cancer in Spain, *Am. J. Epidemiol.*, 139, 466, 1994.

153. La Vecchia, C., Ferraroni, M., D'Avanzo, B., Decarli, A. and Franceschi, S., Selected micronutrient intake and the risk of gastric cancer, *Cancer Epidemiol. Biomarkers Prev.*, 3, 393, 1994.

154. Negri, E., La Vecchia, C., Franceschi, S., Decarli, A. and Bruzzi, P., Attributable risks for oesophageal cancer in northern Italy, *Eur. J. Cancer*, 28A, 1167, 1992.

155. Tavani, A., Negri, E., Franceschi, S. and La Vecchia, C., Risk factors for esophageal cancer in lifelong nonsmokers, *Cancer Epidemiol. Biomarkers Prev.*, 3, 387, 1994.

156. La Vecchia, C., Negri, E., Decarli, A., D'Avanzo, B. and Franceschi, S., A case-control study of diet and gastric cancer in northern Italy, *Int. J. Cancer*, 40, 484, 1987.

157. Boeing, H., Frentzel-Beyme, R., Berger, M., et al., Case-control study on stomach cancer in Germany, *Int. J. Cancer*, 47, 858, 1991.

158. Risch, H. A., Jain, M., Choi, N. W., et al., Dietary factors and the incidence of cancer of the stomach, *Am. J. Epidemiol.*, 122, 947, 1985.

159. Tuyns, A. J., Protective effect of citrus fruit on esophageal cancer, *Nutr. Cancer*, 5, 195, 1983.

160. Buiatti, E., Palli, D., Decarli, A., et al., A case-control study of gastric cancer and diet in Italy, *Int. J. Cancer*, 44, 611, 1989.

161. Cornee, J., Pobel, D., Riboli, E., Guyader, M. and Hemon, B., A case-control study of gastric cancer and nutritional factors in Marseille, France, *Eur. J. Epidemiol.*, 11, 55, 1995.

162. Correa, P., Fontham, E., Pickle, L. W., Chen, V., Lin, Y. P. and Haenszel, W., Dietary determinants of gastric cancer in south Louisiana inhabitants, *J. Natl. Cancer Inst.*, 75, 645, 1985.

163. Demirer, T., Icli, F., Uzunalimoglu, O. and Kucuk, O., Diet and stomach cancer incidence. A case-control study in Turkey, *Cancer*, 65, 2344, 1990.

164. Guo, W., Blot, W. J., Li, J. Y., et al., A nested case-control study of oesophageal and stomach cancers in the Linxian nutrition intervention trial, *Int. J. Epidemiol.*, 23, 444, 1994.

165. Hu, J. F., Zhang, S. F., Jia, E. M., et al., Diet and cancer of the stomach: a case-control study in China, *Int. J. Cancer*, 41, 331, 1988.

166. Jedrychowski, W., Wahrendorf, J., Popiela, T. and Rachtan, J., A case-control study of dietary factors and stomach cancer risk in Poland, *Int. J. Cancer*, 37, 837, 1986.

167. Kono, S., Ikeda, M., Tokudome, S. and Kuratsune, M., A case-control study of gastric cancer and diet in northern Kyushu, Japan, *Jpn. J. Cancer Res.,* 79, 1067, 1988.

168. Li, J. Y., Ershow, A. G., Chen, Z. J., et al., A case-control study of cancer of the esophagus and gastric cardia in Linxian, *Int. J. Cancer,* 43, 755, 1989.

169. Nakachi, K., Imai, K., Hoshiyama, Y. and Sasaba, T., The joint effects of two factors in the aetiology of oesophageal cancer in Japan, *J. Epidemiol. Community Health,* 42, 355, 1988.

170. Trichopoulos, D., Ouranos, G., Day, N. E., et al., Diet and cancer of the stomach: a case-control study in Greece, *Int. J. Cancer,* 36, 291, 1985.

171. Victora, C. G., Munoz, N., Day, N. E., Barcelos, L. B., Peccin, D. A. and Braga, N. M., Hot beverages and oesophageal cancer in southern Brazil: a case-control study, *Int. J. Cancer,* 39, 710, 1987.

172. Yu, M. C., Garabrant, D. H., Peters, J. M. and Mack, T. M., Tobacco, alcohol, diet, occupation, and carcinoma of the esophagus, *Cancer Res.,* 48, 3843, 1988.

173. Edes, T. E. and McDonald, P. S., Retinol and retinol-binding protein in lung cancer screening, *Cancer Detect. Prev.,* 15, 341, 1991.

174. Chow, W. H., Schuman, L. M., McLaughlin, J. K., et al., A cohort study of tobacco use, diet, occupation, and lung cancer mortality, *Cancer Causes Control,* 3, 247, 1992.

175. Shibata, A., Paganini-Hill, A., Ross, R. K. and Henderson, B. E., Intake of vegetables, fruits, beta-carotene, vitamin C and vitamin supplements and cancer incidence among the elderly: a prospective study, *Br. J. Cancer,* 66, 673, 1992.

176. Connett, J. E., Kuller, L. H., Kjelsberg, M. O., et al., Relationship between carotenoids and cancer. The Multiple Risk Factor Intervention Trial (MRFIT) Study, *Cancer,* 64, 126, 1989.

177. Friedman, G. D., Blaner, W. S., Goodman, D. S., et al., Serum retinol and retinol-binding protein levels do not predict subsequent lung cancer, *Am. J. Epidemiol.,* 123, 781, 1986.

178. Shekelle, R. B., Lepper, M., Liu, S., et al., Dietary vitamin A and risk of cancer in the Western Electric study, *Lancet,* 2, 1186, 1981.

179. Wang, L. D. and Hammond, E. C., Lung cancer, fruit, green salad and vitamin pills, *Chin. Med. J. (Engl.),* 98, 206, 1985.

180. Kromhout, D., Essential micronutrients in relation to carcinogenesis, *Am. J. Clin. Nutr.,* 45, 1361, 1987.

181. Knekt, P., Jarvinen, R., Seppanen, R., et al., Dietary antioxidants and the risk of lung cancer, *Am. J. Epidemiol.,* 134, 471, 1991.

182. Ziegler, R. G., Mason, T. J., Stemhagen, A., et al., Carotenoid intake, vegetables, and the risk of lung cancer among white men in New Jersey, *Am. J. Epidemiol.,* 123, 1080, 1986.

183. Shekelle, R. B., Tangney, C. C., Rossof, A. H. and Stamler, J., Serum cholesterol, beta-carotene, and risk of lung cancer, *Epidemiology,* 3, 282, 1992.

184. Shibata, A., Paganini-Hill, A., Ross, R. K., Yu, M. C. and Henderson, B. E., Dietary beta-carotene, cigarette smoking, and lung cancer in men, *Cancer Causes Control,* 3, 207, 1992.

185. Ocke, M. C., Kromhout, D., Menotti, A., et al., Average intake of anti-oxidant (pro)vitamins and subsequent cancer mortality in the 16 cohorts of the Seven Countries Study, *Int. J. Cancer,* 61, 480, 1995.

186. Knekt, P., Aromaa, A., Maatela, J., et al., Serum selenium and subsequent risk of cancer among Finnish men and women, *J. Natl. Cancer Inst.,* 82, 864, 1990.

187. Ziegler, R. G., Mason, T. J., Stemhagen, A., et al., Carotenoid intake, vegetables, and the risk of lung cancer among white men in New Jersey, *Am. J. Epidemiol.,* 123, 1080, 1986.

188. Bostick, R. M., Potter, J. D., McKenzie, D. R., et al., Reduced risk of colon cancer with high intake of vitamin E: the Iowa Women's Health Study, *Cancer Res.,* 53, 4230, 1993.

189. Wu, A. H., Paganini-Hill, A., Ross, R. K. and Henderson, B. E., Alcohol, physical activity and other risk factors for colorectal cancer: a prospective study, *Br. J. Cancer,* 55, 687, 1987.

190. Heilbrun, L. K., Nomura, A., Hankin, J. H. and Stemmermann, G. N., Diet and colorectal cancer with special reference to fiber intake, *Int. J. Cancer,* 44, 1, 1989.

191. Criqui, M. H., Bangdiwala, S., Goodman, D. S., et al., Selenium, retinol, retinol-binding protein, and uric acid. Associations with cancer mortality in a population-based prospective case-control study, *Ann. Epidemiol.,* 1, 385, 1991.

192. Hunter, D. J., Manson, J. E., Colditz, G. A., et al., A prospective study of the intake of vitamins C, E, and A and the risk of breast cancer, *N. Engl. J. Med.,* 329, 234, 1993.

193. Rohan, T. E., Howe, G. R., Friedenreich, C. M., Jain, M. and Miller, A. B., Dietary fiber, vitamins A, C, and E, and risk of breast cancer: a cohort study, *Cancer Causes Control,* 4, 29, 1993.

194. Hsing, A. W., McLaughlin, J. K., Schuman, L. M., et al., Diet, tobacco use, and fatal prostate cancer: results from the Lutheran Brotherhood Cohort Study, *Cancer Res.,* 50, 6836, 1990.

195. Zheng, W., Sellers, T. A., Doyle, T. J., Kushi, L. H., Potter, J. D. and Folsom, A. R., Retinol, antioxidant vitamins, and cancers of the upper digestive tract in a prospective cohort study of postmenopausal women, *Am. J. Epidemiol.,* 142, 955, 1995.

196. Zhang, L., Zhao, L. and Ma, J., Relationship between serum micronutrients and precancerous gastric lesions, *Chung Hua Yu Fang I Hsueh Tsa Chih,* 29, 198, 1995.

197. Chyou, P. H., Nomura, A. M., Hankin, J. H. and Stemmermann, G. N., A case-cohort study of diet and stomach cancer, *Cancer Res.,* 50, 7501, 1990.

198. Atukorala, S., Basu, T. K. and Dickerson, J. W. T., Vitamin A, zinc and lung cancer, *Br. J. Cancer,* 40, 927, 1979.

199. Tominaga, K., Saito, Y., Mori, K., et al., An evaluation of serum microelement concentrations in lung cancer and matched non-cancer patients to determine the risk of developing lung cancer: a preliminary study, *Jpn. J. Clin. Oncol.,* 22, 96, 1992.

200. Scali, J., Astre, C., Segala, C. and Gerber, M., Relationship of serum cholesterol, dietary and plasma beta-carotene with lung cancer in male smokers, *Eur. J. Cancer Prev.,* 4, 169, 1995.

201. Stahelin, H. B., Vitamins and cancer: results of a Basel study, *Soz Praventivmed,* 34, 75, 1989.

202. Berta, J. L., Coste, T., Rautureau, J., Guilloud-Bataille, M. and Pequignot, G., Diet and rectoco-lonic cancers. Results of a case-control study, *Gastroenterol Clin. Biol.,* 9, 348, 1985.

203. Nelson, R. L., Davis, F. G., Sutter, E., et al., Serum selenium and colonic neoplastic risk, *Dis. Colon Rectum,* 38, 1306, 1995.

204. Drozdz, M., Gierek, T., Jendryczko, A., Piekarska, J., Pilch, J. and Polanska, D., Zinc, vitamins A and E, and retinol-binding protein in sera of patients with cancer of the larynx, *Neoplasma,* 36, 357, 1989.

205. Ibrahim, K., Jafarey, N. A. and Zuberi, S. J., Plasma vitamin A and carotene levels in squamous cell carcinoma of oral cavity and oro-pharynx, *Clin. Oncol.,* 3, 203, 1977.

206. Zaridze, D. G., Blettner, M., Trapeznikov, N. N., et al., Survey of a population with a high incidence of oral and oesophageal cancer, *Int. J. Cancer,* 36, 153, 1985.

207. Audisio, M., Mastroiacovo, P., Martinoli, L., et al., Serum values of vitamins A, E, C and carotenoids in healthy adult subjects and those with breast neoplasia, *Boll. Soc. Ital. Biol. Spe.,* 65, 473, 1989.

208. Basu, T. K., Hill, G. B., Ng, D., Abdi, E. and Temple, N., Serum vitamins A and E, beta-carotene, and selenium in patients with breast cancer, *J. Am. Coll. Nutr.,* 8, 524, 1989.

209. Nunez Martin, C. and Ortiz de Apodaca y Ruiz, A., Ascorbic acid in the plasma and blood cells of women with breast cancer. The effect of the consumption of food with an elevated content of this vitamin, *Nutr. Hosp.,* 10, 368, 1995.

210. Gerber, M., Cavallo, F., Marubini, E., et al., Liposoluble vitamins and lipid parameters in breast cancer. A joint study in northern Italy and southern France, *Int. J. Cancer,* 42, 489, 1988.

211. Gerber, M., Richardson, S., Salkeld, R. and Chappuis, P., Antioxidants in female breast cancer patients, *Cancer Invest.,* 9, 421, 1991.

212. Overvad, K., Gron, P., Langhoff, O., Tarp, U., Foldspang, A. and Thorling, E. B., Selenium in human mammary carcinogenesis: a case-referent study, *Eur. J. Cancer Prev.,* 1, 27, 1991.

213. van 't Veer, P., van der Wielen, R. P., Kok, F. J., Hermus, R. J. and Sturmans, F., Selenium in diet, blood, and toenails in relation to breast cancer: a case-control study, *Am. J. Epidemiol.,* 131, 987, 1990.

214. Meyer, F., Verreault, R., van 't Veer, P., et al., Erythrocyte selenium and breast cancer risk, *Am. J. Epidemiol.,* 125, 917, 1987.

215. Prasad, M. P., Krishna, T. P., Pasricha, S., Krishnaswamy, K. and Quereshi, M. A., Esophageal cancer and diet — a case-control study, *Nutr. Cancer,* 18, 85, 1992.

216. Jendryczko, A., Drozdz, M., Pardela, M., Kozlowski, A. and Drozdz, M., Vitamins A and E and vitamin A-binding proteins in the blood serum of patients with esophageal cancer, *Przegl. Lek.,* 46, 632, 1989.

217. Wald, N., Idle, M., Boreham, J. and Bailey, A., Low serum-vitamin-A and subsequent risk of cancer. Preliminary results of a prospective study, *Lancet,* 2, 813, 1980.

218. Knekt, P., Aromaa, A., Maatela, J., et al., Serum vitamin A and subsequent risk of cancer: cancer incidence follow-up of the Finnish Mobile Clinic Health Examination Survey, *Am. J. Epidemiol.,* 132, 857, 1990.

219. Stahelin, H. B., Gey, K. F., Eichholzer, M., et al., Plasma antioxidant vitamins and subsequent cancer mortality in the 12-year follow-up of the prospective Basel Study, *Am. J. Epidemiol.,* 133, 766, 1991.

220. Nomura, A. M., Stemmermann, G. N., Heilbrun, L. K., Salkeld, R. M. and Vuilleumier, J. P., Serum vitamin levels and the risk of cancer of specific sites in men of Japanese ancestry in Hawaii, *Cancer Res.,* 45, 2369, 1985.

221. Comstock, G. W., Helzlsouer, K. J. and Bush, T. L., Prediagnostic serum levels of carotenoids and vitamin E as related to subsequent cancer in Washington County, Maryland, *Am. J. Clin. Nutr.,* 53, 260S, 1991.

222. Eichholzer, M., Stahelin, H. B. and Gey, K. F., Inverse correlation between essential antioxidants in plasma and subsequent risk to develop cancer, ischemic heart disease and stroke respectively: 12-year follow-up of the Prospective Basel Study, *Exs,* 62, 398, 1992.

223. Menkes, M. S., Comstock, G. W., Vuilleumier, J. P., Helsing, K. J., Rjder, A. A. and Brookmeyer, R., Serum beta-carotene, vitamins A and E, selenium, and the risk of lung cancer, *N. Engl. J. Med.,* 315, 1250, 1986.

224. Stahelin, H. B., Rosel, F., Buess, E. and Brubacher, G., Cancer, vitamins, and plasma lipids: prospective Basel study, *J. Natl. Cancer Inst.,* 73, 1463, 1984.

225. Stahelin, H. B., Gey, F. and Brubacher, G., Preventive potential of antioxidative vitamins and carotenoids on cancer, *Int. J. Vitam. Nutr. Res. Suppl.,* 30, 232, 1989.

226. Knekt, P., Vitamin E and smoking and the risk of lung cancer, *Ann. N.Y. Acad. Sci.,* 686, 280, 1993.

227. Nomura, A., Heilbrun, L. K., Morris, J. S. and Stemmermann, G. N., Serum selenium and the risk of cancer, by specific sites: case-control analysis of prospective data, *J. Natl. Cancer Inst.,* 79, 103, 1987.

228. Schober, S. E., Comstock, G. W., Helsing, K. J., et al., Serologic precursors of cancer. I. Prediagnostic serum nutrients and colon cancer risk, *Am. J. Epidemiol.,* 126, 1033, 1987.

229. Zheng, W., Blot, W. J., Diamond, E. L., et al., Serum micronutrients and the subsequent risk of oral and pharyngeal cancer, *Cancer Res.,* 53, 795, 1993.

230. Russell, M. J., Thomas, B. S. and Bulbrook, R. D., A prospective study of the relationship between serum vitamins A and E and risk of breast cancer, *Br. J. Cancer,* 57, 213, 1988.

231. Wald, N. J., Boreham, J., Hayward, J. L. and Bulbrook, R. D., Plasma retinol, beta-carotene and vitamin E levels in relation to the future risk of breast cancer, *Br. J. Cancer,* 49, 321, 1984.

232. Hsing, A. W., Comstock, G. W., Abbey, H. and Polk, B. F., Serologic precursors of cancer. Retinol, carotenoids, and tocopherol and risk of prostate cancer, *J. Natl. Cancer Inst.,* 82, 941, 1990.

233. Reichman, M. E., Hayes, R. B., Ziegler, R. G., et al., Serum vitamin A and subsequent development of prostate cancer in the first National Health and Nutrition Examination Survey Epidemiologic Follow-up Study, *Cancer Res.,* 50, 2311, 1990.

234. Knekt, P., Aromaa, A., Maatela, J., et al., Serum vitamin E, serum selenium and the risk of gastrointestinal cancer, *Int. J. Cancer,* 42, 846, 1988.

Chapter 6

ANTIOXIDANT NUTRIENTS AND LUNG CANCER

Susan T. Mayne and Regina G. Ziegler

Contents

I. Introduction to Lung Cancer 67

II. Observational Studies of Antioxidant Nutrients and Lung Cancer 68

III. Intervention Trials of Antioxidant Nutrients and Lung Cancer 69

IV. Interpretation 82

V. Conclusions and Recommendations 84

References 85

I. INTRODUCTION TO LUNG CANCER

Lung cancer is the most common tumor worldwide.[1] In the U.S., it has been the leading cause of cancer death in men since the early 1950s and in women since 1987. The American Cancer Society estimates that in 1996, 177,000 Americans will be diagnosed with lung cancer and 158,700 will die of the disease.[2] The three cornerstones for reducing cancer-related morbidity and mortality are prevention, early detection, and treatment. Early detection of lung cancer has not been realized; only 15% of lung cancers are discovered when the disease is still localized.[2] The lack of success in treatment for lung cancer is evident given that the 5-year relative survival rate for lung cancer is only 13%.[2] These data emphasize the importance of prevention for reducing lung cancer morbidity and mortality.

A large body of literature has established cigarette smoking as the dominant risk factor for lung cancer; 90.3% of lung cancer deaths in U.S. men and 78.5% in U.S. women are attributable to cigarette smoking.[3] In the U.S., cigarette use among men has declined. A corresponding decline in lung cancer incidence has been observed in U.S. males, from a high of 87 new cases of lung cancer/100,000 in 1984 to 81 cases in 1992.[2] However, many individuals have difficulty quitting, and even those who quit face an increased risk of lung cancer relative to nonsmokers. In most studies, the risk of lung cancer among former smokers remained elevated above the risk in never smokers, even in the longest periods of abstinence evaluated.[4] Thus,

0-8493-8509-1/97/$0.00+$.50
© 1997 by CRC Press LLC

an active area of cancer prevention research is the search for interventions to reduce the risk for lung cancer in current and former smokers.

The gas phase of cigarette smoke is known to be highly oxidative, possessing an array of free radical species.[5] Other exposures involved in lung carcinogenesis, such as asbestos (which contains iron, a catalyst of lipid oxidation), ozone, environmental tobacco smoke, and air pollution, may also involve oxidative mechanisms. This suggests a potential role for antioxidant nutrients in the prevention of lung cancer. As detailed below, many descriptive studies, case-control studies, cohort studies, and intervention trials of antioxidant nutrients and lung cancer have been published. The following summarizes and integrates this literature.

II. OBSERVATIONAL STUDIES OF ANTIOXIDANT NUTRIENTS AND LUNG CANCER

Observational studies of lung cancer have examined the association between antioxidant nutrient intake and disease incidence or between blood or tissue levels of antioxidant nutrients and disease incidence. One type of observational study is prospective, with the antioxidant intake and/or status measured before the clinical diagnosis of lung cancer. Another type of observational study is retrospective, wherein individuals with lung cancer and comparable controls are asked to recall usual dietary intake prior to the development of the disease (cases) or prior to interview (controls). Retrospective studies of nutrients and lung cancer typically rely on recalled dietary intake rather than blood nutrient levels to assess exposure, as altered blood nutrient status could easily be a consequence, rather than a cause, of the disease.

A comprehensive review of the literature on nutrition and lung cancer has been published recently,[6] with considerable attention given to the observational studies. Perhaps the most striking finding to emerge from the observational studies of lung cancer is the apparent protective effect of fruits and vegetables, i.e., persons who consume greater quantities of fruits and vegetables are far less likely to develop lung cancer than persons who consume lesser quantities of fruits and vegetables. The prospective studies of dietary factors and lung cancer risk are summarized in Table 6.1, and the retrospective studies of dietary factors and lung cancer risk are summarized in Table 6.2. Table 6.3 summarizes results of prospective studies of blood micronutrient levels and lung cancer risk. As shown in the tables, intake of fruits and vegetables and/or carotenoids (a marker of consumption of fruits and vegetables) was associated with reduced lung cancer risk in 8 of 8 prospective studies and 18 of 20 retrospective studies reviewed.[6] The reduced risk is observed in men and women, in various countries, in current smokers, ex-smokers, and never-smokers, and for all histologic types of lung cancer.

Fruits and vegetables are known to contain numerous substances with purported antioxidant activity including carotenoids, vitamin C, and other phytochemicals such as polyphenols.[7] What specific role these substances/groups of substances play in lung cancer prevention is unknown. As detailed in the tables, many studies have examined the association of lung cancer risk with total carotenoid intake and/or blood β-carotene levels, with vitamin C intake and/or blood levels, with vitamin E intake and/or blood levels, and with selenium status as measured biochemically. Individual studies suggest protective effects for each of these nutrients, although the totality of the evidence is not convincing at present for any one of these antioxidant micronutrients.[6]

There is clearly more information to be gleaned from observational studies of nutrition and lung cancer. For example, a recent analysis of intake of fruits and vegetables and lung cancer risk in a large population of nonsmoking (never and former smokers) men and women indicated that the lung cancer risk reduction was greater for fruits and vegetables typically consumed in a raw form, as compared to those typically cooked or processed in some manner.[8] Cooking appears to increase the bioavailability of some substances in fruits and vegetables, such as α- and β-carotene;[9] however, other substances in fruits and vegetables are heat labile, including vitamin C[10] and some of the xanthophyllic carotenoids.[11,12] Epidemiologic studies that specifically address the effects of cooking/processing of fruits and vegetables on lung cancer risk are needed, along with laboratory studies of effects of food preparation on levels of other phytochemicals in foods. Also, future epidemiological studies are needed to identify specific fruits and vegetables, if any, that are associated consistently with lung cancer risk reduction.

Observational epidemiologic studies of specific dietary components depend upon food composition data, which are generally adequate for most of the macronutrients and vitamins found in foods. However, data regarding the concentrations of various phytochemicals in foods are lacking. The U.S. Department of Agriculture recently released an individual carotenoid database, which includes levels of the five major carotenoids found in foods.[13] The release of this database has facilitated new research studies of the association between dietary intake of individual carotenoids and lung cancer risk. Le Marchand and colleagues found that dietary intake of α-carotene, β-carotene, and lutein was associated with reduced lung cancer risk in both men and women.[14] Ziegler and colleagues also found significant inverse trends for dietary α- and β-carotene, and a marginally significant effect for lutein.[15] It is notable that in both studies, high intake of a variety of vegetables was more strongly associated with reduced risk than high intake of the individual carotenoids. A food composition database for some of the major phytochemical classes is being developed; this will open new avenues of investigation for observational studies of dietary antioxidants and lung cancer.

III. INTERVENTION TRIALS OF ANTIOXIDANT NUTRIENTS AND LUNG CANCER

Intervention trials of antioxidant nutrients and lung cancer prevention consist predominantly of β-carotene trials, with some trials using β-carotene as a single agent, and others using it in combination with other antioxidant nutrients. Beginning with trials using premalignant endpoints (see Table 6.4), the Tyler (Texas) Chemoprevention Trial randomized 755 asbestos workers to receive β-carotene (50 mg/day) and retinol (25,000 IU every other day) vs. placebo to see if the combination of the two nutrients could reduce the prevalence of atypical cells in sputum. After a mean intervention period of 58 months, the prevalence of sputum atypia was nonsignificantly

TABLE 6.1

Prospective Studies of Vegetable, Fruit, Carotenoid, and Micronutrient Intake and Lung Cancer [a,b,c]

Study	Year	Location/population	No. of cases[d]	Years of follow-up	Dietary assessment	Vegetables + fruits	Vegetables	Fruits
Bjelke et al.	1975	Norway	M + F: 153	9 to 12	FFQ		→	0
Kvale et al.	1983							↓? ↓↓
Shekelle et al.	1981	Chicago, IL	M: 33	19	DH		↓?	↓↓↓
Kromhout et al.	1987	Netherlands	M: 63	25	DH		←	→ ↓↓
Paganini-Hill et al.	1987	Los Angeles, CA, U.S.	M: 125	8	FFQ	←	↓↓	
Shibata et al.	1992	Retirement community	F: 70			→		↓↓↓
Shibata et al.	1992							
Fraser et al.	1991	California, U.S. Seventh-day Adventists	M: 61	6	FFQ			
Knekt et al.	1991	Finland	M: 117	14-20	DH		↓?	↓?
Chow et al.	1992	U.S. White Lutherans	M: 219	20	FFQ		↑	→
Steinmetz et al.	1993	Iowa, U.S. 55+ years old	F: 138	4	FFQ	↓↓↓	↓↓↓	↓↓

Study	Dark green vegetables	Yellow-orange vegetables	Carotenoids	Retinol	Vitamin A	Vitamin C	Total vitamin C	Vitamin E	Total vitamin E
Bjelke et al.					↓↓↓	0			
Kvale et al.		↓↓							
Shekelle et al.			↓↓↓	0		↓?			
Kromhout et al.			0	0		↓↓↓			
Paganini-Hill et al.	↑	→					0		
Shibata et al.	↓↓	↓↓	↓↓			0	0		0
Shibata et al.						↓↓	↓↓		↓↓
Fraser et al.	0								
Knekt et al.		↓?	↓?	↑?	↑?	0		0	
Chow et al.		→	0	0	0	→			
Steinmetz et al.	↓↓↓	→	→			0	0		

From Ziegler, R. G., Mayne, S. T., and Swanson, C. A., *Cancer Causes and Control, 7, 157, 1996.*

a To be included, studies had to assess diet in sufficient detail for the intake of several food groups and/or micronutrients to be evaluated. When sequential analyses of one cohort have been published, results based on the largest number of lung cancer cases or deaths are used.

b ↓↓↓ (and ↑↑↑) indicate inverse (and positive) associations with statistically significant trends. ↓↓ (and ↑↑) indicate inverse (and positive) associations with marginally significant trends or apparent trends that do not reach statistical significance. ↓ (and ↑) indicate inverse (and positive) associations with no evidence of a trend. ↓? (and ↑?) indicate inverse (and positive) associations with insufficient data presented to evaluate trend. 0 indicates no association.

c None of these studies assessed folate or fiber intake. Carotenoids, retinol, vitamin A, vitamin C, and vitamin E refer to intake from foods. Total vitamin C and total vitamin E refer to combined intake from foods and supplements.

d M, males; F, females.

e FFQ, food frequency questionnaire; DH, diet history.

TABLE 6.2
**Retrospective Studies of Vegetable, Fruit, Carotenoid,
and Micronutrient Intake and Lung Cancer** [a,b,c]

Study	Year	Location/ population	No. of cases[d]	Study design[e]	Dietary assessment[f]
Mettlin et al.	1979	Buffalo, NY, U.S.	M: 427	Hos	FFQ
Byers et al.	1984				
Hinds et al.	1984	Hawaii, U.S.	M: 261	Pop	DH
Kolonel et al.	1985	Multi-ethnic	F: 103		
Ziegler et al.	1984	New Jersey, U.S.	WM: 736	Pop	FFQ
Ziegler et al.	1986	Whites and Blacks	WF: 860		
Dorgan et al.	1993		BM: 269		
			BF: 86		
Samet et al.	1985	New Mexico, U.S.	WM + F: 322	Pop	FFQ
		Whites and Hispanics	HM + F: 125		
Wu et al.	1985	Los Angeles, CA, U.S.	W: 210	Com	FFQ
		Whites			
Byers et al.	1987	Western New York, U.S.	M: 296	Pop	FFQ
			F: 154		
Gao et al.	1987	Shanghai, China	F: 672	Pop	FFQ
Pastorino et al.	1987	Milan, Italy	F: 47	Hos	FFQ
Fontham et al.	1988	Louisiana, U.S.	M + F: 1253	Hos	FFQ
		Whites and Blacks			
Koo et al.	1988	Hong Kong Chinese	F: 88	Com	FFQ
		Never-smokers			
Le Marchand et al.	1989	Hawaii, U.S.	M: 230	Pop	DH
		Multi-ethnic	F: 102		
Dartiques et al.	1990	France	M + F: 143	Hos	FFQ
Jain et al.	1990	Toronto, Canada	M + F: 839	Pop	DH
Kalandidi et al.	1990	Athens, Greece	F: 91	Hos	FFQ
		Never-smokers			
Wu-Williams et al.	1990	Northeast China	F: 963	Pop	FFQ
		Air pollution			
Harris et al.	1991	Oxford, U.K.	M: 96	Hos	FFQ
Candelora et al.	1992	Florida, U.S.	F: 124	Pop	FFQ
		Never-smokers			
Forman et al.	1992	Yunnan, China	M: 428		FFQ
Swanson et al.	1992	Tin miners			
Alavanja et al.	1993	Missouri, U.S.	F: 429	Pop	FFQ
		Nonsmokers			
Mayne et al.	1994	New York State, U.S.	M: 201	Pop	FFQ
		Nonsmokers	F: 212		

increased, not reduced, in the subjects receiving supplements.[16] In a 14-week randomized intervention trial in the Netherlands, however, heavy smokers who received supplemental β-carotene (20 mg/day) had a significant reduction in sputum micronuclei.[17] Micronuclei are indicative of DNA damage/chromosomal breakage; however, the relevance of a short-term effect on micronuclei to lung carcinogenesis, which is thought to take decades to develop, is unknown. Notably, in the same trial, β-carotene was not found to reduce *in vivo* oxidation as measured by urinary excretion

TABLE 6.2 (Continued)

Vegetables + fruits	Vegetables	Fruits	Dark green vegetables	Yellow-orange vegetables	Carotenoids	Retinol
					↓?	↓?
					↓?	
					↑?	
↓↓↓	↓↓↓	↓	↓↓↓	↓↓↓	↓↓	↑
	↓↓↓	↓↓↓			↓↓↓	
	0	↑↑↑			↑	
	↓	↑			↑↑	
					↓↓	0
					↑	0
					↓?	0
					↓↓↓	
					0	
			↓?		↑	
					↓?	↓?
↓↓↓	↓↓	↓↓↓			0	0
		↓↓↓	↓	↓		
	↓↓↓	0	↓↓↓	↓↓↓	↓↓↓	0
	↓↓↓	0	↓↓↓	↓↓↓	↓↓↓	0
					↓	↓
	↓↓↓	0			↓	0
	0	↓↓			0	↑?
0		↑				
↓↓			0	↓↓	↓↓↓	↑
	↓↓↓	↓↓↓		↓?	↓↓↓	0
		0	↓↓↓	0		
0	0				0	0
↓↓↓E	0	↓			↓?	0
↓↓↓E	↓↓↓	↓↓			↓?	0

of 8-oxo-7,8-dihydro-2′deoxyguanosine, suggesting that antioxidant activity was not responsible for the reduction in micronuclei.[18]

Two trials of antioxidant nutrients that had lung cancer as a primary endpoint have now been completed (see Table 6.4). The Alpha-Tocopherol Beta-Carotene (ATBC) trial[19] involved 29,133 males age 50 to 69 years old from Finland, who were heavy cigarette smokers at entry (average one pack/day for 36 years). The study design was a two-by-two factorial with participants randomized to receive

TABLE 6.2 (Continued)

Study	Year	Location/ population	No. of cases[d]	Study design[e]	Dietary assessment[f]
Mettlin et al.	1979	Buffalo, NY, U.S.	M: 427	Hos	FFQ
Byers et al.	1984				
Hinds et al.	1984	Hawaii, U.S.	M: 261	Pop	DH
Kolonel et al.	1985	Multi-ethnic	F: 103		
Ziegler et al.	1984	New Jersey, U.S.	WM: 736	Pop	FFQ
Ziegler et al.	1986	Whites and Blacks	WF: 860		
Dorgan et al.	1993		BM: 269		
			BF: 86		
Samet et al.	1985	New Mexico, U.S.	WM + F: 322	Pop	FFQ
		Whites and Hispanics	HM + F: 125		
Wu et al.	1985	Los Angeles, CA, U.S.	W: 210	Com	FFQ
		Whites			
Byers et al.	1987	Western New York, U.S.	M: 296	Pop	FFQ
			F: 154		
Gao et al.	1987	Shanghai, China	F: 672	Pop	FFQ
Pastorino et al.	1987	Milan, Italy	F: 47	Hos	FFQ
Fontham et al.	1988	Louisiana, U.S.	M + F: 1253	Hos	FFQ
		Whites and Blacks			
Koo et al.	1988	Hong Kong Chinese	F: 88	Com	FFQ
		Never-smokers			
Le Marchand et al.	1989	Hawaii, U.S.	M: 230	Pop	DH
		Multi-ethnic	F: 102		
Dartiques et al.	1990	France	M + F: 143	Hos	FFQ
Jain et al.	1990	Toronto, Canada	M + F: 839	Pop	DH
Kalandidi et al.	1990	Athens, Greece	F: 91	Hos	FFQ
		Never-smokers			
Wu-Williams et al.	1990	Northeast China	F: 963	Pop	FFQ
		Air pollution			
Harris et al.	1991	Oxford, U.K.	M: 96	Hos	FFQ
Candelora et al.	1992	Florida, U.S.	F: 124	Pop	FFQ
		Never-smokers			
Forman et al.	1992	Yunnan, China	M: 428		FFQ
Swanson et al.	1992	Tin miners			
Alavanja et al.	1993	Missouri, U.S.	F: 429	Pop	FFQ
		Nonsmokers			
Mayne et al.	1994	New York State, U.S.	M: 201	Pop	FFQ
		Nonsmokers	F: 212		

either supplemental vitamin E (50 mg/day), β-carotene (20 mg/day), the combination, or placebo for 5 to 8 years. Unexpectedly, participants receiving β-carotene (alone or in combination with vitamin E) had a significantly higher incidence of lung cancer (RR = 1.18; 95% CI = 1.03 to 1.36) and total mortality (RR = 1.08, 95% CI = 1.01 to 1.16) than participants receiving placebo. Supplemental β-carotene had no significant effect on the incidence of other major cancers occurring in this population (prostate, bladder, colon/rectum, stomach). Tumor site-specific data were not presented regarding the effects of supplemental β-carotene on less common cancers. Within the placebo group, higher β-carotene intake and higher serum

TABLE 6.2 (Continued)

Vitamin A	Vitamin C	Total vitamin C	Vitamin E	Total vitamin E	Folate	Fiber
↓?	0					0
↓?		↓?				
0		↑?				
0						
↓↓↓						
0						
0						
↓	↓	↓		↓		↓↓↓
0	0	0		0		↓
↓?						
	↓↓↓					
↓↓↓	↓↓↓	↓↓↓			↓↓	↓↓
↓↓	0	↑			↓↓	↓↓
0	0					0
0	↓	↓				
↓↓	↓↓↓					
	0	0	↑↑	↑		↓
				↓		
				↓		

β-carotene concentrations at baseline were each associated with a lower subsequent lung cancer incidence, consistent with the observational literature.

The finding of an increased incidence of lung cancer in β-carotene supplemented smokers has now been replicated in another major trial.[20] The Carotene and Retinol Efficacy Trial (CARET) was a multicenter lung cancer prevention trial of supplemental β-carotene (30 mg/day) plus retinol (25,000 IU/day) vs. placebo in asbestos workers and smokers. The CARET vitamin combination was terminated nearly 2 years early because interim analyses of the data indicated that should the trial have continued for its planned duration, it was highly unlikely that the intervention would

TABLE 6.2 (Continued)

From Ziegler, R. G., Mayne, S. T., and Swanson, C. A., *Cancer Causes and Control*, 7, 157, 1996.

a   To be included, studies had to assess diet in sufficient detail for the intake of several food groups and/or micronutrients to be evaluated. When several analyses of one study population have been published, results based on the largest number of lung cancer cases or deaths are used.
b   ↓↓↓ (and ↑↑↑) indicate inverse (and positive) associations with statistically significant trends. ↓↓ (and ↑↑) indicate inverse (and positive) associations with marginally significant trends or apparent trends that do not reach statistical significance. ↓ (and ↑) indicate inverse (and positive) associations with no evidence of a trend. ↓? (and ↑?) indicate inverse (and positive) associations with insufficient data presented to evaluate trend. 0 indicates no association.
c   Carotenoids, retinol, vitamin A, vitamin C, vitamin E, folate, and fiber refer to intake from foods. Total vitamin C and total vitamin E refer to combined intake from foods and supplements.
d   M, males; F, females; W, Whites; B, Blacks.
e   Hos, hospital-based; Pop, population-based; Com, community-based.
f   FFQ, food frequency questionnaire; DH, diet history.
g   Trends were seen for raw vegetables and fruits.

have been found to be beneficial, given the results as of late 1995. Furthermore, the interim results indicated that the supplemented group was developing more lung cancer, not less, consistent with the results of the Finnish trial. Overall, lung cancer incidence was increased by 28% in the supplemented subjects (RR = 1.28; 95% CI = 1.04 to 1.57) and total mortality was also increased (RR = 1.17; 95% CI = 1.03 to 1.33). Nonlung cancers were distributed nearly evenly between the two groups. While the *p*-value for the lung cancer increase ($p = 0.032$) is less than the conventional *p*-value of 0.05, it cannot be concluded that this trial provided statistically significant evidence of harm. Interim analyses, particularly if done repeatedly, could occasionally indicate a treatment difference ($p < 0.05$) even when one does not truly exist, just due to random fluctuations in the data.[21] Thus, in order to preserve an overall significance level of 0.05, interim analyses typically have very stringent significance levels ($p = 0.007$ for the 1995 CARET analysis).

The CARET investigators reported that baseline serum β-carotene levels were inversely correlated with the subsequent incidence of lung cancer in both the placebo and β-carotene groups.[20] CARET results also suggested effect modification by smoking status. Supplemental β-carotene increased lung cancer risk significantly in the participants who were smoking at the time of randomization (RR = 1.42; 95% CI = 1.07 to 1.87). In contrast, supplemental β-carotene was nonsignificantly protective in those smokers who had given up smoking prior to randomization (RR = 0.80; 95% CI = 0.48 to 1.31).[20] Risk estimates for lung cancer in former smokers are not available from the ATBC study, which restricted eligibility to current smokers.

Major findings of one additional trial, the Physicians' Health Study of supplemental β-carotene vs. placebo in 22,071 male U.S. physicians, were also published[22] along with the CARET results. There was no significant effect — positive or negative — of 12 years of supplementation of β-carotene (50 mg every other day) on cancer or total mortality. With regard to lung cancer, there was no indication of excess lung cancer in the β-carotene supplemented individuals, even among smokers. The relative risk for lung cancer in current smokers randomized to β-carotene was 0.90 (95% CI = 0.58 to 1.40). Among nonsmokers, the relative risk was 0.78 (0.34 to

1.79). The apparent lack of an effect of long-term supplementation of β-carotene on lung cancer incidence, even in baseline smokers who took the supplements for up to 12 years, is noteworthy. While only 11% of the participants were current smokers at entry, an additional 39% were former smokers. As discussed further below, the lack of effect of supplemental β-carotene on lung cancer in this trial may be an important clue in trying to understand the overall relationship between β-carotene and lung cancer.

The findings of the Physicians' Health Study illustrate the potential problems involved in overinterpreting results based upon interim analyses. After 9 years of intervention, an interim analysis was done to look at any cancers that developed during years 5 to 9 of the intervention. Discounting the first few years of intervention is typical and reasonable, as cancers that develop shortly after randomization were probably pre-existing yet undiagnosed. When this analysis was completed, the β-carotene supplemented group had 500 total cancers vs. 567 in the placebo group ($p = 0.03$).[22] Rather than closing the trial at this point, the finding of benefit was used as a grounds for continuation. At the conclusion of the trial, the reduction in total cancer was no longer statistically significant or clinically relevant in the total study population. This highlights why caution must be used in interpreting results obtained from trials before their planned conclusion.

Two other trials involving antioxidant nutrients were not designed as lung cancer prevention trials; nonetheless, their results are of relevance to the topic of lung cancer prevention. The first was a trial of selected nutrient combinations in the prevention of esophageal and gastric cancers in China.[23] The trial was conducted in residents from the general population of Linxian County, a population with several micronutrient deficiencies. Nearly 30,000 men and women aged 40 to 69 took part in the study, which tested the efficacy of four different nutrient combinations at inhibiting the development of esophageal and gastric cancers. The nutrient combinations included retinol plus zinc, riboflavin plus niacin, ascorbic acid plus molybdenum, and the combination of β-carotene, selenium, and vitamin E. After a 5-year intervention period, those who were given the combination of β-carotene, vitamin E, and selenium had a 13% reduction in cancer deaths (RR = 0.87; 95% CI = 0.75 to 1.00), a 9% reduction in total deaths (RR = 0.91; 95% CI = 0.84 to 0.99), a 4% reduction in esophageal cancer deaths (RR = 0.96; 95% CI = 0.78 to 1.18), and a 21% reduction in gastric cancer deaths (RR = 0.79; 95% CI = 0.64 to 0.99).[23] None of the other nutrient combinations reduced gastric or esophageal cancer deaths significantly in this trial. As for lung cancer, this trial had limited statistical power with only 31 total lung cancer deaths.[24] However, the relative risk of death from lung cancer was 0.55 (95% CI = 0.26 to 1.14) among those receiving the combination of β-carotene, α-tocopherol, and selenium. The smoking prevalence, including individuals who had ever smoked cigarettes for 6 months or more, was 30% in this study population.

Another study was a decade-long, double-blind trial of a daily oral supplement of selenium-enriched yeast (200 μg selenium/person/day) vs. placebo in 1300 older Americans. The study, designed as a skin cancer prevention trial, observed a significant reduction in the incidence of total cancer (RR = 0.59; $p = 0.0004$) and that of several cancer sites, including lung cancer (RR = 0.54; $p = 0.04$).[25] The reduction in lung cancer risk, while intriguing, was not a prior hypothesis and is presumably

TABLE 6.3
Prospective Studies of Blood Micronutrient Levels and Lung Cancer [a,b]

Study	Year	Location/ population	No. of cases[c]	Years of follow-up	β-Carotene	Vitamin A	Vitamin E	Vitamin C	Selenium
Stahelin et al.	1984	Basel, Switzerland	M: 68	12-14	↓↓↓	↓[d]	↓	0	0
Stahelin et al.	1991								
Stahelin et al.	1991								
Nomura et al.	1985	Hawaii, U.S.	M: 74	~10	↓↓↓	0	0		0
Nomura et al.	1987	Japanese							
Menkes et al.	1986	Washington County, MD, U.S.	M + F: 99	9	↓↓↓	0	↓↓↓		↑↑
Wald et al.	1986	London, U.K.	M: 50	3-10	↓↓↓	0	0		
Wald et al.	1987								
Wald et al.	1988								
Friedman et al.	1986	San Francisco-Oakland, CA, U.S.	M + F: 151	7-14		0			
Virtamo et al.	1987	Finland 55+ years old	M: 38	9	↓↓	0	↓		↓?
Connett et al.	1989	22 centers in U.S.	M: 66	10	↓↓	0	→		0

Knekt et al.	1988	Finland	M: 144	5-9	0	↓?	↑?	↓↓↓
Knekt et al.	1990							
Knekt et al.	1990							
Criqui et al.	1991	10 centers in U.S.	M + F: 27	8.5	0	0		0
Van den Brandt et al.	1993	Netherlands	M: 285	3				↓↓↓[e]
		55+ years old	F: 32					↓↓↓[e]
Kabuto et al.	1994	Japan	M + F: 77	11-13				0
Garland et al.	1995	U.S.	F: 47	3.5				↑↑[e]

From Ziegler, R. G., Mayne, S. T., and Swanson, C. A., *Cancer Causes and Control*, 7, 157, 1996.

[a] Only analyses with at least 25 lung cancer cases or deaths are included. When sequential analyses of one cohort have been published, results based on the largest number of lung cancer cases or deaths are used.

[b] ↓↓↓ (and ↑↑↑) indicate inverse (and positive) associations with statistically significant trends. ↓↓ (and ↑↑) indicate inverse (and positive) associations with marginally significant trends or apparent trends that do not reach statistical significance. ↓ (and ↑) indicate inverse (and positive) associations with no evidence of a trend. ↓? (and ↑?) indicate inverse (and positive) associations with insufficient data presented to evaluate trend. 0 indicates no association.

[c] M, males; F, females.

[d] Only observed in men 60+ years of age.

[e] Selenium was measured in toenails.

TABLE 6.4
Chemoprevention Trials Relevant to Antioxidant Nutrients and Lung Cancer

Study, year	Population	Daily intervention	Total subjects	Endpoint	Result
		Premalignant Endpoints			
McLarty et al., 1995	Male asbestos workers	50 mg β-carotene + 25,000 IU Vitamin A[a]	755	Sputum atypia	OR = 1.24 (CI = 0.78 to 1.96)
Van Poppel et al., 1992	Male smokers	20 mg β-carotene	114	Sputum micronuclei	27% decrease (CI = 9 to 41%)
		Primary Prevention — Completed			
ATBC, 1994	Finnish male smokers	20 mg β-carotene ± 50 mg Vitamin E	29,133	Lung cancer	BC: RR = 1.18 (CI = 1.03 to 1.36) Vit. E: RR = 0.98 (CI = 0.86 to 1.12)
CARET, 1996	Smokers/asbestos workers	30 mg β-carotene + 25,000 IU Vitamin A	18,314	Lung cancer	RR = 1.28 (CI = 1.04 to 1.57)
Physicians' Health Study, 1996	Male physicians	50 mg β-carotene[a] ± 325 mg Aspirin[a]	22,071	Cancer Lung cancer[b]	RR = 0.98 (CI = 0.91 to 1.06) RR = 0.90 (CI = 0.58 to 1.40)
Blot et al., 1994	General population Linxian, China	15 mg β-carotene + 30 mg Vitamin E + 50 μg Selenium	29,584	Lung cancer[c]	RR = 0.55[c] (CI = 0.26 to 1.14)
Clark et al., in press	Older Americans	200 μg Selenium	>1300	Lung cancer[c]	RR = 0.54[c] (p = 0.04)

Study	Population	Dose	N	Endpoint	Findings
Primary Prevention — Ongoing					
Women's Antioxidant Cardiovascular Study	High-risk women	500 mg Vitamin C ± 600 IU Vitamin E[a] + 50 mg β-carotene[a]	8000	Cancer, CHD	
Heart Protection Study	High-risk CHD U.K.	20 mg β-carotene+ 600 mg Vitamin E+ 250 mg Vitamin C	20,000+	Cancer, CHD	
Secondary Prevention — Completed					
Pastorino et al., 1993	Stage I non-small cell lung cancer patients	300,000 IU Vitamin A	307	Second cancer	Longer time to second cancer (p = 0.045)
Secondary Prevention — Ongoing					
EUROSCAN	Oral, larynx, lung cancer patients	300,000 IU Vitamin A 600 mg N-acetylcysteine	2000	Second cancer	
Mayne et al.	Oral, pharynx, larynx cancer patients	50 mg β-carotene	264	Second cancer (incl. lung)	
Toma et al.	Oral, pharynx, larynx cancer patients	75 mg β-carotene[d]	211	Second cancer (incl. lung)	

Note: OR = odds ratio; CI = 95% confidence interval; RR = relative risk; BC = β-carotene; Vit. E. = vitamin E.

[a] The dose listed was taken every other day. All others are daily doses.
[b] Lung cancer in smokers only (overall RR = 0.93 for β-carotene).
[c] Lung cancer not a primary endpoint of the trial; results based upon relatively few lung cancer cases.
[d] Given in 4-month cycles of three months on medication followed by one month off medication.

based upon relatively small numbers (number of lung cancers not stated). Thus, this finding must be interpreted cautiously.

IV. INTERPRETATION

As detailed above, there is a lack of concordance between the observational studies of antioxidant nutrients and lung cancer and the trials, at least with regard to β-carotene. Even within the trials, there are discordant findings regarding β-carotene and lung cancer. This section will attempt to reconcile and discuss some of these inconsistencies.

Beginning with a comparison of the trials, the CARET and ATBC trial both found an excess of lung cancer in the active intervention group, but it must be noted that the interventions were not the same. The CARET used a combination of β-carotene plus retinol; in contrast the ATBC trial used β-carotene alone or in combination with α-tocopherol in a factorial design, allowing for an evaluation of the independent effect of β-carotene. Since both trials found adverse effects, this has led to the widespread conclusion that the β-carotene must necessarily be the agent responsible for the increased lung cancer incidence. However, as previously noted, the Physicians' Health Study used β-carotene by itself and for a longer duration, and did not see any evidence of an increase in lung carcinogenesis, even among smokers. How does one explain this? Several issues can be considered, including baseline nutrient status, bioavailable dose, smoking interactions, and single nutrients vs. nutrient combinations.

Baseline nutrient status: Plasma β-carotene levels in participants in the Chinese trial, which showed a benefit with antioxidant nutrient supplementation, were low as expected (approximately 0.06 µg/mL).[23] These levels compare to median levels of 0.17 µg/mL in CARET[20] and in ATBC,[19] and even higher levels in the Physicians' Health Study (0.30 µg/mL reported in the placebo group[22]). Based upon the Chinese data, pre-randomization blood nutrient levels could be important in predicting efficacy. Some, but not all, observational studies of dietary β-carotene and lung cancer risk find that the majority of the reduction in lung cancer risk associated with increasing dietary β-carotene intake occurs between the first and second quartiles of intake. For example, in a recent study of lung cancer risk in nonsmokers (where residual confounding by active smoking is not problematic), the odds ratios for lung cancer risk in males dropped from 1.0 for the lowest dietary quartile of raw fruits and vegetables to 0.52 in the second quartile. Improving intake to the third and fourth quartiles had only a marginal additional benefit (odds ratios 0.51 and 0.41, respectively).[8] A recent analysis of total mortality, cancer mortality, and cardiovascular mortality as a function of baseline plasma β-carotene showed notably more deaths in the lowest quartile of plasma β-carotene.[26] For example, 101 persons in the lowest quartile died during the follow-up period, compared to 71, 55, and 58 in the next 3 quartiles of plasma β-carotene. It is thus possible that more moderate doses of supplemental β-carotene (see below), or preferably increasing intake of fruits and vegetables, might have more favorable effects on lung cancer and total mortality if given to populations with low β-carotene intake at baseline.

Bioavailable dose: Another possibility worthy of consideration surrounds the dosing regimen, formulation, and actual exposure as estimated by plasma β-carotene levels. The Physicians' Health Study gave 50 mg β-carotene (BASF formulation) every other day, a regimen that elevated plasma β-carotene levels only fourfold relative to the placebo group, to a level of 1.2 µg/mL (unclear if this value is for mean or median).[22] In contrast, the ATBC intervention (20 mg β-carotene per day, Hoffmann La Roche formulation) elevated median β-carotene levels nearly 18-fold, to a very high level of 3.0 µg/mL postsupplementation.[19] The CARET intervention, consisting of 30 mg β-carotene/day (Hoffmann La Roche formulation) plus retinyl palmitate, elevated median plasma β-carotene levels approximately 12-fold, to 2.1 µg/mL.[20] Blood levels in participants in the Chinese trial were elevated 15-fold, to 0.9 µg/mL with the 15 mg supplemental β-carotene.[23] Thus, the two trials with adverse outcomes had the highest blood β-carotene levels, suggesting that toxicity had been reached. It is possible that there may be a threshold plasma level below which adverse effects are not seen. In the absence of supporting mechanistic data, future trials of β-carotene, should they be undertaken, would be well-advised to use populations with low β-carotene status at entry and/or select doses/formulations that produce plasma β-carotene levels lower and more physiologic than those achieved in CARET and in the ATBC trial.

Smoking interactions: Smoking status is another potential explanation for the differences in results between the trials. The beneficial results seen in the Chinese trial may reflect a low total prevalence of smoking (30% ever smoking). This is in contrast to 50% ever smoking prevalence in the Physicians' Health Study, nearly 100% in CARET, and 100% in the ATBC trial. CARET smokers given supplemental β-carotene, who had a greater risk for lung cancer than smokers in ATBC given supplemental β-carotene, reported smoking more cigarettes per day than participants in ATBC (24 vs. 20 cigarettes/day). Other trials of β-carotene should examine their data for possible effect modification by smoking status and intensity.

Single nutrients vs. combinations: Alternatively, the beneficial results seen in the Chinese trial may have been due to the selenium, the α-tocopherol, or the combination of the three nutrients, particularly in a micronutrient deficient population. The one trial that used supplemental selenium as a single agent did find beneficial effects on lung cancer,[25] although that was not the primary endpoint of the trial. Another explanation for the beneficial effects observed in the Chinese trial is that a combination of antioxidants may have greater efficacy with regard to cancer prevention than isolated antioxidant nutrients. Experimentally, antioxidant nutrients are known to interact. For example, β-carotene in oil has been shown to be oxidized rapidly in the absence of α-tocopherol; however, it is relatively stable when combined with α-tocopherol.[27] Several ongoing trials (see Table 6.4) are using combinations of antioxidants, the results of which will help clarify the value of combination approaches vs. single agent approaches for cancer prevention. Examples include the British Heart Protection study, a large trial (goal = 20,000) of cholesterol-lowering medication and antioxidant nutrients in a factorial design, the U.S. Women's Antioxidant Cardiovascular Disease Study, and others.

V. CONCLUSIONS AND RECOMMENDATIONS

The vast majority of lung cancer is caused by tobacco, the smoke of which is known to be highly oxidative. Furthermore, individuals who consume more fruits and vegetables, rich sources of many phytochemicals, including antioxidant nutrients, are far less likely to develop lung cancer. Recently, completed trials of antioxidant nutrients and lung cancer prevention, however, indicate that high-dose antioxidant nutrient supplements do not seem to be of value for lung cancer prevention, with the possible exception of selenium, in well-nourished populations. The efficacy of antioxidant nutrient supplementation for lung cancer prevention in micronutrient deficient populations is unknown, as there are too little data available to comment. What, then, is a reasonable course of action for studies of antioxidant nutrients and lung cancer prevention? There are multiple avenues of research that would help to unravel the complexities of this research area. A few suggestions are as follows.

A wealth of new information from additional analyses of completed and ongoing trials will be forthcoming. Some of the subgroup analyses may suggest mechanisms that could then be evaluated for biological plausibility in metabolic or laboratory studies. Such research should help to explain whether or not β-carotene is causally associated with lung cancer risk and the generalizability of the effect. Some mechanisms to explain the adverse effects have been suggested;[28,29] careful evaluation of these hypotheses is needed.

A greater emphasis on the exploration of subgroups in observational studies as well as in trials to determine which subgroups are more likely to benefit from a given intervention is needed. The promising results obtained in the Linxian County, China trial suggest that subgroups with deficiencies of various micronutrients may be of particular interest. The public health approach of identifying populations with nutrient deficiencies and supplementing them to adequacy in order to prevent disease has been used successfully for decades, and should continue to be explored for the purposes of cancer prevention.

The beneficial effects observed in the Linxian County trial with the combination of three antioxidant nutrients — β-carotene, α-tocopherol, and selenium — suggest that further attention should also be given to combinations of nutrients, both in the observational studies as well as in the trials. Several observational studies of antioxidant nutrients and chronic disease have attempted to create an "antioxidant index," to take into account a person's dietary intake and/or blood nutrient status of several antioxidant nutrients, including β-carotene, vitamin C, vitamin E, and selenium. While intuitively appealing, there is no consistent approach used for generating antioxidant indices, nor have any of the indices been validated as being predictive of some meaningful measure of total antioxidant capacity. A challenge for the antioxidant/chronic disease field is to develop and validate meaningful biomarkers of oxidative damage and antioxidant status. This is perhaps more difficult than what might seem at first glance, given the fact that antioxidant capacity has been found to be a function of the initiating (reactive oxygen) species involved.[30] Since we do not know at this point what reactive oxygen species are involved in the pathogenesis of various diseases such as lung cancer, the predictive value of any measure of antioxidant capacity is thus unknown. The reactive oxygen species involved in the pathogenesis of some diseases are better characterized; for example, erythropoietic protoporphyria is known to involve singlet oxygen.[31] β-Carotene's well-known therapeutic value in the treatment of this disease[31] most likely relates to the fact that β-carotene is one of the most efficient quenchers of singlet oxygen. This also implies that measures of resistance to singlet oxygen-induced oxidation would be predictive with regard to that disease. Cancer, in contrast, is far more complex, likely involving multiple reactive oxygen species, potentially at multiple steps in the disease process (initiation, promotion, progression). This must be considered by those attempting to develop/validate antioxidant measures for observational studies of cancer etiology, as well as those designing antioxidant-based interventions for cancer prevention clinical trials.

REFERENCES

1. Kabat, G. C., Recent developments in the epidemiology of lung cancer, *Semin. Surg. Oncol.*, 9, 73, 1993.
2. American Cancer Society, *Cancer Facts and Figures 1996*, Atlanta, GA.
3. Shopland, D. R., Eyre, H. J., and Pechacek, T. F., Smoking-attributable cancer mortality in 1991: is lung cancer now the leading cause of death among smokers in the United States? *J. Natl. Cancer Inst.*, 83, 1142, 1991.
4. U.S. Department of Health and Human Services, *The Health Benefits of Smoking Cessation: A Report of the Surgeon General*, Public Health Service, Centers for Disease Control, Center for Chronic Disease Prevention and Health Promotion, Office of Smoking and Health, Rockville, MD, 1990, 110.
5. Church, D. F. and Pryor, A. W., Free radical chemistry of cigarette smoke and its toxicological implications, *Environ. Health Perspect.*, 64, 111, 1985.
6. Ziegler, R. G., Mayne, S. T., and Swanson, C. A., Nutrition and lung cancer, *Cancer Causes and Control*, 7, 157, 1996.
7. Dragsted, L. O., Strube, M., and Larsen, J. C., Cancer protective factors in fruits and vegetables: Biochemical and biological background, *Pharmacol. Toxicol.*, 72(suppl), s116, 1993.
8. Mayne, S. T., Janerich, D. T., Greenwald, P., Chorost, S., Tucci, C., Zaman, M. B., et al., Dietary beta carotene and lung cancer risk in U.S. nonsmokers, *J. Natl. Cancer Inst.*, 86, 33, 1994.
9. Olson, J. A., Needs and sources of carotenoids and vitamin A, *Nutr. Rev.*, 52, 67, 1994.
10. Guthrie, H. A., *Introductory Nutrition*, 4th Edition, C. V. Mosby, St. Louis, 1979, 279.
11. Micozzi, M. S., Beecher, G. R., Taylor, P. R., and Khachik, F., Carotenoid analyses of selected raw and cooked foods associated with a lower risk for cancer, *J. Natl. Cancer Inst.*, 82, 282, 1990.
12. Khachik, F., Goli, M. B., Beecher, G. R., Holden, J. H., Lusby, W. R., Tenorio, M. D., et al., Effect of food preparation on qualitative and quantitative distribution of major carotenoid constituents of tomatoes and several green vegetables, *J. Agric. Food Chem.*, 40, 390, 1992.
13. Mangels, A. R., Holden, J. M., Beecher, G. R., Forman, M. R., and Lanza, E., Carotenoid content of fruits and vegetables: an evaluation of analytic data, *J. Am. Diet. Assoc.*, 93, 284, 1993.
14. Le Marchand, L., Hankin, J. H., Kolonel L. N., Beecher, G. R., Wilkens, L. R., and Zhao, L. P., Intake of specific carotenoids and lung cancer risk, *Cancer Epidemiol., Biomarkers Prev.*, 2, 183, 1993.
15. Ziegler, R. G., Colavito, E. A., Hartge, P., McAdams, M. J., Schoenberg, J. B., Mason, T. J., et al., The importance of alpha-carotene, beta-carotene, and other phytochemicals in the etiology of lung cancer, *J. Natl. Cancer Inst.*, 88, 612, 1996.

16. McLarty, J. W., Holiday, D. B., Girard, W. M., Yanagihara, R. H., Kummet, T. D., and Greenberg, S. D., Beta-carotene, vitamin A and lung cancer chemoprevention: results of an intermediate endpoint study, *Am. J. Clin. Nutr.,* 62(Suppl), 1431S, 1995.

17. Van Poppel, G., Kok, F. J., and Hermus, R. J., Beta-carotene supplementation in smokers reduces the frequency of micronuclei in sputum, *Br. J. Cancer,* 66, 1164, 1992.

18. Van Poppel, G., Poulsen, H., Loft, S., and Verhagen, H., No influence of beta-carotene on oxidative DNA damage in male smokers, *J. Natl. Cancer Inst.,* 87, 310, 1995.

19. The Alpha-Tocopherol, Beta Carotene Cancer Prevention Study Group, The effect of vitamin E and beta carotene on the incidence of lung cancer and other cancers in male smokers, *N. Engl. J. Med.,* 330, 1029, 1994.

20. Omenn, G. S., Goodman, G. E., Thornquist, M. D., Balmes, J., Cullen, M. R., Glass, A., et al., Effects of a combination of beta carotene and vitamin A on lung cancer and cardiovascular disease, *N. Engl. J. Med.,* 334, 1150, 1996.

21. Pocock, S. J., *Clinical Trials: A Practical Approach,* John Wiley and Sons, New York, 1983.

22. Hennekens, C. H., Buring, J. E., Manson, J. E., Stampfer, M., Rosner, B., Cook, N. R., et al., Lack of effect of long-term supplementation with beta carotene on the incidence of malignant neoplasms and cardiovascular disease, *N. Engl. J. Med.,* 334, 1145, 1996.

23. Blot, W. J., Li, J.-Y., Taylor, P. R., Guo, W., Dawsey, S., Wang, G.-Q., et al., Nutrition intervention trials in Linxian, China: supplementation with specific vitamin/mineral combinations, cancer incidence, and disease-specific mortality in the general population, *J. Natl. Cancer Inst.,* 85, 1483, 1993.

24. Blot, W. J., Li, J-Y., Taylor, P. R., and Li, B., Lung cancer and vitamin supplementation, Letter to the editor, *N. Engl. J. Med.,* 331, 614, 1994.

25. Combs, G. F., Jr., Selenium and cancer prevention, in *Antioxidants and Disease Prevention,* ch 8 of this volume.

26. Greenberg, E. R., Baron, J. A., Karagas, M. R., Stukel, T. A., Nierenberg, D. W., Stevens, M. M., et al., Mortality associated with low plasma concentration of beta carotene and the effect of oral supplementation, *J. Am. Med. Assoc.,* 275, 699, 1996.

27. Terao, J., Yamauchi, R., Murakami, H., and Matsushita, S., Inhibitory effects of tocopherols and beta-carotene on singlet oxygen-initiated photooxidation of methyl linoleate and soybean oil, *J. Food Process. Preserv.,* 4, 79, 1980.

28. Mayne, S. T., Handelman, G. J., and Beecher, G., Beta-carotene and lung cancer promotion: A plausible relationship?, *J. Natl. Cancer Inst.,* 88, 1513, 1996.

29. Olson, J. A., Benefits and liabilities of vitamin A and carotenoids, *J. Nutr.,* 126(suppl.), 1208S, 1996.

30. Halliwell, B. and Gutteridge, J. M. C., The definition and measurement of antioxidants in biological systems, Letter to the Editor, *Free Rad. Biol. Med.,* 18, 125, 1995.

31. Mathews-Roth, M. M., Carotenoids in erythropoietic protoporphyria and other photosensitivity diseases, *Ann. N.Y. Acad. Sci.,* 691, 127, 1993.

Chapter 7

ANTIOXIDANT NUTRIENTS
AND ORAL CAVITY CANCER

Harinder S. Garewal

Contents

I. Introduction 87

II. Oral Cavity Cancer 88

III. Epidemiologic Evidence 89

IV. Premalignant Lesions of the Oral Cavity 90

V. β-Carotene and Vitamin E Studies in Oral Leukoplakia 91

VI. Future Directions 92

References 94

I. INTRODUCTION

Oxidative damage, alternatively referred to as free radical induced injury, is now widely accepted as a common mechanism whereby disease-producing changes occur in cells and tissues. Mechanisms have been described that produce altered subcellular components, proteins, lipids, and nucleic acids, which contribute to various diseases, including cardiovascular disease and cancer, the two commonest causes of death in the U.S. Even though successful treatment of the final stages of these diseases is important, eventual control of the tremendous morbidity and mortality produced by them will depend on success in prevention. Since the contributing etiologies for these chronic, life-shortening diseases are almost certainly multifactorial, prevention will involve the application of different modalities, each making its own contribution to the overall goal. For example, cardiovascular disease can be prevented to some extent with blood pressure control, exercise, discontinuing tobacco, and management of cholesterol, to name a few of the best described approaches. Similarly, prevention of many cancers will result from steps such as tobacco control, attention to diet, and reduced sun exposure. Attempts at limiting oxidative damage by proper intake of nutritional agents is another avenue for disease prevention that should be considered in the context of a contribution to the overall effort, rather than as a specific entity

0-8493-8509-1/97/$0.00+$.50
© 1997 by CRC Press LLC

to be applied in the absence of other health promoting recommendations. It has become increasingly clear that one single approach is not going to prevent all malignancies or even all cases of a single type of cancer. Given the likelihood of multifactorial etiology, this is no surprise. Instead, the most likely to succeed approach toward decreasing the overall morbidity and mortality from cancer by prevention will depend on identification and application of different interventions, that together will result in significant reductions in incidence of the disease. Using nutrition and nutritional agents must be viewed in this context. In this chapter, the current state of evidence, supporting the importance of the so-called antioxidant nutritional agents in oral cavity cancer prevention, is reviewed.

The review will focus on β-carotene and vitamin E. The significance of a specific agent, or agents, depends on the population being considered. From a disease prevention standpoint, it is likely that maximum benefit from a nutritional agent is attained when the intake and tissue level of that agent is increased to a certain threshold level. For example, for the vitamins, deficiency states are prevented by intake at levels close to those defined by the Recommended Dietary Allowances (RDAs). Clearly, teleologic considerations of the evolution of human diets would suggest that any additional disease-preventive activity is likely to be achieved by intakes that are only a fewfold, perhaps 2- to 3-fold, greater than the RDA. This point is perhaps better appreciated by considering blood and tissue levels. There must exist a threshold level, exceeding which adds no additional benefit and perhaps may even be harmful. Raising levels to this threshold, whether by altering diet or using supplements, would be a reasonable test strategy with the likelihood of benefit depending on the baseline intake and levels in the population being studied. Recent negative clinical trials with β-carotene in lung cancer prevention in well-nourished Western populations stand in contrast to the positive results in a Chinese population with lower baseline levels.[1-3] Such considerations also suggest that vitamin E, rather than β-carotene, may be the more important supplemental agent in overall disease prevention in western societies, since increasing vitamin E intake to raise its blood level 2 to 3 fold by dietary modification alone is impractical.

II. ORAL CAVITY CANCER

Oral cavity cancer is a common, morbid, and lethal disease. Although not infrequent in the U.S., very high rates are encountered in developing countries, where it is frequently the commonest cancer encountered.[4,5] Its incidence is very closely related to identified etiologies, the principal ones being tobacco and alcohol. Tobacco, chewed or smoked, probably contributes to more than 75% of cases of this malignancy. Heavy alcohol use is an independent risk factor that synergies with tobacco use. The highest risk with tobacco occurs with the chewed form of this carcinogen. In fact, increasing use of chewing tobacco, particularly among younger individuals, is a serious cause of concern in western countries.[6] In developing countries, in addition to chewing carcinogenic substances, other noxious habits, such as "reverse smoking" (putting the lighted end in the mouth) account for a majority of cases. Despite considerable effort, cure rates for oral cavity cancer have not changed significantly over the past three decades.[7] This again points to the need for effective prevention for eventual control of this disease.

The natural history and underlying biology of oral cavity cancer make it an excellent target for chemoprevention. The latter term refers to the use of specific chemicals to try and inhibit carcinogenesis. This cancer, like most other malignancies, develops through a multistep process that occurs over years. The entire oral mucosa, together with the upper aerodigestive tract, is affected by this disease process, a phenomena often referred to as "field cancerization."[8] The advantage of oral cavity cancer as a model lesion over other malignancies lies in the easy accessability of this region for study. Mucosal samples, premalignant lesions, and other tissues are easily obtained and observed. Consequently, this site has received major attention in recent years as a target for chemoprevention research.

One group of compounds that has attracted significant recent interest is the retinoids. Retinoids are important in numerous cellular functions including differentiation. The activity of these agents in reversing oral premalignant changes has been known for nearly three decades. Initially, this was demonstrated with high dose vitamin A itself.[9] However, the well-known serious toxicities of vitamin A precluded efforts at using these agents in oral cavity cancer prevention. Since then more than 1500 synthetic analogs of vitamin A have been developed, with the goal of reducing toxicity and maintaining efficacy. Although this goal has been realized to varying degrees in the form of specific synthetic retinoids, all of them still have significant side effects. Consequently, their potential for making any meaningful reduction in oral cavity cancer incidence is virtually nonexistent. Presently, the most studied retinoid in this context is 13-cis-retinoic acid. Although previously shown to be active in reversing oral premalignant lesions, interest in this activity resurfaced with its confirmation in the mid 1980s.[10,11] Nevertheless, its toxicity has limited its applicability in any significant clinical context, including recent efforts by oral surgeons who are most likely to encounter premalignant lesions in the oral cavity.[12] Consequently, although such activity continues to have biologic interest, its applicability to reducing oral cavity incidence remains severely limited.

Clearly, nutritional, nontoxic agents have tremendous advantages over synthetic, toxic drugs from the standpoint of eventual usage. Any benefit or activity of such agents is immediately transferable to general use. Consequently, from a worldwide public health standpoint, if oral cavity cancer incidence can be reduced by increasing intake of specific nutritional agents, this would have very practical implications for disease prevention.

A large body of laboratory and animal model evidence exists in support of a carcinogenesis inhibitory activity of the antioxidant agents.[13-16] This will not be discussed in detail in this chapter, which will focus primarily on human clinical and epidemiology studies. The hamster cheek pouch model of oral carcinogenesis is an important system, however, that has been used extensively to identify potential agents and to study the mechanisms involved.[15,16]

III. EPIDEMIOLOGIC EVIDENCE

As is true for a number of cancers, numerous studies have shown an inverse link between fruit and vegetable intake and oral cavity cancer.[17] These foods are rich in carotenoids, including β-carotene. Nevertheless, epidemiologic studies alone cannot extend these associations to identification of a single compound or group of compounds as being responsible for risk reduction. Dietary studies also suggest significant risk reduction with increasing intake of vitamin E.[18,19] Recently reported studies have suggested an effect of supplemental vitamin E, rather than intake based on diet alone.[19]

IV. PREMALIGNANT LESIONS OF THE ORAL CAVITY

The multistep process of carcinogenesis has been extensively studied in many laboratory and animal model systems. Stages such as initiation, promotion, and progression have been characterized by identifying cellular and subcellular changes that occur with each step. Such studies have clearly established that the process of carcinogenesis is highly dependent on the system being used, i.e., the carcinogen as well as the animal species. Furthermore, the earlier stages of carcinogenesis, although accompanied by chemical and/or cellular changes, do not have an associated gross, clinically visible lesion by which an affected tissue can be identified. Premalignant lesions are, in fact, the first clinically identifiable lesions that indicate that an organ or tissue has been affected by carcinogenesis. Such lesions have now been recognized for most human malignancies. An important strategy in cancer prevention research is to look for reversal of premalignant lesions as an endpoint. It should be emphasized that all premalignant lesions are not equivalent, and in general, most such lesions are associated with rather low frequency of conversion to overt cancer. Consequently, when targeting such lesions for screening agents for cancer preventive activity, it is important to balance the toxicity of the agent vs. the risk posed by the premalignant lesion. These points are illustrated below using oral leukoplakia, the premalignant lesion for oral cavity cancer, as an example.

Leukoplakia is defined as a white patch that cannot be removed by scraping and cannot be clinically classified as another disease entity. A biopsy is usually needed to confirm the diagnosis and to assess the risk of cancer by judging the degree of dysplasia. Axell et al. have recently reported the conclusions of an international collaborative group which met to describe the various types of oral leukoplakic lesions and their malignancy risk.[20] If a reddish component is present, the lesion is called erythroplakia, which is associated with greater degrees of dysplasia and cancer risk. The risk of cancer in leukoplakia varies from very low (less than 1% per year) or undetermined to greater than 10% per year if high grades of dysplasia are present.[21,22] In general, particularly in Western societies, the majority of leukoplakic lesions are low risk lesions, which is not different from premalignant lesions at other sites. For example, most colonic adenomas, the premalignant lesion for colon cancer, fall into the small or diminutive polyp category, which is a very low risk lesion.

The standard treatments for leukoplakia depend on its etiology, size, and risk of malignancy. An attempt should always be made to eliminate any identifiable etiology. Excision, cryosurgery, and other such local modalities are applicable to the smaller lesion that can be completely treated in this manner. Regular follow-up, usually by an oral surgeon, is important to observe for any changes suggesting transformation. Finally, agents such as topical bleomycin have been used with success.[23]

From a cancer prevention standpoint, the objective of trials in leukoplakia is not to develop another treatment modality, but rather to use activity in leukoplakia as an indication of potential for oral cancer prevention. As mentioned above, retinoids, including vitamin A itself, can produce clinical reversions in oral leukoplakia. However, because of their toxicity, these drugs are not suitable for prevention purposes.

V. β-CAROTENE AND VITAMIN E STUDIES IN ORAL LEUKOPLAKIA

A number of studies have now been conducted using β-carotene and/or vitamin E, either alone or in combination with other agents, in oral leukoplakia. The rationale for these studies was based on the preclinical evidence, the known activity of retinoids, and the lack of toxicity of the nutritional agents. Stich and colleagues have reported a series of trials, conducted in India, using vitamin A and β-carotene. In one study, intervention consisted of 180 mg/week β-carotene (group I), β-carotene plus vitamin A 100,000 IU/week (group II), or placebo (group III) given in twice weekly doses for 6 months.[24] These authors report complete response rates only, which were 15% in group I and 27.5% in group II, compared with only 3% in the placebo group. A strong inhibition of new lesions was also reported. In a subsequent trial using 200,000 IU of vitamin A alone per week for 6 months, Stich and colleagues reported a 57% complete response rate with total suppression of new lesions.[25] In a more recent study in India, Krishnaswamy and colleagues studied reverse smokers, supplementing 150 subjects with vitamin A, riboflavin, zinc, and selenium.[26] In contrast to a complete remission rate of 8% in a placebo group, the intervention group had a 57% complete response rate. It should be emphasized that the study populations in India differ from those in Western countries in that the lesions in India are caused primarily by chewing of betel nuts and other carcinogenic substances as well as habits such as reverse smoking. Additionally, a degree of vitamin A deficiency may also be present at baseline.

Several studies have now been reported from Western populations also. Our group conducted a pilot trial of β-carotene alone at a dose of 30 mg/day for 3 to 6 months.[27] An overall response rate of 71% (complete and partial response) was found in 24 treated patients. Malaker et al. conducted a study in Canada with a response rate of about 50% with β-carotene.[28] Kaugars and colleagues used a combination of β-carotene, vitamin C, and vitamin E.[29] Clinical improvement of the oral lesion was noted in 55.7% with responses more frequently noted in patients who reduced alcohol or tobacco use also. Incidently, Kaugars and Silverman have also reported their experience with 13-cis-retinoic acid with the initial observations showing only three of ten patients responding, but with major difficulties related to retinoid toxicity.[12]

In a trial conducted in Italy, Toma et al. reported a response rate of 44% in 18 evaluable subjects using a β-carotene dose of 90mg/day.[30] Once again, in contrast to their experience with retinoids, side effects were not a problem even at this relatively high dose of β-carotene.

Most recently, we have completed a multicenter trial involving the University of California (Irvine), University of Connecticut (Farmington), and the University of Arizona.[31] In this study, all patients were treated with 60 mg/day of β-carotene for 6 months (induction phase) followed by randomization of the responders to continue β-carotene or placebo for another 12 months. The goals were to confirm the response rate to β-carotene in a multicenter setting and to determine whether continued treatment is necessary for maintenance of the response. The results of the induction phase of this study have been analyzed and show a response rate of 52% (95% confidence interval 38 to 66%) in 50 evaluable patients. This rate is very comparable to those reported for the toxic retinoids in larger, multicenter studies.

Zaridze and colleagues adopted a somewhat different strategy in a population-based, prospective, placebo-controlled, randomized trial conducted in males in Uzbekistan (Central Asia). In this region, use of nass, a mixture of tobacco, ash, cotton oil, and lime placed in the mouth is a major cause of the lesion and oral cancers. The treatment group received β-carotene (40mg/day), retinol (100,000 IU/week), and vitamin E (80 mg/week) for 6 months.[32] They found a significant reduction in the prevalence of oral leukoplakia in the treatment group vs. control.

Interest in testing vitamin E alone is more recent. From a disease prevention standpoint, especially in Western societies, vitamin E will probably be one of the more important supplemental agents because of its activity in a number of conditions. To date, only a single trial has been reported with vitamin E alone in oral leukoplakia. Benner et al. conducted a multicenter study showing a response rate of 45% (95% confidence interval 32 to 61%) in 43 subjects treated with 400 IU of vitamin E twice daily for 24 weeks.[33] The response rate for this study was 65% if calculated on the basis of evaluable patients, of which there were 31. Vitamin E was extremely well tolerated with no unusual or unexpected toxicities being encountered.

VI. FUTURE DIRECTIONS

Numerous lines of evidence suggest a possible role for antioxidant nutritional agents in the prevention of oral cavity cancer. Nevertheless, it must be emphasized that all the evidence comes from indirect approaches. Clearly, the most convincing way to show that an agent prevents a particular malignancy would be to do a randomized, controlled, blinded study in the right population with the endpoint being the cancer of interest. However, such studies are simply not possible to do for most malignancies because of the insurmountable practical and logistic problems involved. Individual types of cancers are relatively uncommon events in healthy populations. Therefore, impossibly large numbers of subjects would have to be involved for decades in order to achieve a conclusive result. The easy availability, lack of toxicity, and possibility of benefit in other conditions all mitigate against successfully maintaining a treatment and placebo control group for such long periods of time. Consequently, the only reasonable way to come to a conclusion would be for individuals to consider indirect lines of evidence as has been attempted in this chapter. Rather than placebo-controlled trials with oral cavity cancer as an endpoint, it may, at some date, be more feasible to undertake population-based intervention studies as demonstration projects in countries where the disease is extremely common.

Other indirect type of evidence would involve the use of intermediate markers of cancer risk as endpoints. This is an area of active investigation with numerous biomarkers being proposed. Such endpoint studies are clearly shorter and more practical. However, their interpretation will depend on the reliability and validity of the marker. Unfortunately, at this time there is no marker that has been proven to be a reliable intermediate endpoint. In one sense, premalignant lesions, such as oral leukoplakia, can be considered to be intermediate markers themselves. However, because of their clinical importance, they are often not classified with other proposed biomarkers. One biomarker that has been tested in the context of clinical trials is the frequency of micronuclei in exfoliated oral cavity cells. An increase in the frequency of micronuclei has been proposed as a marker of genetic damage and has been linked with the presence of cancers and premalignant lesions. In studies conducted in India, Stich et al. have reported reduction in micronucleus frequency with β-carotene and/or vitamin A intervention.[34] In our experience, however, in Western populations, micronuclei frequency is not increased in patients with oral leukoplakia compared to controls, unless chewing tobacco is involved.[35] Furthermore, the actual frequency of these micronuclei is too low to undertake modulation experiments by putative chemopreventive agents.

Another group of subjects that has been utilized in testing chemopreventive approaches is patients who have been cured of one head and neck cancer. These patients are at a high risk for developing a second primary malignancy of the aerodigestive tract.[36,37] This most likely reflects a "field cancerization" defect underlying the entire aerodigestive mucosa, most probably produced by exposure to carcinogens, such as tobacco.

A small, initial study that involved all stages of cancer planned to use high doses of 13-cis-retinoic acid.[38] A significant reduction in second primary cancers was reported. Even in this relatively high-risk setting, the very significant toxicity of high-dose retinoids was a major problem with a large number of subjects not being able to complete the planned treatment duration. More recently, a larger, prospective, randomized, placebo-controlled European trial that included early stage patients and used etretinate showed no effect on survival or second primary cancers.[39] Etretinate is a synthetic retinoid somewhat less toxic than 13-cis-retinoic acid, but with equivalent activity against oral leukoplakia in previous studies. Despite being less toxic than 13-cis-retinoic acid, retinoid toxicity was still a serious problem. At this time, no studies with β-carotene or vitamin E have been reported in the context of prevention of second malignancies. Such studies are presently underway in Canada and in the U.S.

Finally, it is important to consider the findings in oral cavity cancer in the context of overall disease prevention, morbidity reduction, and extension of life in the targeted population. These nutritional agents will play different roles in different populations. Their potential for prevention of a number of diseases, such as heart disease and eye disease, would make them viable options for disease prevention if the studies continue to hold promise. In developing countries, one or both of these agents, together with other compounds under study such as vitamin C and selenium, may all have a role to play. In Western countries, vitamin E may turn out to be the more important agent, given its promise in cardiovascular disease prevention. Nevertheless, additional studies are of great interest simply because these agents, if they prove useful, are highly suited for general supplementation. This is in contrast to other drugs, such as the retinoids, which even if they inhibit cancer in one model system or another are unlikely to find use except in very limited circumstances where their toxicity could be justified.

REFERENCES

1. The Alpha-tocopherol, Beta-carotene cancer prevention study group. The effect of vitamin E and beta-carotene on the incidence of lung cancer and other cancers in male smokers. *N. Engl. J. Med.* 1994, 330, 1029.
2. Omenn, G.S., Goodman, G.E., Thornquist, M.D., et al. Effects of a combination of beta-carotene and vitamin A on lung cancer and cardiovascular disease. *N. Engl. J. Med.* 1996, 334, 1150.
3. Blot, W.J., Li, J.Y., Taylor, R.R., et al. Nutrition intervention trials in Linxian, China: supplementation with specific vitamin/mineral combinations, cancer incidence and disease-specific mortality in the general population. *J. Natl. Cancer Inst.* 1993, 85, 1483.
4. Parkin, S.M., Laara, E., and Muir, C.S. Estimates of the worldwide frequency of sixteen major cancers. *Int. J. Cancer* (Phila). 1988, 41, 184.
5. Boring, C.C., Squires, T.S., and Tong, T. Cancer statistics, 1993 *Cancer J. Clin.* 1993, 43, 7.
6. U.S. Dept. of Health and Human Services Smoking and Tobacco control Monograph 2, Smokeless Tobacco or Health, An International Perspective, NIH Publication No. 93-3461, May 1993.
7. Cancer Statistics Review (1973-87), NCI Division of Cancer Prevention and Control Surveillance Program, Publication No. 90-2789 (U.S. Dept of Health and Human Services), PHS, NCI, NIH, Bethesda, MD; 1990.
8. Slaughter, D.P., Douthwich, H.W., and Smejkal, W. Field cancerization in oral stratified squamous epithelium: clinical implications of multicentric origin. *Cancer* (Phila). 1953, 5, 963.
9. Silverman, S., Eisenberg, E., and Renstrap, G. A study of the effects of high doses of vitamin A on oral leukoplakia (hyperkeratosis), including toxicity, liver function and skeletal metabolism. *J. Oral Ther. Pharmacol.* 1965, 2, 9.
10. Koch, H.F. Biochemical treatment of precancerous oral lesions: the effectiveness of various analogues of retinoic acid. *J. Maxillofac. Surg.* 1978, 6, 59.
11. Hong, W.K., Endicott, J., Itri, L.M., et al. 13-cis-retinoic acid in the treatment of oral leukoplakia. *N. Engl. J. Med.* 1986, 315, 1501.
12. Kaugars, G. and Silverman, S. The use of 13-cis-retinoic acid in the treatment of oral leukoplakia: short-term observations. *Oral Surg. Med. Pathol.* 1995, 79, 264.
13. Som, S., Chatterjee, M., and Bannerjee, M.R. Beta-carotene inhibition of DMBA-induced transformation of murine mammary cells *in vitro. Carcinogenesis.* 1984, 5, 937.
14. Stich, H.F. and Dunn, B.P. Relationship between cellular levels of beta-carotene and sensitivity to genotoxic agents. *Int. J. Cancer.* 1987, 38, 713.
15. Schwartz, J., Suda, D., and Light, G. Beta-carotene is associated with the regression of hamster buccal pouch carcinoma and induction of tumor necrosis factor in macrophages. *Biochem. Biophys. Res. Commun.* 1987, 136, 1130.
16. Shklar, G. Oral mucosal carcinogenesis in hamsters: inhibition by vitamin E. *J. Natl. Cancer Inst.* 1982, 68, 791.
17. Block, G., Patterson, B., and Subar, A. Fruit, Vegetables and Cancer Prevention: a review of the epidemiologic evidence. *Nutr. Cancer.* 1992, 18, 1.
18. Barone, J., Taioli, E., Hebert, J.R., and Wynder, E.L. Vitamin Supplement Use and Risk for Oral and Esophageal Cancer. *Nutr. Cancer.* 1992, 18, 31.
19. Gridley, G., McLaughlin, J.K., Block, G., Blot, W.J., Gluch, M., and Fraumeni, J.F. Vitamin Supplement Use and Reduced Risk of Oral and Pharyngeal Cancer. *Am. J. Epidemiology.* 1992, 135, 1083.

20. Axell, T., Pindborg, J.J., Smith, C.J., van der Waal, I. and an International Collaborative Group on Oral White Lesions. Oral white lesions with special reference to precancerous and tobacco-related lesions: conclusions of an international symposium held in Upsala, Sweden, May 18-21, 1994. *J. Oral Pathol. Med.* 1996, 25, 49.
21. Silverman, S. and Shillitoe, E.J. *Etiology and Predisposing Factors in Oral Cancer.* S. Silverman. Ed.: 7-39 3rd Edition. American Cancer Society New York; 1990.
22. Hansen, L.S., Olson, J.A., and Silverman, S. Proliferative verrucous leukoplakia. A long-term study of thirty patients. *Oral Surg. Med. Pathol.* 1985, 60, 285.
23. Wong, R., Epstein, J., and Millner, A. Treatment of oral leukoplakia with topical bleomycin. *Cancer* (Phila). 1989, 64, 361.
24. Stich, H.F., Rosin, M.P., and Hornby, A.P. Remission of oral leukoplakias and micronuclei in tobacco/betel quid chewers treated with beta-carotene and with beta-carotene plus vitamin A. *Int. J. Cancer.* 1988, 42, 195.
25. Stich, A.F., Hornby, A.P., Mathew, B., et al. Response of oral leukoplakia to the administration of vitamin A. *Cancer Lett.* 1988, 40, 93.
26. Krishnaswamy, K., Prasad, M.P.R., Krishna, T.P., Annapurna, V.V., and Reddy, A.G. A case study of nutrient intervention or oral precancerous lesions in India. Oral Oncol. *Eur. J. Cancer* 1995, 31B, 41.
27. Garewal, H.S., Meyskens, F.L., and Killen, D. Response of oral leuko-plakia to beta-carotene. *J. Clin. Oncol.* 1990, 8, 1715.
28. Malaker, K., Anderson, B.J., Beecroft, W.A., and Hodson, D.I. Management of oral mucosal dysplasia with beta-carotene retinoic acid: a pilot crossover study. *Cancer Det. and Prev.* 1991, 15, 335.
29. Kaugars, G., Silverman, S., Lovas, J.G.L., et al. A clinical trial of antioxidant supplements in the treatment of oral leukoplakia. *Oral. Surg. Med. Pathol.* 1994, 78, 462.
30. Toma, S., Benso, S., Albanese, E., Palumbo, R., Nicolo, G., and Mangiante, P. Response of oral leukoplakia to β-carotene treatment. Pennington Symposium "Vitamins and Cancer Prevention." Louisiana State University Press. Baton Rouge, Louisiana; 1991.
31. Garewal, H.S., Meyskens, F., Katz, R.V., Friedman, S., Morse, D.E., Alberts, D., and Girodias, K. Beta-carotene produces sustained remissions in oral leukoplakia: results of a 1 year randomized controlled trial. Proceedings of American Society of Clinical Oncology (31st Annual Meeting) 1995; 1173.
32. Zaridze, D., Evstifeeva, T., and Boyle, P. Chemoprevention of oral leukoplakia and chronic esophagitis in an area of high incidence of oral and esophageal cancer. *Ann. Epidemiol.,* 1993, 3, 225.
33. Benner, S.E., Winn, R.W., Lippman, S.M., Poland, J., Hansen, K.S., Luna, M.A., and Hong, W.K. Regression of oral leukoplakia with alpha-tocopherol: a community clinical oncology program chemoprevention study. *J. Natl. Cancer Inst.* 1993, 85, 44.
34. Stich, H.F., Stich, W., Rosin, M.P., and Vallejera, D.M. Use of the micronucleus test to monitor the effect of vitamin A, beta-carotene and canthaxanthin on the buccal mucosa of betel nut/tobacco chewers. *Int. J. Cancer.* 1990, 34, 745.
35. Garewal, H.S., Ramsey, L., Boyle, J., and Kaugars, G. Clinical experience with the micronucleus assay. *J. Cell. Biochem.* 1993, 17F, 206.
36. Kotwall, C., Razack, M.S., Sako, K., and Rao, U. Multiple primary cancers in squamous cell cancers of the head and neck. *J. Surg. Oncol.* 1990, 40, 97.
37. Shapshay, W., Hong, W.K., and Fried, M. Simultaneous carcinomas of the esophagus and upper aerodigestive tract. Otolaryngol. *Head, Neck Surg.* 1980, 88, 373.
38. Hong, W.K., Lippman, S.M., Itri, L.M., et al. Prevention of second primary tumors with isotretinoin in squamous cell carcinoma of the head and neck. *N. Engl. J. Med.* 1990, 323, 795.
39. Bolla, M., Lefur, R., Ton Van, J., Domenge, C., Badet, J.M., Koskas, Y., and Laplanche, A. Prevention of second primary tumors with etretinate in squamous cell carcinoma of the oral cavity and oropharynx. Results of a multicenter double-blind randomized study. *Eur. J. Cancer* 1994, 30A, 767.

Chapter 8

SELENIUM AND CANCER PREVENTION

Gerald F. Combs, Jr.

Contents

I. Introduction 97

II. Epidemiology of Selenium and Cancer 97

III. Animal Model Studies of Selenium and Carcinogenesis 102

IV. Hypotheses for the Mechanisms of Anticarcinogenic Actions of
Selenium 103

V. Chemopreventative Potential of Selenium 106

References 107

I. INTRODUCTION

That the nutritionally essential trace element selenium (Se) may have anticarcinogenic activities was first proposed by Shamberger and Frost,[1] who observed that cancer mortality rates in the U.S. were inversely associated with the geographic distribution of Se in forage crops. Shamberger and Willis[2] then observed that cancer mortality rates were negatively correlated with blood Se level in selected urban communities, a logical finding in light of the direct relationship of blood and forage Se levels in the same areas.[3] Over the ensuing quarter-century, a substantial body of research has yielded insight into the function of Se both in supporting normal health and in affecting cancer risk.[4,5] This chapter reviews the more recent research in this area and discusses the major issues relevant to the consideration of Se-compounds in cancer chemoprevention.

II. EPIDEMIOLOGY OF SELENIUM AND CANCER

Geographical studies of the relationship of Se status and cancer incidence in human populations have indicated inverse associations of Se status and cancer mortality. For example, Shamberger and Willis[2] found that mortality due to lymphomas and cancers of the gastrointestinal tract, peritoneum, lung, and breast were lower for both males and females residing in areas of the U.S. that can be classified, on

0-8493-8509-1/97/$0.00+$.50
© 1997 by CRC Press LLC

the basis of the Se contents of local forage crops, as being either moderate (0.06 to 0.10 μg/g Se, air dry basis) or high (>0.10 μg/g Se) in the element. Schrauzer et al.[6] also found that, in over 27 developed countries, overall cancer mortality rates, as well as age-corrected mortality rates due to leukemia and cancers of the colon, rectum, breast, ovary, and lung, correlated inversely with estimated per capita intakes of Se in those countries. Age-adjusted mortality rates within the U.S. for cancers of the breast, colon, rectum, and lung were also found to be inversely related to whole blood Se concentrations as estimated on the basis of average values obtained from blood bank samples. Similar results were reported by Yu et al.[7] in a study conducted in 24 locations in a total of 8 provinces in China: a significant negative correlation was observed between age-adjusted total cancer mortality rate and whole blood Se concentration. Further, in a county with a particularly high incidence of hepatoma (Qidong County, Jiangsu), the geographic distribution of liver cancer incidence was inversely related to blood Se level and Se contents of local food grains.

Clark et al.[8] found a significant inverse association between colorectal cancer mortality rates and local forage Se status in the U.S.; this association would appear to relate to the dietary Se environment. Their analysis indicated that cancer mortality rates were significantly lower in intermediate- and high-Se counties, in comparison to low-Se counties, for cancers in both sexes at all sites combined as well as for cancers of the lung, colon, rectum, bladder, esophagus, and pancreas. They also found inverse associations of Se exposure for females with cancers of the breast, ovary, and cervix; in contrast, cancers of the liver and stomach, Hodgkin's disease, and leukemia were positively correlated with Se exposure in both sexes.

A number of cross-sectional case-control studies have been conducted to examine the hypothesis that Se status is related to cancer risk in human populations. Results support that hypothesis and tend to show that cancer patients are generally of lower Se status than healthy controls (Table 8.1). However, the careful evaluation of these types of results necessitates determining whether the controls were actually drawn from the same population as the cancer cases, and whether the indices of Se status may have been affected by the process of carcinogenesis. The difficulty in making these determinations for the majority of published studies limits their usefulness; however, some have been designed in ways that avoid problems with confounding effects and are useful tests of the hypothesis. Prospective studies offer the advantage of having prediagnostic sampling; however, they tend to be of limited size and usually have limited statistical power for individual sites of cancer.

Our group[9,10] conducted prospective studies of Se status and cancer incidence. We found, in a cohort of some 1738 free-living Americans followed for over 10 years, that plasma Se concentration predicted subsequent risks to both nonmelanoma skin cancer (basal and/or squamous cell carcinoma) and colonic adenomatous polyps. Patients with plasma Se levels less than the population median (128 ng/g) were 4 times more likely to have one or more adenomatous polyps and had 3.5 times more polyps per patient. Eight cohort studies have examined the association of plasma Se level and colorectal/gastrointestinal cancer risk,[11-18] and although none achieved statistical significance, each showed patients who developed cancer to have had lower initial plasma Se levels than controls.

TABLE 8.1
Cancer Case-Control Comparisons of Selenium Status[a] Reported Since 1985

Cancer site	Country	Specimen	Controls (ng/g)	Cases (ng/g[b])	References
Cancer deaths	Finland pre-'84	serum	61	54	98
All cancers	Finland pre-'84	serum, M	63 ± 15	59 ± 18*	99
		serum, W	64 ± 14	64 ± 17	99
	U.S., HI	serum	125 ± 19	123 ± 20	16
	U.S., MD	serum	110 ± 16	113 ± 18	20
	U.S.	plasma	149 ± 26	150 ± 27	100

Site-Specific Cancers

Cancer site	Country	Specimen	Controls (ng/g)	Cases (ng/g[b])	References
Brain	Finland pre-'84	serum	72	65	101
Breast, primary	France	serum	88 ± 21	93 ± 16	102
	Japan	whole blood	286 ± 21	195 ± 57*	103,104
	Netherlands	plasma	93 ± 15	89 ± 14	105
	Sweden	plasma	110 ± 20	103 ± 23*	106
	U.S., CA	whole blood	191 ± 23	167 ± 32*	103,104
	U.S., KY	serum	157 ± 8[c]	125 ± 4[c]*	107
			183	164 ± 39	104
	U.S.,OH	whole blood	229 ± 35	245 ± 48	108
	Croatia	serum	80	48*	109
Breast, recurr.	Japan	whole blood	286 ± 21	188 ± 61*	103,102
	U.S., CA	whole blood	191 ± 23	162 ± 38*	103
			183	164 ± 39	104
Colon	U.S., HI	serum	125 ± 19	123 ± 19	16
	Finland	serum	67	62	17
	U.S., NY	plasma	59 ± 13	57 ± 11	100
	Croatia	serum	64 ± 12	47 ± 11	111
Rectal	U.S., HI	serum	125 ± 19	125 ± 23	16
	Finland	serum	66	65	17
	Finland	serum	61	54	12
		serum	54	48	12
		serum	55	54	14
		serum	67	62	17
		serum	66	65	17
	Norway	whole blood	129	123	18
	U.S., GA	serum	115 ± 21	116 ± 22	13
	U.S., HI	serum	125 ± 19	123 ± 19	16
		serum	125 ± 19	125 ± 23	16
	U.S., KY	serum	148 ± 7	114 ± 8*	112
	U.S., MD	serum	115 ± 21	110 ± 15	15
	U.S., NY	plasma	59 ± 13	57 ± 11	110
Colon polyps	U.S., AZ	plasma	135 ± 28	125 ± 26	9
	U.S., NY	plasma	59 ± 13	61 ± 10	110
Stomach	Finland pre-'84	serum	65 ± 13	58 ± 15*	99
	Japan	plasma	141 ± 30[c]	118 ± 46[c]	112
	U.S., HI	serum	125 ± 19	122 ± 14	16
Cervical	Finland pre-'84	serum	95 ± 2[c]	72 ± 3[c]	113
Endometrial	Finland pre-'84	serum	95 ± 2[c]	84 ± 2[c]	113
Ovarian	Finland pre-'84	serum	95 ± 2[c]	79 ± 2[c]	113
	Finland post-'84[d]	serum	126 ± 3	103 ± 3*	115

TABLE 8.1 (Continued)
Cancer Case-Control Comparisons of Selenium Status[a] Reported Since 1985

Cancer site	Country	Specimen	Controls (ng/g)	Cases (ng/g[b])	References
Esophageal	Finland pre-'84	serum	72	60	101
Oral/pharyngeal	Finland pre-'84	serum	61	65	101
	Finland pre-'84	serum	68	62	101
Liver	England	serum	88 ± 21	77 ± 18	116
	Finland pre-'84	serum	62	60	101
Leukemia	Belgium	serum	97 ± 35	82 ± 33*	117
Lung	Finland post-'84[d]	serum	61	57*	117
	Poland	serum	89 ± 47	81 ± 13	119
	U.S., HI	serum	125 ± 19	125 ± 22	16
Melanoma	Finland pre-'84	serum	61	60	101
Pancreas	Finland pre-'84	serum	63 ± 14	53 ± 12*	99
	Japan	plasma	132 ± 14	102 ± 36	120
	U.S., MD	serum	141	125	121
Bladder	Finland pre-'84	serum	70	74	101
	U.S., HI	serum	125 ± 19	121 ± 21	16
Renal	Finland pre-'84	serum	64	58	101

[a] Mean or mean ± standard deviation.
[b] Reported as significantly different from control value ($p < 0.05$).
[c] Standard error.
[d] In 1984, Finland initiated the country-wide use of Se-supplementation to agricultural fertilizers.

Salonen et al.[19] conducted a prospective case-control study to evaluate the relationship of serum Se concentration and total cancer mortality in a random population sample of 8113 residents of two counties in eastern Finland. The subjects were among a larger population that was examined in 1972; persons free of cancer were entered into the study and were followed for 6 years. During that period, each cancer death was paired with a control matched for age, gender, tobacco use, and serum cholesterol level at entry to the study. The analysis of 128 such matched pairs revealed that mean serum Se concentration was significantly lower in cancer cases than in controls, with a logistic estimate of the adjusted odds ratio of 3.1 ($p < 0.01$). Another prospective case-control study in the same cohort[12] showed that 51 terminal cancer cases had a mean serum Se that was 12% lower than matched controls. The adjusted relative risk for cancer-related death was 5.8 for subjects in the low vs. high tertiles of serum Se level. A significant interactive effect of Se and vitamin E status was detected: subjects in the low tertiles for both serum Se and α-tocopherol levels had an adjusted relative risk of fatal cancer of 11.4 compared to subjects in the high tertiles for those parameters.

The retrospective case-control study of Willet et al.[11] followed more than 11,000 cancer-free hypertensives over a 5-year period. A total of 111 cancer cases that were diagnosed after entry to the study were matched with 210 controls. Those investigators found a relative risk of 2.0 for cancer in subjects in the lowest (<115 ng/g) vs. highest (>154 ng/g) quintiles of serum baseline Se level. Peleg et al.[13] conducted another retrospective case-control study, finding no significant differences in serum Se levels between 130 cancer cases and an equal number of age- and gender-matched controls (mean serum Se: 116 ng/g). These discrepant results suggest different sets of environmental confounders between the two studies.

Menkes et al.[20] conducted a retrospective case-control study of the relationship of Se, vitamins A and E, and β-carotene status to the risk of lung cancer in a cohort (Washington County, MD) that consisted of 25,802 subjects followed from 1975 to 1983. During that time, 99 subjects diagnosed with primary lung cancer were compared with 196 controls matched for age, gender, race, month of blood donation, and tobacco use. Those investigators noted inverse associations of serum β-carotene and α-tocopherol levels and risk of lung cancer, but they found no significant differences in serum Se levels between cases (113 ng/g) and controls (110 ng/g). On the basis of histological examinations of 93 cases, the risk of squamous cell carcinoma of the lung was greater for subjects in the high tertile of serum Se and the low tertile of serum α-tocopherol. Schober et al.[15] also used a retrospective case-control design to study the relationship of Se and vitamin A and E status to risk of colon cancer in the Washington County cohort. They compared of 72 cases and 143 matched controls and found no significant independent or interactive effects of serum levels of Se, retinol, β-carotene, or α-tocopherol on the risk of colon cancer.

Kok et al.[21] reported the results of a prospective case-control study involving 10,532 Dutch subjects. They collected and archived sera at entry to the study in 1975 and followed the subjects for 8 years. They observed a total of 69 cancer deaths, occurring at least 1 year after entry to the study, which they compared to 164 matched controls. The results showed that among males the mean serum Se level of cases (116.7 ± 4.0 ng/g) was significantly less than that of controls (126.4 ± 3.1 ng/g), whereas among females the mean levels of cases and controls were similar (130.6 ± 6.0 ng/g vs. 129.3 ± 4.3 ng/g). For males in the lowest quintile of serum Se level compared to the other quintiles, the adjusted (by a multiple logistic model) relative risk of cancer death was 2.7 ($p = 0.05$). Two other nested case-control studies in the Washington County cohort revealed that individuals with low plasma Se levels had increased risk of bladder cancer (RR = 2.06).[22,23]

Several studies have used the Se contents of toenails as parameters of nutritional Se status. In the Netherlands, individuals in the lowest quartile of toenail Se were 2.5 times more likely to develop lung cancer than those in the highest quartile.[24] The level of Se among cases by histological type suggested that males with squamous cell carcinomas had higher toenail Se levels (0.541 μg/g) than those with adenocarcincoma (0.518 μg/g), small cell carcinomas (0.520 μg/g), or large cell or other carcinomas (0.517 μg/g). The same group investigated gastrointestinal cancers in this cohort; after excluding cases diagnosed in the first year, they found no significant associations between toenail Se and cancers of the stomach, colon, or rectum.[25] Similar results were reported for the predictive value of low toenail Se and risk to oral cancer.[26] Garland et al.,[27] however, found higher toenail Se levels to be associated with slightly increased risk to cancers in a cohort of nurses. The interpretation of that study has been questioned[28] on the basis of possible overadjustment for the major risk factor smoking, which may also affect nutritional Se status. Clearly, the fundamental premise implicit in the use of toenail Se as a measure of Se status, that it is related in a first-order way to a metabolically relevant Se pool, has not been tested.

Two other studies also failed to detect significant associations between Se status, as indicated by serum Se concentration, and risk to total cancers[29] or cancers of the bladder, colon-rectum, lung, or stomach.[16] However, low plasma Se was found to be associated with increased risk to thyroid cancer (RR = 7.7, lowest vs. highest tertiles).[30]

On balance, these epidemiological studies support the hypothesis that Se status can be inversely related to the risk to at least some kinds of cancer in human populations. That not all studies have demonstrated relationships of Se status and cancer risk may indicate that low Se status may be a risk modifier rather than an effector per se of carcinogenesis. The effect of a risk modifier, by definition, would be influenced by levels of exposure to the primary carcinogenic agents as well as to other risk modifiers. The results of several studies suggest that such a role of Se may relate to other factors including antioxidant nutrient status (e.g., vitamins A, C, and E, and the trace elements zinc, copper, and manganese).

III. ANIMAL MODEL STUDIES OF SELENIUM AND CARCINOGENESIS

Selenium compounds have been found to be capable of inhibiting and/or retarding tumorigenesis in a variety of experimental animal models.[5] Of more than 100 studies in which tumor production and/or preneoplastic changes have been monitored in more than two dozen animal models, two thirds have shown reductions in tumor incidence. In half of these studies, dramatic reductions (50% or more) in tumorigenesis were produced. Only an eighth of these studies have not shown Se to affect tumorigenesis; few[31] have employed levels of Se exposure that are within or only slightly above the nutritional range.

The few animal model studies that have measured histological parameters of preneoplastic change (e.g., esophageal dysplasia in the methylbenzylnitrosamine-treated rat, formation of γ-glutamyl transpeptidase-staining foci in livers or pancreases of carcinogen-treated rats) rather than, or in addition to, frank tumor expression, have yielded less consistent results. Half of available studies indicate that Se may retard early stages of tumorigenesis,[32-34] whereas half have failed to detect significant effects of Se.[32,35] None have shown high levels of Se to enhance the process.

Four animal tumor model studies have shown high levels of Se to enhance tumorigenesis at some sites. Dorado et al.[36] found that dietary exposure of either 4 or 6 µg/g Se (as Na_2SeO_3) to rats treated with diethylnitrosamine after partial hepatectomy and later promoted with phenobarbital produced modest reductions in the incidence of hepatic tumors, but nearly doubled the incidence of renal tumors. Perchellet et al.[37] found that when Se (40 µg Na_2SeO_3) was administered with α-tocopherol (40 µmoles) i.p. to mice treated topically with 7,12-dimethyl-benz[a]anthracene, the treatment did not affect skin tumors resulting from a single high dose of the carcinogen; however, it nearly doubled the incidence of papillomas among mice given smaller multiple doses of the carcinogen. Ankerst and Sjoegren[38] found Se treatment of rats to increase the incidence of 1,2-dimethylhydrazine-induced tumors of the small intestine, while decreasing the incidence of tumors of the large intestine. They also found Se-treatment to increase the incidence of virally induced mammary tumors in the rat.

With the exceptions of the four cases cited above, the preponderance of available information from controlled animal tumor model studies involving the induction of tumors by chemical or viral agents or by transplantation indicates that high-level exposure to at least some Se-compounds can be antitumorigenic. It should be noted that almost all of these studies have involved Na_2SeO_3 as the source of Se; the extent to which these effects can be extended to other sources of the element is open to question. While reduction in tumorigenesis by Se in animal tumor model systems has, in most cases, been demonstrated at subtoxic levels of the element, the effectiveness of Se appears to occur *only* at high supranutritional levels, i.e., greater than approximately 1 mg/kg in the diet or approximately 0.7 mg/l in drinking water.* Because these levels are considerably higher that those experienced by almost all free-living people, it is appropriate to consider the specific effects of Se exposures more closely approximating those of human populations, i.e., nutritional levels of the element.

Relatively few studies have been conducted in such ways as to test the hypothesis that nutritionally limiting levels of Se can effect tumorigenesis. Of some two dozen studies that have employed low-Se (<0.05 mg/kg) semi-purified diets in some 13 animal tumor models, comparison of the tumor responses of animals fed unsupplemented diets to those of animals treated with Se (in every case this has been Na_2SeO_3) have yielded inconsistent results. Ten studies have indicated that nutritional Se-deficiency can enhance tumorigenicity; seven of these have involved models of mammary carcinogenesis. In contrast, five studies have found Se-deficiency to reduce tumorigenesis, although this effect has not been observed in mammary tumor models. Nine studies have failed to demonstrate any effects of Se-deficiency. Four other animal tumor model studies have tested the effects of nutritional Se-deficiency on preneoplastic histological signs, i.e., the formation of γ-glutamyl transpeptidase-positive foci in the livers[33,34,39] of aflatoxin B_1-treated rats. Two of these[33,34] showed no effects of low Se status on this indicator of tumorigenesis, whereas one[39] found Se-deficiency to enhance this indicator in animals fed diets high in polyunsaturated fat (20% corn oil).

Present evidence concerning the effects of nutritionally deficient levels of Se in animal tumor models is compatible with the hypothesis generated in human epidemiological studied, i.e., that low-Se status can increase cancer risk. However, research in this area has not been extensive.

IV. HYPOTHESES FOR THE MECHANISMS OF ANTICARCINOGENIC ACTIONS OF SELENIUM

Several mechanisms have been proposed as hypotheses for the inhibition of tumorigenesis by supranutritional levels of Se:[40-42] alteration in carcinogen

---

* The dietary requirements of most species for Se are estimated to be 0.1 to 0.2 mg/kg; those of humans are 50 to 70 µg/day.

metabolism by Se, protection against oxidative damage by Se, and cytotoxicity of metabolites formed under high-Se conditions, affecting antioxidant protection, and affecting apoptosis. Several studies[43-56] have examined the effects of Se on carcinogen metabolism. Some indicate that the constitutive activities of cytochrome P_{450} and at least certain hepatic mixed-function oxygenases (e.g., aryl hydrocarbon hydroxylase) may be enhanced by Se;[46,47] however, there is little evidence to suggest that induced activities are affected.[43,45,46] Studies of carcinogen metabolism have yielded varying results concerning the effects of Se. For example, comparable dietary levels of Se (2 mg/kg as Na_2SeO_3) reduced the formation of covalent adducts of aflatoxin metabolites and DNA in the chick,[45] but increased the process in the rat.[44] Treatment with Se has been shown to shift the metabolism of 2-acetylaminofluorene away from N-hydroxylation towards ring-hydroxylation,[51,57] thus reducing its activation to the carcinogenic form. Studies using Ames-type *Salmonella* tester systems have shown Se-supplementation of rats to reduce the hepatic microsomal production of mutagenic metabolites of several carcinogens: N,N-dimethylanaline,[48] dimethylbenzanthracene,[53,54,58,59] 2-acetylaminofluorene,[46,50] and benzo(*a*)pyrene.[60] These reports indicate that, while high level Se supplementation can affect carcinogen metabolism, this effect is not universal with respect to either carcinogen or host species.

In view of the findings that Se can be inhibitory to both chemically and viral-induced tumors, that inhibition appears to involve both initiation as well as post-initiation events, and since the effects of Se appear to be reversible, Medina[61] suggested that the antitumorigenic effects of Se result from endocrinologically/immunologically based cellular responses. Selenite-treatment had no effects on the estrous cycle or on blood prolactin or estrogen levels in mice;[62] however, it is now clear that Se plays essential roles in thyroid hormone metabolism, where it is an essential component (as selenocysteine) in thyroidal and extrathyroidal iodothyronine 5'-deiodinases.[63] There is also reason to consider Se as an affecter of immune function, as Se-deficient animals have been found to have impaired humoral immune responses.[4] Because such responses are dependent upon the function of T-cells, macrophages, and B-cells, it is possible that humoral effects may involve roles of Se in immune cells, which have also been documented.[4]

It is not clear whether the chemopreventative effects of high-level Se are tumorigenesis phase-specific. Temple and Basu[64] found dietary selenite (1 mg Se/kg) to reduce dimethylhydrazine-induced colonic tumors in mice only when it was given during the initiation phase, whereas Reddy et al.[65] found a higher dietary level of selenite (2.5 mg Se/kg) to protect against azoxymethane-induced colonic tumors only during the postinitiation phase. Studies in another model (dimethylbenzanthracene/rat mammary tumor) indicate that the anti-tumorigenic effects of high-level Se may not be highly specific: Se was effective both during the initiation and promotion phases of carcinogenesis, with maximal inhibition achieved by continuous Se-treatment.[66]

Griffin[67] suggested that Se may be anti-carcinogenic through its role as an essential component of the Se-dependent glutathione peroxidase (GPX, of which several have now been identified), which is important in the metabolic protection from oxidant stress. Support for this hypothesis comes from the mutagenicity and carcinogenicity of malonyldialdehyde, a scission product of the peroxidative degradation of linoleic acid, which is presumed to be formed in conditions of Se (hence, GPX)-deficiency. That antioxidant protection may be relevant to colorectal carcinogenesis is suggested by several findings: dimethylhydrazine-enhanced lipid peroxidation in colonocyte mitochondrial membranes;[68] high levels of reactive oxygen species in colon cancer tissues;[69] trends toward fewer dimethylhydrazine-induced colon tumors in rats fed the antioxidant vitamin E;[70] and improved survival of colon cancer patients treated with the free radical scavengers.[71]

Whereas correction of cellular GPX deficiencies would account for the action of Se supplements to deficient animals, it should be noted that most studies that have examined tumor responses to Se in this range have not produced positive results. A GPX response is not relevant to the responses to supplemental Se by animals fed Se-adequate diets; animals show maximal GPX activities in most tissues at dietary levels of approximately 0.2 mg/kg. Further, the findings that antitumorigenic amounts of Se (e.g., 1.5 mg/kg) reduced tissue lipid peroxidation potential only slightly[72] or not at all[73] suggest that those effects are independent of the function of GPX in cellular antioxidant systems. Therefore, it is probable that antitumorigenic effects of high levels of Se involve mechanisms unrelated to the activities of these selenoenzymes.

It is likely, however, that the antitumorigenic effect of Se involves the perturbation of normal metabolism and/or production of cytotoxic metabolites due to the presence of large amounts of Se-metabolites. Le Boeuf and Hoekstra[74] proposed that high levels of selenite-Se alter intracellular levels of reduced (GSH) and oxidized (GSSG) glutathione by the catalytic oxidation of GSH by selenite. They showed that chronic feeding of a high-Se diet (6 mg/kg as Na_2SeO_3) to rats resulted in increased hepatic concentrations of both GSH and GSSG with a decreased GSH to GSSG ratio. The same high-Se treatment increased hepatic activities of glutathione reductase and glucose-6-phosphate dehydrogenase, which the authors interpreted as adaptive responses to selenite-induced GSH oxidation. Similar biochemical changes were seen in cultured hepatoma cells treated with high levels of selenite, and Se-treatment was found to retard cell doubling time. The authors suggested that the Se-induced increase in GSSG affected the process of protein synthesis. They pointed out that GSSG is known to activate a protein kinase which inactivates, through phosphorylation, eukaryotic initiation factor 2,[75,76] which was inactivated by selenite[77] or its dithiol derivative selenodiglutathione (GSSeSG).[78] Vernie et al.[79] found that the inhibition of the elongation factor was associated with inhibition of tumor growth in mice implanted with malignant lymphoblasts, and Poirier and Milner[80] found GSSeSG to be more effective in inhibiting the growth of Ehrlich ascites tumors in mice than either the inorganic or amino acid forms of Se. These results suggest that, under conditions of excessive selenite exposure, abnormally high levels of the reductive metabolite, GSSeSG, are produced which inhibit protein synthesis, presumably preferentially affecting the proliferative response. The problem with this hypothesis is that GSSeSG is unstable; at physiological GSSG to GSH ratios (<1:4), it breaks down to GSSeH and H_2Se. Thus, it is unlikely that intracellular concentrations of GSSeSG are ever great enough to affect protein synthesis.

The anticarcinogenicity of high levels of Se may involve the formation of other, more stable selenotrisulfides, such as those of proteins, which impair tumor cell metabolism. Evidence for such an effect comes from the studies of Ganther and Corcoran,[81] who found Se to inhibit bovine pancreatic ribonuclease by forming an intramolecular selenotrisulfide bridge in the place of the normal disulfide one. A similar effect was shown by Donaldson,[82] i.e., selenotrisulfide formation involving the sulfhydryl groups of chick hepatic fatty acid synthase resulted in the inhibition of enzymic activity. These results, as well as findings of inhibition by selenite of Na,K-ATPase,[83] suggest that high levels of selenite can inhibit important sulfhydryl-sensitive enzymes.

Studies by Ip and Ganther[84-88] provide strong evidence that the antitumorigenic effects of Se in the dimethylbenzanthracene/rat mammary tumor model are mediated by the methylated Se-metabolites (e.g., methylselenol, dimethylselenide). They suggested that methylated Se-metabolites may be antitumorigenic by occupying hydrophobic sites to protect critical macromolecules, by forming methylselenylated bases in nucleic acids, or by being directly cytotoxic to transformed cells. El-Bayoumy et al.[89,90] have demonstrated antitumorigenic activities for synthetic organoseleium compounds (e.g., 1,4-phenylenebis[methylene]selenocyanate), and these effects were related to apoptotic responses.[90] These findings are significant in that they demonstrate anticarcinogenic potential of normal products of Se-metabolism levels, which may be expected to increase under conditions of high-level intakes of *either* inorganic *or* organic forms of the trace element. They may also inform the development of Se-compounds as cancer chemopreventive agents.

In summary, it is possible that the antitumorigenic action of Se may be mediated through one or more of several mechanisms which have been shown to be plausible. At the present time, however, it is not clear which, if any, of these possibilities relates to the antitumorigenic effects demonstrated in animal models. Further, the extent to which any of these possibilities may be generalized to include forms of Se other than Na_2SeO_3 is also not clear. What is apparent, however, is that supranutritional levels of at least some forms of Se can impair metabolism in several fundamental ways, each of which would be expected to have great effects on proliferating cells.

V. CHEMOPREVENTATIVE POTENTIAL OF SELENIUM

While the potential for Se to be useful in cancer chemotherapy would appear clear, many questions remain concerning the types of tumors that may be affected, the chemical forms of Se that may be effective, and the dose regimens that may be appropriate. Animal tumor model studies have shown that Se can be effective as a chemopreventative agent; however, tests of its chemotherapeutic potential have yielded mixed results. Several studies with transplanted tumors have shown high levels of Se to retard tumor growth,[91-93] while others have failed to demonstrate significant effects of Se.[94,95] The prospects of Se-compounds as possible cancer chemopreventative agents are strengthened by the convergent results of studies both with animal tumor models and basic metabolism.

Evidence concerning the effects of Se supplementation on cancer incidence in humans is only presently emerging. An intervention trial that employed combinations of several vitamins and/or minerals in an area of China (Linxian, Henan) with high prevalence of esophageal cancer yielded results suggestive of a modest protective effect of the treatment that contained Se (plus vitamin E and β-carotene) against cancer mortality.[96] Our study[97] showed a stronger cancer-protective effect in an uncomplicated design. In a decade-long, double-blind, placebo-controlled, clinical intervention trial with over 1300 older Americans, we found the use of a daily oral supplement of Se-enriched yeast (200 µg Se/person/day) to produce significant reductions, in comparison to gender-matched controls, in the incidence of total cancer (RR = 0.59, p = 0.0004), total carcinomas (RR = 0.54, p = 0.0001), cancers of the lung (RR = 0.54, p = 0.040), colon-rectum (RR = 0.36, p = 0.017) and prostate (RR = 0.31, p = 0.0004), as well as as cancer mortality rate (RR = 0.49, p = 0.0013).

The results of these recent clinical intervention trials must be viewed against a background of epidemiology that supports the plausibility of Se as a risk factor in human cancers, and a very substantial body of experimental data from a variety of animal tumor models that establishes that Se can be antitumorigenic. Determining the role of Se in cancer chemoprevention will necessitate more extensive studies of the metabolism and toxicology of various forms of the element. Specifically, information is needed concerning the Se-metabolite(s) that discharge the antitumorigenic effects, and the efficacies and risks of particular oral/dietary Se-compounds as precursors to those active metabolites. While information to date is encouraging that at least forms of Se (e.g., Se-enriched yeast) can reduce cancer risk, the minimum effective dose levels must be determined in light of the element's nutritional essentiality as well as its potential toxicity.

REFERENCES

1. Shamberger, R. J. and Frost, D. V. Possible protective effect of selenium against human cancer. *Can. Med. Assoc. J.* 104, 82, 1969.
2. Shamberger, R. J. and Willis, C. E. Selenium distribution of human cancer mortality. *CRC Crit. Rev. Clin. Lab Sci.* 2, 211, 1971.
3. Allaway, W. H., Kubota, J., Losee, F. and Roth, M. Selenium, molybdenum and vanadium in human blood. *Arch. Environ. Health* 16, 342, 1968.
4. Combs, Jr., G. F. *The Role of Selenium in Nutrition*, Academic Press, New York, 535 pp., 1986.
5. Combs, G. F., Jr. Selenium. in *Nutrition and Cancer Prevention*. (Moon, T. and Micozzi, M., Eds.), Marcel Dekkar, NY, pp. 389, 1989.
6. Schrauzer, G. N., White, D. A., and Schneider, C. J. Cancer Mortality correlation studies. III. Statistical association with dietary selenium intakes. *Bioinorg. Chem.* 7, 23, 1977.
7. Yu, S. Y., Chu, Y. J., Gong, X. L., Hou, C., Li, W. G., Gong, H. M., and Xie, J. R. Regional variation of cancer mortality incidence and its relation to selenium levels in China, *Biol. Trace Elem. Res.* 7, 21, 1985.
8. Clark, L. C., Cantor, K. P., and Allaway, W. H. Selenium in forage crops and cancer mortality in U.S. counties. *Arch. Environ. Health* 46, 37, 1981.
9. Clark, L. C., Combs, G. F., Jr., Hixon, L., Deal, D. R., Moore, J., Rice, J. S., Dellasega, M., Rogers, A., Woodard, J., Schurman, B., Curtis, D., and Turnbull, B. W. Low plasma selenium predicts the prevalence of colorectal adenomatous polyps in a cancer prevention trial. *FASEB J.* 7, A65, 1993.

10. Clark, L., Hixon, L., Combs, G. F. Jr., Reid, M., Turnbull, B. W., and Sampliner, R. Plasma selenium concentration predicts the prevalence of colorectal adenomatous polyps. *Cancer Epidemiol. Biomarkers Prev.* 2, 41, 1993.

11. Willett, W., Polk, B., Morris, S., Stampfer, M., Preissel, S., Rosner, B., Taylor, J., Schneider, K., and Hames, C. Prediagnostic serum selenium and risk of cancer. *Lancet* 2, 130, 1983.

12. Salonen, J. T., Salonen, R., Lappeteläinen, R., Mäenpää, P. H., Alfthan, G., and Puska, P. Risk of cancer in relation to serum concentrations of selenium and vitamins A and E: matched case-control analysis of prospective data. *Br. Med. J.* 290, 417, 1985.

13. Pelag, I., Morris, S., and Hames, C. G. Is serum selenium a risk factor for cancer? *Med. Oncol. Tumor Pharmacother.* 2, 157, 1985.

14. Virtamo, J., Valkeila, E., Alfthan, G., Punsar, S., Huttunen, J. K., and Karvonen. M. J. Serum selenium and risk of cancer. A prospective follow-up of nine years. *Cancer* 60, 145, 1987.

15. Schober, S. E., Comstock, G. W., Helsing, K. J., Salkeld, R. M., Morris, J. S., Rider, A. A., and Brookmeyer, R. Serologic precursors of cancer. I. Prediagnostic serum nutrients and colon cancer risk. *Am. J. Epidemiol.* 126, 1033, 1987.

16. Nomura, A., Heilbrun, L. K., Morris, J. S., and Stemmermann, G. N. Serum selenium and the risk of cancer, by specific sites: Case-control analysis of prospective data. *J. Natl. Cancer Inst.* 79, 103, 1987.

17. Knekt, P., Aromaa, A., Maatela, J., Alfthan, G., Aaran, R. K., Teppo, L., and Hakama, M. Serum vitamin E, serum selenium and the risk of gastrointestinal cancer. *Int. J. Cancer* 42, 846, 1988.

18. Ringstad, J., Jacobsen, B. K., Tretli, S., and Thomassen, Y. Serum selenium concentration associated with risk of cancer. *J. Clin. Pathol.* 41, 454, 1988.

19. Salonen, J. T., Alfthan, G., Huttunen, J. K., and Puska, P. Association between serum selenium and the risk of cancer. *Am. J. Epidemiol.* 120, 342, 1984.

20. Menkes, M. S., Comstock, G. W., Vuilleumier, J. P., Helsing, K. J., Rider, A. A., and Brookmeyer, R. P. Serum beta-carotene, vitamins A and E, selenium, and the risk of lung cancer. *New Engl. J. Med.* 315, 1250, 1986.

21. Kok, F. J., De Bruijn, A. M., Hofman, A., Vermeeren, R., and Valkenburg, H. A. Is serum selenium a risk factor for cancer in men only? *Am. J. Epidemiol.* 125, 12, 1987.

22. Helzlsour, K. J., Comstock, G. W., Morris, J., S. Selenium, lycopene, alpha-tocopherol, beta-carotene, retinol and subsequent bladder cancer. *Cancer Res.* 49, 6144, 1989.

23. Helzlsour, K. J., Alberg, A. J., Norkus, E. P., Morris, J. S., Hoffman, S. C., and Comstock, G. W., Prospective study on serum micronutrients and ovarian cancer. *J. Natl. Cancer Inst.* 88, 32-37, 1995.

24. van den Brandt, P., Goldbohm, R., van't Veer, P., Bode, P., Dorant, E., Hermus, R., and Sturmans, F. A prospective cohort study of toenail selenium levels and risk of gastrointestinal cancer. *J. Natl. Cancer Inst.* 85, 224, 1993.

25. van den Brandt, P. A., Goldbohm, R. A., Veer, P. V., Bode, P., Durant, E., Hermus, R. J., and Sturmans, F. A prospective cohort study on selenium status and risk of lung cancer. *Cancer Res.* 53, 4860, 1993.

26. Rogers, M. A. M., Thomas, D. B., Davis, S., Weiss, N. S., Vaughan, T. L., and Nevissi, A. E. A case-control study of oral cancer and pre-diagnostic concentrations of selenium and zinc in nail tissue. *Int. J. Cancer Res.* 48, 182, 1991.

27. Garland, M., Morris, J. S., Stampfer, M. J., Colditz, G. A., Spate, V. L., Basket, C. K., Rosner, B., Speizer, F. E., Willet, W. C., and Hunter, D. J., Prospective study of toenail selenium levels and cancer among women. *J. Natl. Cancer Inst.* 87, 497, 1995.

28. Clark, L. C. and Alberts, D. S. Selenium and cancer: risk or protection? *J. Natl. Cancer Inst.* 87, 473, 1995.

29. Coates, R. J., Weiss, N. S., Daling, H. J., Morrism S. J., and Labbe, R. E. Serum levels of selenium and retinol and the subsequent risk of cancer. *Am. J. Epid.* 128, 515, 1988.

30. Glattre, E., Thomassen, Y., Thoresen, S. O., Haldorsen, T., Lund-Lasen, P. G., Theodorsen, L., and Aaseth, J. Prediagnostic serum selenium in a case-control study of thyroid cancer. *Int. J. Epidemiol.* 18, 45, 1994.

31. Shamberger, R. J. Relationship of selenium to cancer. I. Inhibitory effect of selenium on carcinogenesis. *J. Natl. Cancer Inst.* 44, 931, 1970.

32. Le Boeuf, R. A., Laishes, B. A., and Hoekstra, W. G. Effects of dietary selenium concentration on the development of enzyme-altered liver foci and hepatocellular carcinoma by diethyl-nitrosamine of N-acetylaminoflurene in rats. *Cancer Res.* 45, 5489, 1985.
33. Baldwin, S. and Parker, R. S. Influence of dietary fat and selenium in initiation and promotion of aflatoxin B_1-induced preneoplastic foci in rat liver. *Carcinogen.* 8, 101, 1986.
34. Milks, M. M., Wilt, S. R., Ali, I. I., and Couri, D. The effects of selenium on the emergence of aflatoxin B_1-induced enzyme-altered foci in rat liver. *Fund. Appl. Toxicol.* 5, 320, 1985.
35. Bogden, J. D., Chung, H. B., Kemp, F. W., Holding, K., Bruening, K. S., and Naveh, Y. Effect of selenium and molybdenum on methylbenzylnitrosamine-induced esophageal lesions and tissue trace metals in the rat. *J. Nutr.* 116, 2432, 1986.
36. Dorado, R. D., Porta, E., A., and Aquino, T. M. Effects of dietary selenium on hepatic and renal tumorigenesis induced in rats by diethylnitrosamine. *Hepatology* 5, 1201, 1985.
37. Perchellet, J. P., Abney, N. L., Thomas, R. M., Guislain, Y. L., and Perchellet, E. M. Effects of combined treatments with selenium, glutathione, and vitamin E on glutathione peroxidase activity, ornithine decarboxylase induction, and complete and multistage carcinogenesis in mouse skin. *Cancer Res.* 47, 477, 1987.
38. Ankerst, J. and Sjogren, H. Effect of selenium on the induction of breast fibroadenomas by adenovirus type 9 and 1,2-dimethylhydrazine-induced bowel carcinogenesis in rats. *Int. J. Cancer* 29, 707, 1982.
39. Baldwin, S. and Parker, R. S. The effects of dietary fat and selenium on the development of preneoplastic lesions in rat liver. *Nutr. Cancer.* 8, 273, 1987.
40. Milner, J. A. Effect of selenium on virally induced and transplantable tumor models. *Fed. Proc.* 44, 2568, 1985.
41. Ip, C. and Medina, D. Current concept of selenium and mammary tumorigenesis, in *Cellular and Molecular Biology of Breast Cancer* (Medina, D., Kidwell, W., Heppner, G., and Anderson, E. P., Eds.) Plenum Press, New York, pp. 479, 1987.
42. El-Bayoumy, K. The role of selenium in cancer prevention. in *Practice of Oncology*, 4th edition (DeVita, V. T., Hellman, S., and Rosenberg, S. S., Eds.), Lippincott, Philadelphia, pp. 1-15, 1991.
43. Thompson, H. J. Selenium as an anticarcinogen. *J. Agric. Food Chem.* 32, 422, 1984.
44. Chen, J., Goetchius, M. P., Campbell, C., and Combs, Jr., G. F. Effects of dietary selenium and vitamin E on hepatic mixed-function oxidase activities and *in vivo* covalent binding of aflatoxin B_1 in rats. *J. Nutr.* 112, 324, 1982.
45. Chen, J., Goetchius, M. P., Combs, Jr., G. F., and Campbell, C. Effects of dietary selenium and vitamin E on covalent binding of aflatoxin to chick liver cell macromolecules. *J. Nutr.* 112, 350, 1982.
46. Chow, C. K. and Gairola, G. C. Influence of dietary vitamin E and selenium on metabolic activation of chemicals to mutagens. *J. Agric. Food Chem.* 32, 443, 1984.
47. Capel, I. D., Jenner, M., Darrell, H. M., and Williams, D. C. The influence of selenium on some hepatic carcinogen metabolizing enzymes of rats. *IRCS Med. Sci. Libr. Compend.* 8, 382, 1980.
48. Olsson, U., Onfelt, A., and Beije, B. Dietary selenium deficiency causes decreased N-oxygenation of N,N-diethylaniline and increased mutagenicity of dimethylnitrosamine in the isolated rat liver/cell culture system. *Mutation Res.* 126, 73, 1984.
49. Wortzman, M. S., Besbris, H. J., and Cohen, A. M. Effect of dietary selenium on the interaction between 2-acetylaminofluorene and rat liver DNA *in vivo*. *Cancer Res.* 40, 2670, 1980.
50. Gairola, C. and Chow, C. K. Dietary selenium, hepatic arylhydrocarbon hydroxylase and mutagenic activation of benzo(a)pyrene, 2-aminoanthracene and 2-aminofluorene. *Toxicol. Letts.* 11, 281, 1982.
51. Besbris, H. J., Wortzman, M. S., and Cohen, A. M. Effect of dietary selenium on the metabolism and excretion of 2-acetylaminofluorene in the rat. *J. Toxicol. Environ. Health* 9, 63, 1982.
52. Hughes, D. A. and Bjeldanes, L. F. Influence of selenium-supplemented torula yeast diets on liver-mediated mutagenicity of aflatoxin B_1. *J. Food Sci.* 48, 759, 1983.
53. Schillaci, M., Martin, S. E., and Milner, J. A. The effects of dietary selenium on the biotransformation of 7,12-dimethylbenz(a)anthracene. *Mutation Res.* 101, 31, 1982.
54. Martin, S. E. and Schillaci, M. Inhibitory effects of selenium on mutagenicity. *J. Agric. Food Chem.* 32, 426, 1984.

55. Burguera, J. A., Edds, G. T., and Osuna, O. Influence of selenium and aflatoxin B₁ or crotalaria toxicity in turkey poults. *Am. J. Vet. Res.* 44, 1714, 1983.
56. Skaare, J. U. and Nafstad, I. Interaction of vitamin E and selenium with the hepatotoxic agent dimethylnitrosamine. *Acta Pharmacol. Toxicol.* 43, 119, 1978.
57. Harr, J. R., Exon, J. H., Whanger, P. D., and Weswig, P.H. Effect of dietary selenium on N-2-fluorenyl acetamide (FFA)-induced cancer in vitamin E-supplemented, selenium-depleted rats. *Clin. Toxicol.* 5, 187, 1972.
58. Tsen, C. C. and Tappel, A. L. Catalytic oxidation of glutathione and other sulfhydryl compounds by selenite. *J. Biol. Chem.* 233, 1230, 1958.
59. Jacobs, M. Inhibitory effects of selenium on 1,2-dimethylhydrazine and methylazoxymethanol colon carcinogenesis. Cerrelative studies on selenium effects on the mutagenicity and sister chromatid exchange rates of selected carcinogens. *Cancer* 40, 2557, 1977.
60. Teel, R. W. and Kain, S. R. Selenium modified mutagenicity and metabolism of benzo(a) pyrene in an S9-dependent system. *Mutation Res.* 127, 9, 1984.
61. Medina, D. Mechanisms of selenium inhibition of tumorigenesis. *J. Am. Coll. Toxicol.* 5, 21, 1986.
62. Ip, C. Factors influencing the anti-carcinogenic efficacy of selenium in demthylbenz[a]-anthracene-induced mammary tumorigenesis in rats. *Cancer Res.* 41, 2683, 1981.
63. Larsen, R. P. and Berry, M. J. Nutritional and hormonal regulation of thyroid hormone deiodinases. *Ann. Rev. Nutr.* 15, 323, 1995.
64. Temple, N. J. and Basu, T. K. Selenium and cabbage and colon carcinogenesis in mice. *J. Natl. Cancer Inst.* 79, 1131, 1987.
65. Reddy, B. S., Sugie, S., Maruyama, H., and Marra, P. Effect of dietary excess of inorganic selenium during initiation and post-initiation phases of colon carcinogenesis in F344 rats. *Cancer Res.* 48, 1777, 1988.
66. Tempero, M. A., Deschner, E. E., and Zedeck, M. S. The effect of selenium on cell proliferation in liver and colon. *Biol. Trace Elem. Res.* 10, 145, 1986.
67. Griffin, A. C. Role of selenium in the chemoprevention of cancer. *Adv. Cancer Res.* 29, 419, 1979.
68. Rana, R. S., Stevens, R. H., Oberley, L, Loven, D. P., Graves, J. M., Cole, D. A., and Meck, E. S., Evidence for a defective mitochondrial membrane in 1,2-dimethylhyrdazine-induced colon adenocarcinoma in rat: enhanced lipid peroxidation potential *in vitro. Cancer Lett.* 9, 237, 1980.
69. Kashavarzian, A., Zapeda, D., List, T., and Mobarhan, S. High levels of reactive oxygen metabolites in colon cancer tissue: analysis by chemiluminescence probe. *Nutr. Cancer* 17, 243, 1992.
70. Chester, J., Gaissert, H., Ross, J., Malt, R., and Weitsman, S. Augmentation of 1,2-dimethyl hydrazine-induced colon cancer by experimental colitis in mice: role of dietary vitamin E. *J. Natl. Cancer Inst.* 76, 939, 1986.
71. Salim, A. S. Scavengers of oxygen-derived free radicals prolong survial in advanced colonic cancer. A new approach. *Tumor Biol.* 14, 9, 1993.
72. Lane, H. W. and Medina, D. Mode of action of selenium inhibition of 7,12-demethylbenz (a)anthracene-induced mouse mammary tumorigenesis. *J. Natl. Cancer Inst.* 75, 675, 1985.
73. Horvath, P. M. and Ip, C. Synergistic effect of vitamin E and selenium in the chemoprevention of mammary carcinogenesis in rats. *Cancer Res.* 43, 5335, 1983.
74. Le Beouf, R. A. and Hoekstra, W.G. Adaptive changes in hepatic glutathione metabolism in response to excess dietary selenium. *J. Nutr.* 113, 845, 1983.
75. Jacobs, M. M., Jansson, B., and Griffin, A. C. Inhibitory effects of selenium on 1,2-dimethyl hydrazine and methylazoxymethanol acetate induction of colon tumors. *Cancer Letters* 2, 133, 1977.
76. Jacobs, M. M., Matney, J. S., and Griffin, A. C. Inhibitory effects of selenium on the mutagenicity of 2-acetylaminofluorene (AAF) and AAF derivatives. *Cancer Letts.* 2, 319, 1977.
77. Safer, B., Jagus, B., and Crouch, D. Indirect inactivation of eukaryotic initiation factor 2 in reticulocyte lysates by selenite. *J. Biol. Chem.* 255, 6913, 1980.
78. Vernie, L. N. Inhibition of protein synthesis and anticarcinogenicity of selenium compounds, in *Proceedings of the Third International Symposium on Selenium in Biology and Medicine* (Combs, G.F., Jr., Spallholz, J.E., Levander, O.A., and Oldfield, J.E., eds.), AVI Publ. Co., Westport, Conn., vol. B, p. 1074, 1987.

79. Vernie, L. N., Hamburg, C. J., and Bont, W. S. Inhibition of the growth of milignant mouse lymphoid cells by selenodiglutathione and selenocystine. *Cancer Letts.* 14, 303, 1981.
80. Poirier, K. A. and Milner, J. A. Factors influencing the antitumorigenic properties of selenium in mice. *J. Nutr.* 113, 2147, 1983.
81. Ganther, H. E. and Corcoran, C. Selenotrisulfides. II. Cross-linking of reduced pancreatic ribonuclease with selenium. *Biochemistry* 8, 2557, 1969.
82. Donaldson, W. E. Selenium inhibition of avian fatty acid synthase complex. *Chem.-Biol. Interact.* 17, 313, 1977.
83. Bergad, P. L. and Rathbun, W. B. Inhibition of Na,K-ATPase by sodium selenite and reversal by glutathione. *Curr. Eye Res.* 5, 919, 1986.
84. Ip, C. and Ganther, H. Activity of methylated forms of selenium in cancer prevention. *Cancer Res.* 50, 1206, 1990.
85. Ip, C. and Ganther, H. Combination of blocking agents and suppressing agents in cancer prevention. *Carcinogen.* 12, 365, 1991.
86. Ip, C. and Ganther, H. Novel strategies in selenium cancer chemoprevention research. Chapt. 9 in *Selenium in Biology and Human Health* (Burk, R. F., Ed.), Springer-Verlag, New York, pp.170, 1993.
87. Ip, C. and Ganther, H. E. Comparison of selenium and sulfur analogs in cancer prevention. *Carcinogenesis* 13, 1167, 1992.
88. Vadhanavikit, S., Ip, C., and Ganther, H. E. Metabolism of selenite and methylated selenium compounds administered at cancer chemopreventive levels in rats. *Xenobiotica* 23, 731, 1983.
89. El-Bayoumy, K., Chae, Y. H., Upadhyaya, P., Mescher, C., Cohen, L. A., and Reddy, B. S. Selenium in chemoprevention of carcinogensis II. Inhibition of 7,12-dimethylbenz[a]-anthracene-induced tumors and DNA adduct formation in the mammary glands of female Sprague-Dawley rats by the synthetic organoselenium compound 1,4-phenylenebis(methylene)seleno-cyanate. *Cancer Res.* 52, 2402, 1992.
90. Thompson, H. J., Wilson, A., Lu, J., Singh, M., Jiang, C., Upadhyaya, P., El-Bayoumy, K., and Ip, C. Comparison of the effects of an organic and inorganic form of selenium on a mammary carcinoma cell line. *Carcinogenesis* 15, 183, 1994.
91. Watrach, A. M., Milner, J. A., and Watrach, M. A. Effect of selenium on growth rate of canine mammary carcinoma cells in athymic nude mice. *Cancer Letts.* 15, 137, 1982.
92. Greeder, G. A. and Milner, J. A. Factors influencing the inhibitory effect of selenium on mice inoculated with Ehrlich ascites tumor cells. *Science* 209, 825, 1980.
93. Milner, J. A. and Hsu, C. Y. Inhibitory effects of selenium on the growth of L1210 leukemic cells. *Cancer Res.* 41, 1652, 1982.
94. Medina, D. and Lane, H. W. Stage specificity of selenium-mediated inhibition of mouse mammary tumorigensis. *Biol. Trace Elem. Res.* 5, 297, 1994.
95. Schrauzer, G. N., McGuinness, J. E., and Kuehn, K. Effects of temporary selenium supple mentation on the genesis of spontaneous mammary tumors in inbred female C₃H/St mice. *Carcinogenesis* 1, 199, 1980.
96. Blot, W. J., Li, J. Y., Taylor, P. R., Guo, W., Dawsey, S., Wang, G. Q., Yang, C. S., Zheng, S. F., Gail, M., Li, G. Y., Liu, B. Q., Tangrea, J., Sun, Y. H., Liu, F., Fraumeni, Jr., F., Zhang, Y. H., and Li, B. Nutrition intervention trials in Linxian, China: supplementation with specific vitamin/mineral combinations, cancer incidence, and diesease-specific mortality in the general population. *J. Natl. Cancer Inst.* 85, 1483, 1993.
97. Clark, L. C., Combs, Jr., G. F., Turnbull, B. W., Slate, E., Alberts, D., Abele, D., Allison, R., Bradshaw, J., Chalker, D., Chow, J., Curtis, D., Dalen, J., Davis, L., Deal, R., Dellasega, M., Glover, R., Graham, G., Gross, E., Hendrix, J., Herlong, J., Knight, F., Krongrad, A., Lesher, J., Moore, J., Park, K., Rice, J., Rogers, A., Sanders, B., Schurman, B., Smith, C., Smith, E., Taylor, J., and Woodward, J., The Nutritional Prevention of Cancer with Selenium 1983-1993: a Randomized Clinical Trial. *J. Am. Med. Assoc.* (in press), 1997.
98. Salonen, J. T., Salonen, R., Penttilä, I., Herranen, J., Jauhiainen, M., Kantola, M., Lappeteläinen, R., Mäenpää, P., Alfthan, G., and Puska, P. Serum fatty acids, apolipoproteins, selenium and vitamin antioxidants and the risk of death from coronary artery disease. *Am. J. Cardiol.* 56, 226, 1985.

99. Knekt, P., Aromaa, A., Maatela, J., Alfthan, G., Aaren, R. K., Hakama, M., Hakulinen, T., Peto, R., and Teppo, L. Serum selenium and subsequent risk of cancer among Finnish men and women. *J. Natl. Cancer Inst.* 82, 864, 1990.

100. Criqui, M.H., Bangdiwala, S., Goodman, D. S., Blaner, W. S., Morris, J. S., Kritchevsky, S., Lippel, K., Mebane, I., and Tyroler, H. A. Selenium, retinol, retinol-binding protein and uric acid associations with cancer mortality in a population-based prospective case-control study. *Ann. Epidemiol.* 1, 385, 1981.

101. Knekt, P., Aromaa, A., Maatela, J., Alfthan, G., Aaren, R. K., Nikkan, T., Hakama, M., Hakulinen, T., and Teppo, L. Serum micronutrients and risk of cancers of low incidence in Finland. *Am. J. Epidemiol.* 134, 356, 1991.

102. Gerber, M., Richardson, S., and Chappuis, P. Selenium and other antioxidants in breast cancer, in *Selenium in Medicine and Biology* (Nève, J. and Favier, A., Eds.), de Gruyter, New York, p. 263, 1988.

103. Schrauzer, G. N., Molenaar, T., Mead, S., Luehn, K., Yamamoto, H., and Araki, E. Selenium in the blood of Japanese and American women with and without breast cancer and fibrocystic disease. *Jap. J. Cancer Res.* (Gann) 76, 374, 1985.

104. Schrauzer, G. N., Schrauzer, T., Mead, S., Kuehn, K., Yamamoto, H., and Araki, E. Selenium in the blood of Japanese and American women with and without breast cancer and fibrocystic disease. in *Selenium in Biology and Medicine* (Combs, Jr., G. F., Spallholz, J. E., Levander, O. A., and Oldfield, J. E., Eds.), AVI Publ. Co., Westport, Conn., vol. B, p. 1116, 1987.

105. van't Veer, P., van der Weilen, R. P. J, Kok, F. J., Hermus, R. J. J., and Sturmans, F., Selenium in diet, blood and toenails in relation to breast cancer: a case-control study. *J. Epidemiol.* 131, 987, 1990.

106. Hardell, L., Danell, M., Ängqvist, C. A., Marklund, S. L., Fredriksson, M., Zakari, A. L., and Kjellgren, A., Levels of selenium in plasma and glutathione peroxidase in erythrocytes and the risk of breast cancer: A case-control study. *Biol. Trace Elem. Res.* 36, 99, 1993.

107. McConnell, K. P., Jager, R. M., Bland, K. I., and Blotky, A. J. The relationship of dietary selenium and breast cancer. *J. Surg. Oncol.* 15, 67, 1980.

108. Shamberger, R. J., Rukovena, E., Longfield, A. K., Tytko, S. A., Deadbar, S., and Willis, C. E. Antioxidants and Cancer: I. Selenium in the blood of normal and cancer patients. *J. Natl. Cancer Inst.* 50, 863, 1973.

109. Kršnjavi, H. and Beker, D. Selenium in serum as a possible parameter for assessment of breast disease. *Breast Cancer Res. Treat.* 16, 57, 1990.

110. Dworkin, B., Newman, L. J., Berezin, S., Rosenthal, W. S., Schwarz, S. M., and Weiss, L. Low blood selenium levels in patients with cystic fibrosis compared to controls and healthy adults. *J. Parent. Ent. Nutr.* 11, 38, 1987.

111. Mikac-Dević, M., Vukelić, N., and Kljaić, K. Serum selenium level in patients with colorectal cancer. *Biol. Trace Elem. Res.* 33, 87, 1992.

112. McConnell, K. P., Broghamer, W. L., Blotky, A. J., and Harr, O. J. Selenium levels in blood and tissues in health and disease. *J. Nutr.* 105, 1026, 1965.

113. Saito, K., Saito, T., Hosokawa, T., and Ito, K. Blood selenium level and the interaction of copper, zinc and manganese in stomach cancer, in *Selenium in Biology and Medicine* (Combs, Jr., G. F., Spallholz, J. E., Levander, O. A., and Oldfield, J. E., Eds.) AVI Publishing Co., Westport, Conn., vol. B, pp. 1104, 1987.

114. Sundström, H. Annual variation of serum selenium in patients with gynecological cancer during 1978-1983 in Finland, a low selenium area. *Int. J. Vit. Nutr. Res.* 55, 433, 1985.

115. Sundström, H., Yrjanheikke, E. and Kauppila, A. Serum selenium and thromboxane in patients with gynecological cancer. *Carcinogenesis* 5, 1051, 1986.

116. Thuluvath, P. J. and Triger, D. R. Selenium and chronic liver disease. *J. Haematol.* 14, 176, 1992.

117. Beguin, Y., Bours, V., Delbrouck, J. M., Robave, G., Roelands, I., Bury, J., Fillet, G., and Weber, G. Relationship of serum selenium levels to tumor activity in acute and non-lymphocytic leukemia. *Carcinogen.* 10, 2089, 1989.

118. Knekt, P., Alfthan, G., Aromaa, A., Hakama, M., Hakulinen, T., Maatela, J., Peto, R., Saxén, E., and Teppo, L. Low serum selenium level and elevated risk of lung cancer, in *Selenium in Biology and Medicine* (Wendel, A., Ed.), Springer-Verlag, New York, pp. 313, 1993.

119. Masiak, M. and Harzyk, D. Behaviour of microelements in lung cancer patients. *Fres. Z. Anal. Chem.* 317, 661, 1984.
120. Uehara, S., Honjo, K., Hirano, F., Sakai, N., Hirayama, A., and Jin, K. Clinical significance of selenium levels in chronic pancreatitis. *J. Clin. Biochem. Nutr.* 5, 201, 1988.
121. Burney, P. G. J., Comstock, G. W., and Morris, J. S. Serologic precursors of cancer: Serum micronutrients and the subsequent risk of pancreatic cancer. *Am. J. Clin. Nutr.* 49, 895, 1989.

Chapter 9

ANTIOXIDANTS AND LDL OXIDATION

Cindy J. Fuller and I. Jialal

Contents

I. Introduction 115

II. LDL Oxidation and Atherosclerosis 115

III. Effects of Antioxidants on LDL Oxidizability 118

References 123

I. INTRODUCTION

The oxidative modification of low-density lipoprotein (LDL) may be a key early step in atherogenesis. Dietary antioxidants such as α-tocopherol, ascorbate, β-carotene, and flavonoids have been shown to decrease the susceptibility of LDL to oxidation *in vitro*. Supplementation studies in humans have also shown reductions in LDL oxidative susceptibility. Estrogens and ubiquinol-10 also have antioxidant capabilities. This chapter will review the proposed role of oxidized LDL (Ox-LDL) in atherogenesis, laboratory analyses routinely used to detect LDL oxidation, and the effect of antioxidants on LDL oxidizability and atherosclerosis.

II. LDL OXIDATION AND ATHEROSCLEROSIS

The fatty streak is the earliest and most common atherosclerotic lesion. Microscopically, it is comprised of subendothelial aggregates of foam cells. These are cells that contain large cytoplasmic deposits of cholesteryl ester and free cholesterol in lipid droplets. The majority of foam cells are of macrophage origin, with smooth muscle cells comprising the rest. Fatty streaks may regress or progress to fibrous plaques. The fibrous plaque is the most characteristic lesion of advancing atherosclerosis. It usually consists of a fibrous cap made up of smooth muscle cells and dense connective tissue, an underlying cellular layer, and a deeper necrotic core. The major cell type in the fibrous plaque is the smooth muscle cell. The fibrous plaque may undergo changes such as calcification, necrosis, hemorrhage, ulceration, or thrombosis to form a complex lesion. These are the lesions most often associated with the clinical signs of atherosclerosis.

115

A high plasma concentration of LDL is a primary risk factor for atherosclerosis; however, it is unknown how LDL promotes the development of the lipid-laden foam cells that comprise the fatty streak. The classic LDL receptor pathway cannot be responsible for the cholesterol accumulation, as it is down-regulated by an increase in intracellular cholesterol.[1] The macrophage scavenger receptors, in contrast, are able to recognize chemically modified LDL (e.g., acetylated-LDL).[2] The scavenger receptor is not down-regulated by intracellular cholesterol,[1] and LDL taken up by this mechanism can thus result in appreciable cholesteryl ester accumulation.

The most plausible and biologically relevant LDL modification is oxidation. The three main cell types in the arterial wall — endothelial cells, smooth muscle cells, and macrophages — are able to oxidize LDL *in vitro*.[3-5] Numerous chemical changes occur to the lipid phase of LDL as it is oxidized. Under normal conditions, polyunsaturated fatty acids (PUFA) are nonconjugated, i.e., two single bonds separate two double bonds in fatty acid chains. Oxidation of LDL causes rearrangement of the electrons in PUFA to form conjugated double bond systems (conjugated dienes), where two double bonds are separated by only one single bond. The development of conjugated dienes can be monitored spectrophotometrically at 234 nm.[6,7] The PUFA content is reduced, accompanied by an increase in lipid peroxides and aldehydes such as malondialdehyde (MDA).[3,7] Two methods exist to monitor the development of lipid peroxides directly. A rapid and simple method is based on the oxidation of iodide to iodine.[8] In addition, lipid peroxides can be monitored by the oxidation of ferrous to ferric ion in the presence of xylenol orange.[9] With modifications, this method can also be used to analyze plasma or serum lipid peroxides.[10] Aldehydes formed from LDL oxidation can be determined by the thiobarbituric acid-reactive substances (TBARS) assay, which is an indication of MDA formation. The TBARS assay is not specific for MDA. Other aldehydes, sugars, and amino acids also react with thiobarbituric acid. This can complicate interpretation of results in cellular LDL oxidation systems if appropriate blanks are not used. The chromogen formed in this assay can be monitored spectrophotometrically[11] or fluorimetrically.[12]

Cholesterol in LDL can be oxidized to oxysterols, mainly 7-ketocholesterol, which can be detected by gas chromatography.[13] In this study, the investigators found that free cholesterol was only slightly more susceptible to oxidation than were cholesterol esters. The lecithin content of LDL decreases upon oxidation, concomitant with an increase in lysolecithin.[3] This hydrolysis has been attributed to a calcium-independent phospholipase A2 that circulates associated with LDL.[14]

The protein moiety of LDL, apolipoprotein B (apoB), is also affected by LDL oxidation. Extensive oxidation of LDL results in the derivatization of lysine residues on apoB by lipid hydroperoxides or aldehydes such as malondialdehyde, 4-hydroxynonenal, and hexanal, thus increasing its negative charge.[7,15] The increase in negative charge can be monitored by agarose gel electrophoresis at pH 8.6.[16] Aldehydic modification of apoB-100 also generates fluorophores which fluoresce strongly at 430 nm with excitation at 360 nm.[18] Fragmentation of apoB can also occur with extensive oxidative damage.[17] This is detectable by sodium dodecyl sulfate polyacrylamide gel electrophoresis.[19] These changes in apoB decrease LDL uptake by the LDL receptor, but increase its uptake by the macrophage scavenger receptor.[3]

Oxidatively-modified LDL has numerous effects on cultured cells that may promote atherogenesis *in vivo*. Uptake of Ox-LDL via the scavenger receptor stimulates increased cholesterol esterification by macrophages with possible foam cell formation.[1,20,21] The products of LDL oxidation, including oxysterols, are cytotoxic.[14,22-24] These cytotoxic effects could induce endothelial cell dysfunction[25] and may also promote the development of a more advanced lesion.[2]

Mild oxidation of LDL results in the formation of minimally modified LDL (MM-LDL). This species is not taken up by the macrophage scavenger receptor, but by the LDL receptor. The content of TBARS in MM-LDL is <5 nmol/mg protein, whereas the TBARS content of Ox-LDL can be 10 times higher.[26,27] Berliner et al.[26] demonstrated that MM-LDL stimulated binding of monocytes to cultured endothelial cells. In addition, MM-LDL stimulates the production of monocyte chemotactic protein-1 (MCP-1) by endothelial and smooth muscle cells. This results in promotion of monocyte chemotaxis.[28] Navab et al.[5] showed that cocultures of human aortic smooth muscle and endothelial cells could modify LDL sufficiently to stimulate MCP-1 production. Minimally modified LDL and products of LDL oxidation stimulate production of adhesion molecules such as ELAM and VCAM by aortic endothelial cells.[29,30] Liao et al.[31] showed that *in vivo* Ox-LDL infusion into rat mesenteric venules can stimulate neutrophil adhesion, mast cell degranulation, and albumin leakage into the interstitial space. Oxidized LDL itself is a chemoattractant for monocytes;[32] at the same time, it inhibits macrophage chemotaxis.[33] This trapping phenomenon may lead to the formation of foam cells in the subendothelial space. Lysolecithin in Ox-LDL is also chemotactic for human monocytes.[34]

Oxidized LDL also affects secretion of other growth factors and cell signals that can affect the pathogenesis of atherosclerosis. Minimally modified LDL stimulates production of colony-stimulating factors by aortic endothelial cells,[35] which can promote differentiation of monocytes into macrophages. Activation of the macrophage-colony-stimulating factor gene has been shown to require nuclear transcription factor-NF-κB.[36] Interleukin-1 (IL-1) release by mononuclear cells is also stimulated by Ox-LDL,[37] which could promote smooth muscle cell proliferation. Oxidized LDL results in a decrease in platelet-derived growth factor (PDGF) secretion by human macrophages.[38] The significance of this effect remains to be elucidated. Prostacyclin production by human endothelial cells is increased by Ox-LDL,[39] but not by rabbit smooth muscle cells.[40] However, chronic exposure of cultured bovine endothelial cells (20 μg protein/mL for 3 days) to Ox-LDL inhibited prostacyclin release.[41] Mouse peritoneal macrophages were stimulated to produce leukotriene B4 by Ox-LDL, but not by native or acetylated LDL.[42]

Oxidized LDL may also be responsible for reduced fibrinolysis and procoagulant activity by inducing tissue factor expression.[43] Plasminogen activator inhibitor-1 (PAI-1) prevents fibrinolysis. Latron et al.[44] reported that Ox-LDL increased PAI-1 synthesis and secretion by cultured endothelial cells in a dose-related manner. Also, Ox-LDL may have a procoagulant effect by increasing the activity of thromboplastin and, in turn, factor VII,[45] and by activating platelet phospholipase A2/cyclooxygenase.[46] The procoagulant state induced by Ox-LDL may thus provide a bridge between atherosclerosis and thrombosis.[45] In addition, Ox-LDL may promote abnormal vasoreactivity by inhibiting nitric oxide synthesis,[47] a potent vasodilator, and by stimulating secretion of the vasoconstrictor endothelin.[48] In contrast, Jougasaki et al.[49] reported that endothelin secretion was inhibited by Ox-LDL due to the presence of lysolecithin.

Several lines of evidence point to the *in vivo* existence of Ox-LDL. Immunostaining of rabbit and human atherosclerotic lesions show positive reactions with antibodies to epitopes on Ox-LDL.[50] LDLs isolated from human and rabbit atheromas exhibit physicochemical and biological properties of Ox-LDL.[51] Oxidatively modified and fragmented apoB have been isolated from the plasma of normal subjects and from patients with atherosclerosis.[52] Autoantibodies to Ox-LDL epitopes have been isolated from human and rabbit plasma.[53] The presence of autoantibodies against Ox-LDL has been positively correlated with the presence of atherosclerosis, as manifested by carotid artery stenosis in a Finnish study.[54] In addition, Regnström et al.[55] have shown a significant inverse correlation ($r = -0.45$, $p < 0.02$) between the lag phase of LDL oxidation and the severity of coronary atherosclerosis as measured by angiography. Finally, antioxidants such as probucol, α-tocopherol, butylated hydroxytoluene (BHT), or N,N'-diphenyl-phenylenediamine (DPPD) have been shown to decrease the degree of LDL oxidation and the extent of atherosclerosis.[56-58] Although the data are not conclusive, they do provide strong support of the concept of oxidatively modified LDL as an early step in atherogenesis.

III. EFFECTS OF ANTIOXIDANTS ON LDL OXIDIZABILITY

Although BHT and DPPD are effective in the prevention of atherosclerosis in animals, toxicity limits their utility in humans.[59,60] BHT in doses over 1% of the diet can cause hepatic and renal dysfunction, while DPPD is a mutagen. Probucol, a hypolipidemic drug, has been shown to reduce the progression of atherosclerosis in rabbits[56] and reduce the extent of lipoprotein oxidation in diabetic rats.[61] In human studies, probucol decreased the oxidative susceptibility of LDL to oxidation.[62,63] Probucol treatment, however, can result in a drop in high density lipoprotein (HDL) cholesterol.[64] A recent clinical trial failed to show a benefit for probucol therapy.[65] However, the significant reduction in HDL-cholesterol could have been a significant factor since HDL inhibits LDL oxidation. Present in HDL is at least three antioxidants: α-tocopherol, paraoxanase, and platelet activating factor acetyhydrolase.[66]

Given the toxicity of BHT and DPPD, and the potential side effects of probucol, supplementation with antioxidant nutrients may be a better approach in the prevention of atherosclerosis. Doses of vitamins E and C in excess of the recommended dietary allowances (RDA) are well tolerated.[67,68] High doses of β-carotene have been prescribed to patients with the photosensitivity disease erythropoietic protoporphyria without serious adverse reactions.[69]

Much of the antioxidant nutrient work with LDL oxidation has been done with α-tocopherol. α-Tocopherol is the most prevalent and biologically active form of vitamin E. It is the predominant lipophilic antioxidant in tissues and LDL,[70] at a ratio of 6 moles per mole of LDL.[71] α-Tocopherol traps peroxyl free radicals and thus acts as a chain-breaking antioxidant. α-Tocopherol inhibits LDL oxidation *in vitro*. Esterbauer et al.[71] have shown that increasing the LDL α-tocopherol content *in vitro* produced a prolongation of the lag phase of LDL oxidation. Data from some animal studies indicate that dietary α-tocopherol can slow the progression of atherosclerosis.[72-76] In one study, α-tocopherol supplementation resulted in a decreased progression of lesions as assessed by carotid Doppler studies in male monkeys over a 3-year period.[74] However, there was no significant change in lesion formation by histology. Two other studies showed that dietary α-tocopherol increased lipoprotein resistance against *in vitro* oxidation in rabbits.[75,76]

One can reasonably speculate that α-tocopherol can slow the progression of atherosclerosis by reducing LDL oxidative susceptibility. Numerous human studies have shown that α-tocopherol supplementation reduced LDL oxidizability in healthy subjects.[77-78] Dieber-Rotheneder et al.[77] showed that 3 weeks of α-tocopherol supplementation prolonged the lag phase of LDL oxidation, and that LDL α-tocopherol concentrations correlated significantly with the duration of the lag phase. This study had only two subjects in each supplemented group, which precluded statistical analysis. A 12-week placebo-controlled trial[78] focused on the time course of LDL oxidation. The investigators showed a significant prolongation of the lag phase, along with a reduction in the oxidation rate.[79] α-Tocopherol levels correlated significantly with both the lag phase and the oxidation rate. Another study, in which the subjects received α-tocopherol for only 7 days, showed similar results.[80] The minimum dose of α-tocopherol required to reduce LDL oxidizability in healthy men in an 8-week trial was found to be 400 IU/day.[81] Both plasma and LDL α-tocopherol concentrations were significantly correlated with lag phase and oxidation rate. Princen et al.[82] found that the lag phase of LDL oxidation was significantly increased by as little as 25 mg/day; however, it took at least 400 mg/day to show significant reductions in the rate of oxidation. However, this study was not a dose response study in design since the doses were sequentially increased without a washout phase. α-Tocopherol supplementation in normal volunteers decreased LDL oxidation and its cytotoxic effect on endothelial cells.[83] Finally in two studies, high dosages of α-tocopherol (1600 and 1200 IU/day, respectively) significantly reduced LDL oxidative susceptibility in persons with diabetes without having an effect on protein glycation.[84,85]

Three intervention studies indicate that α-tocopherol supplementation may have value in stemming the progression of atherosclerosis. DeMaio et al.[86] reported that α-tocopherol supplementation showed a trend towards reducing the incidence of coronary artery restenosis after angioplasty. Hodis et al.[87] showed that subjects who took >100 IU α-tocopherol/day had reduced arterial lesion progression over a 2-year period as assessed by coronary angiography. The Cambridge Heart Antioxidant Study[88] demonstrated that 400 or 800 IU α-tocopherol/day produced significant reductions in risk of nonfatal myocardial infarction and cardiovascular death in patients with established ischemic heart disease. The median duration of treatment was only 510 days. However, the Alpha-Tocopherol, Beta-Carotene study[89] found no reduction in the incidence of coronary heart disease in male smokers who received 50 mg/day for 5 to 8 years. It is possible that the dosage was insufficient to affect the incidence of cardiovascular disease in this group of long-term smokers. The study also did not control for cardiovascular risk factors, such as diet and weight, since the primary endpoint studied was lung cancer. Thus, the weight of the evidence shows that pharmacological dosages of α-tocopherol may have value in secondary prevention of coronary heart disease.

Ascorbate is a water-soluble, chain-breaking antioxidant that is able to react with superoxide anion, hydroxyl radical, and singlet oxygen.[90] It can also regenerate α-tocopherol from the chromanoxyl radical form.[91] Frei et al.[92] showed that ascorbate was the most powerful antioxidant in plasma when a water-soluble radical initiator was added. Several studies implicate low plasma and tissue ascorbate as a risk factor for atherosclerosis. A significant inverse correlation was found between plasma ascorbate and coronary disease mortality.[93] In addition, ascorbate concentrations are lower in the aortas of patients with atherosclerosis relative to unaffected controls.[94] Smokers, persons with diabetes, and patients with coronary artery disease have lower levels of plasma ascorbate than do controls.[95-97] Mezzetti et al.[98] reported that arterial tissue from smokers undergoing coronary artery bypass graft surgery had significantly lower concentrations of ascorbate than nonsmokers, and that tissue ascorbate was positively correlated with plasma ascorbate.

Ascorbate's solubility in water makes it unlikely that it would reside within the hydrophobic core of the LDL particle; however, Jialal et al.[99] found that physiological concentrations of ascorbate could prevent LDL oxidation by copper or by cultured human monocyte-derived macrophages. By preventing LDL oxidation, ascorbate prevented subsequent uptake and degradation by the macrophage scavenger receptor pathway. In a subsequent study,[62] ascorbate protected the endogenous antioxidants in LDL (β-carotene, α- and γ-tocopherol) against copper-catalyzed oxidation, whereas probucol showed no protective effect. It has been hypothesized that dehydroascorbate or another breakdown product of ascorbate may alter metal-binding sites on the LDL particle, thus increasing the resistance of LDL to oxidation.[100,101] Stait and Leake[102] reported that ascorbate may actually increase the oxidation of minimally modified LDL by macrophages cultured in iron-containing medium. The antioxidant effect of ascorbate is not solely due to its ability to chelate metal ions, as it can also inhibit oxidation by activated neutrophils and U-937 cells, systems that lack transition metal catalysts.[103,104]

Several human studies have established a positive role for ascorbate in the reduction of LDL oxidizability. Harats et al.[105] showed that ascorbate supplementation reduced the oxidation of plasma and LDL induced by an acute bout of smoking (5 to 7 cigarettes in a 90-minute period). Rifici and Khachadurian[106] reported that ascorbate also decreased lipoprotein (mixture of VLDL and LDL) oxidation in nonsmokers. The numbers of subjects tested in these two studies were small, and the time course of LDL oxidation was not studied. A study by Fuller et al.[107] examined the effect of ascorbate supplementation on LDL oxidative susceptibility in smokers in a placebo-controlled, double-blind study. Supplementation of subjects with 1 g ascorbate/day for 4 weeks resulted in a significant increase in the lag phase and reduction in the oxidation rate. The concentrations of LDL α-tocopherol and β-carotene were not affected by supplementation. Another study with smoking subjects[108] showed that a modest amount of ascorbate from orange juice (145 mg/day for 3 weeks) and 18 mg/day β-carotene from carrot juice decreased LDL oxidative susceptibility as measured by the maximum formation of TBARS. LDL oxidation kinetics (lag phase and oxidation rate) were not affected by this level of supplementation.

It thus appears that ascorbate supplementation does have beneficial effects against LDL oxidation.

β-Carotene is a member of the carotenoid family of plant-derived pigments. It is also carried in blood primarily by LDL.[109] Burton and Ingold[110] have demonstrated that β-carotene is an excellent singlet oxygen quencher and antioxidant, particularly at low oxygen pressures. There are little data on the relationship between β-carotene and atherosclerosis. One animal study showed that β-carotene reduced atherosclerosis in cholesterol-fed rabbits.[111] Increased β-carotene intake has been inversely linked to incidence of self-reported angina.[112] Smokers have reduced plasma β-carotene concentrations relative to nonsmokers.[96,113] A European multicenter case-control trial showed that individuals with low adipose tissue β-carotene had a greater risk of myocardial infarction than those with high adipose β-carotene.[114]

It may be that the beneficial effect of β-carotene could be partially due to its inhibitory effect on LDL oxidation. Esterbauer et al.[70] have shown that carotenoids are auxiliary antioxidant defenses in LDL particles after α-tocopherol. *In vitro* studies of the effect of β-carotene on LDL oxidation have shown mixed results. Two studies have shown reductions in LDL oxidation with β-carotene,[115,116] whereas Gaziano et al.[117] saw no protective effect. Cellular LDL oxidation was reduced *in vitro* by β-carotene, while copper-catalyzed oxidation was not, in another study.[118] The results of supplementation studies with β-carotene are similarly mixed. Princen et al.[80] reported a significant, albeit small (6 minutes), increase in the lag phase of LDL oxidation with 20 mg β-carotene/day; however, the rate of oxidation was unaffected. This laboratory has found similar results in a placebo-controlled trial of 30 mg/day β-carotene in nonsmoking males.[118] Other studies have seen no favorable effect of β-carotene supplementation on LDL oxidizability.[111,117,119-121] Two other studies[122,123] have reported that the effect of a supplement containing α-tocopherol, β-carotene, and ascorbate on LDL oxidation could be attributed almost entirely to the α-tocopherol. In one of the studies, combined supplementation was not superior to high dose α-tocopherol alone in inhibiting LDL oxidation.[123] Given the evidence to date, it appears that β-carotene has only a minor inhibitory effect on LDL oxidation. Future studies should examine the effects of other carotenoids such as lycopene, which has been shown to be a better antioxidant than β-carotene *in vitro*.[124]

α-Tocopherol has other effects on risk factors for coronary heart disease other than the prevention of LDL oxidation. Supplementation with α-tocopherol, alone or in combination with ascorbate and β-carotene, has been shown to reduce platelet adhesion.[125,126] In addition, physiologic concentrations of α-tocopherol inhibit smooth muscle cell proliferation and protein kinase C activity.[127,128] Also, enrichment of endothelium with α-tocopherol decreases subsequent adhesion of monocytes.[129] Finally, α-tocopherol may have a role in endothelial vasodilation. Low doses of α-tocopherol increased vasodilator function in arteries from cholesterol-fed rabbits.[130] In a similar study, cholesterol-fed rabbits given 0.2% dietary vitamin E showed partial reversal of impaired endothelium-dependent responses to acetylcholine in the preconstricted perfused ear.[76]

Other compounds other than antioxidant nutrients are being investigated for their effects on LDL oxidation. Ubiquinol-10 (or reduced coenzyme Q10) is a lipophilic compound that is consumed faster than α-tocopherol during LDL oxidation.[70,131] It is able to protect LDL from oxidation in the presence of aqueous or lipophilic free radical generators.[132,133] Mohr et al.[134] showed that supplementation of three individuals with 300 mg/day of ubiquinol 10 for 11 days produced a fourfold increase in plasma and LDL ubiquinol 10 and a reduced susceptibility of LDL to oxidation by an aqueous radical generator. Although these results are intriguing, the small number of subjects tested limits interpretation of the results. These studies require confirmation by other groups.

Flavonoids are a diverse group of polyphenols found in plants. It is believed that these compounds are nontoxic and may have clinical value in a number of conditions.[135] The phenols in red wine have been shown to inhibit LDL oxidation *in vitro*.[136] The results of human supplementation studies, however, are mixed. Fuhrman et al.[137] demonstrated that drinking 400 ml/day red wine, but not white wine, for 2 weeks produced significant reductions in LDL oxidizability, as evidenced by an increased lag phase and reduced content of TBARS, lipid peroxides, and conjugated dienes after oxidation. A crossover study showed that white wine, but not red wine, reduced TBARS concentrations after LDL oxidation.[138] When both red and white wines were drunk in combination, there was no additional reduction in TBARS concentrations. An additional study showed that neither red nor white wine affected LDL oxidizability.[139] The wines drunk by these subjects were reduced in alcohol content to 3.5%, which may have played a role in the disparity in the results seen. Specific flavonoids isolated from foods have also been tested for their ability to reduce LDL oxidation. Myricetin, quercetin, and rutin have been shown to reduce LDL oxidation, as evidenced by reductions in lipid hydroperoxide and TBARS production.[140,141] Flavonoids can also prevent the cytotoxicity of LDL to cell lines.[141,142] However, Rankin et al.[140] noted that myricetin and gossypetin altered LDL in a nonoxidative manner that increased its uptake by mouse macrophages. Upon further investigation, the LDL particles were found to be aggregated in the presence of flavonoids. Clearly, further studies on the bioavailabilities, interactions with other food components, and effects of these compounds *in vivo* are needed.

Finally, estrogens may play a role in LDL oxidation *in vivo*. Mazière et al.[143] showed that estrogens inhibited both copper- and cell-mediated oxidation of LDL *in vitro*. The order of efficacy was estradiol > estriol > estrone. Testosterone had no effect on LDL oxidizability. Also, transdermal estrogen therapy decreases the oxidative susceptibility of LDL to oxidation.[144] In another study, LDL from postmenopausal women with and without hormone-replacement therapy (combined estrogen and progestin) were examined for their oxidizability.[145] The women who received hormone-replacement therapy had reduced mean conjugated diene formation and oxidation rate relative to those who did not receive hormones. Estrogen replacement in postmenopausal women also lowers plasma LDL cholesterol and increases HDL cholesterol,[146,147] even if the estrogen is combined with progestin;[148] thus, hormone-replacement therapy in postmenopausal women has multiple favorable effects that could result in the prevention of coronary heart disease.

Oxidatively modified LDL has numerous characteristics that may contribute to the early stages of atherosclerosis. Antioxidant nutrients, particularly α-tocopherol, have shown promise in protecting LDL against oxidation *in vitro* and in some clinical studies to reduce cardiovascular mortality. Flavonoids and estrogens also may have favorable effects on LDL oxidizability, although data are limited. Much future work remains to be done to establish the utility of antioxidants in the primary and secondary prevention of atherosclerosis.

REFERENCES

1. Brown, M.S. and Goldstein, J.L. Lipoprotein metabolism in the macrophage. *Ann. Rev. Biochem.* 52, 223, 1983.
2. Parthasarathy, S. and Rankin, S.M. Role of oxidized low density lipoprotein in atherogenesis. *Prog. Lipid. Res.* 31, 127, 1992.
3. Steinbrecher, U.P., Parthasarathy, S., Leake, D.S., Witztum, J.L., and Steinberg, D. Modification of low density lipoprotein by endothelial cells involves lipid peroxidation and degradation of low density lipoprotein phospholipids. *Proc. Natl. Acad. Sci. U.S.A.* 81, 3883, 1984.
4. VanHinsbergh, V.W.M., Scheffer, M., Havekes, L., and Kempen, H.J.M. Role of endothelial cells and their products in the modification of low density lipoproteins. *Biochim. Biophys. Acta* 878, 49, 1986.
5. Navab, M., Imes, S.S., Hama, S.Y., Hough, G.P., Ross, L.A., Bork, R.W., Valente, A.J., Berliner, J.A., Drinkwater, D.C., Laks, H., and Fogelman, A.M. Monocyte transmigration induced by modification of low density lipoprotein in cocultures of human aortic wall cells is due to induction of monocyte chemotactic protein 1 synthesis and is abolished by high density lipoprotein. *J. Clin. Invest.* 88, 2039, 1991.
6. Esterbauer, H., Striegl, G., Puhl, H., and Rotheneder, M. Continuous monitoring of *in vitro* oxidation of human low density lipoprotein. *Free Radical Res. Commun.* 6, 67, 1989.
7. Esterbauer, H., Jürgens, G., Quehenberger, O., and Koller, E. Autoxidation of human low density lipoprotein: Loss of polyunsaturated fatty acids and vitamin E and generation of aldehydes. *J. Lipid. Res.* 28, 495, 1987.
8. El-Saadani, M., Esterbauer, H., El-Sayed, M., Goher, M., Nasser, A.Y., and Jürgens, G. A spectrophotometric assay for lipid peroxides in serum lipoproteins using a commercially available reagent. *J. Lipid. Res.* 30, 627, 1989.
9. Jiang, Z.-Y., Hunt, J.V., and Wolff, S.P. Ferrous ion oxidation in the presence of xylenol orange for detection of lipid hydroperoxide in low density lipoprotein. *Anal. Biochem.* 202, 384, 1992.
10. Nourooz-Zadeh, J., Tajaddini-Sarmadi, J., and Wolff, S.P. Measurement of plasma hydroperoxide concentrations by the ferrous oxidation-xylenol orange assay. *Anal. Biochem.* 220, 403, 1994.
11. Buege, J.A. and Aust, S.D. Microsomal lipid peroxidation. *Methods Enzymol.* 52, 302, 1978.
12. Maseki, M., Nishigaki, I., Hagihara, M., Tomoda, Y., and Yagi, K. Lipid peroxide levels and lipid content of serum lipoprotein fractions of pregnant subjects with and without pre-eclampsia. *Clin. Chim. Acta* 115, 155, 1981.
13. Jialal, I., Freeman, D.A., and Grundy, S.M. Varying susceptibility of different low density lipoproteins to oxidative modification. *Arterioscler. Thrombosis.* 11, 482, 1991.
14. Young, S.G. and Parthasarathy, S. Why are low-density lipoproteins atherogenic? *West. J. Med.* 160, 153, 1994.
15. Witztum, J.L. and Steinberg, D. Role of oxidized low density lipoprotein in atherogenesis. *J. Clin. Invest.* 88, 1785, 1991.
16. Jialal, I. and Devaraj, S. Low density lipoprotein oxidation, antioxidants and atherosclerosis:A clinical biochemistry perspective. *Clin. Chem.* 42, 498, 1996.
17. Fong, L.G., Parthasarathy, S., Witztum, J.L., and Steinberg, D. Nonenzymatic oxidative cleavage of peptide bonds in apoprotein B-100. *J. Lipid. Res.* 28, 1466, 1987.
18. Cominacini, L., Garbin, U., Davoli, A., Micciolo, R., Bosello, O., Gaviraghi, G., Scuro, L.A., and Pastorino, A.M. A simple test for predisposition to LDL oxidation based on the fluorescence development during copper-catalyzed oxidative modification. *J. Lipid. Res.* 32, 349, 1991.

19. Laemmli, U.K. Cleavage of structural proteins during the assembly of the head of bacteriophage T4. *Nature* 227, 680, 1970.
20. Gerrity, R.G. The role of the monocyte in atherogenesis. I. Transition of blood-borne monocytes into foam cells in fatty lesions. *Am. J. Pathol.* 103, 181, 1981.
21. Ryu, B.-H., Mao, F.W., Lou, P., Gutman, R.L., and Greenspan, P. Cholesteryl ester accumulation in macrophages treated with oxidized low density lipoprotein. *Biosci. Biotech. Biochem.* 59, 1619, 1995.
22. Morel, D.W., Hessler, J.R., and Chisolm, G.M. Low density lipoprotein cytotoxicity induced by free radical peroxidation of lipid. *J. Lipid. Res.* 24, 1070, 1983.
23. Clare, K., Hardwick, S.J., Carpenter, K.L.H., Weeratunge, N., and Mitchinson, M.J. Toxicity of oxysterol to human monocyte-macrophages. *Atherosclerosis* 118, 67, 1995.
24. Coffey, M.D., Cole, R.A., Colles, S.M., and Chisolm, G.M. *In vitro* cell injury by oxidized low density lipoprotein involves lipid hydroperoxide-induced formation of alkoxyl, lipid, and peroxyl radicals. *J. Clin. Invest.* 96, 1866, 1995.
25. DiCorleto, P.E. and Chisolm, G.M. Participation of the endothelium in the development of the atherosclerotic plaque. *Prog. Lipid. Res.* 25, 365, 1986.
26. Berliner, J.A., Territo, M.C., Sevanian, A., Ramin, S., Kim, J.A., Bamshad, B., Esterson, M., and Fogelman, A.M. Minimally modified low density lipoprotein stimulates monocyte-endothelial interactions. *J. Clin. Invest.* 85, 1260, 1990.
27. Parthasarathy, S., Fong, L.G., Quinn, M.T., and Steinberg, D. Oxidative modification of LDL: comparison between cell-mediated and copper-mediated modification. *Eur. Heart. J.* 11 (suppl. E), 83, 1990.
28. Cushing, S.D., Berliner, J.A., Valente, A.J., Territo, M.C., Navab, M., Parhami, F., Gerrity, R., Schwartz, C.J., and Fogelman, A.M. Minimally modified low density lipoprotein induces monocyte chemotactic protein 1 in human endothelial cells and smooth muscle cells. *Proc. Natl. Acad. Sci. U.S.A.* 87, 5134, 1990.
29. Cybulski, M.I. and Gimbrone, M.A., Jr. Endothelial expression of a mononuclear leukocyte adhesion molecule during atherogenesis. *Science* (Washington, D.C.) 251, 788, 1990.
30. Kume, N., Cybulski, M.I., and Gimbrone, M.A., Jr. Lysophosphatidylcholine, a component of atherogenic lipoproteins, induces mononuclear leukocyte adhesion molecules in cultured human and rabbit arterial endothelial cells. *J. Clin. Invest.* 90, 1138, 1992.
31. Liao, L., Aw, T.Y., Kvietys, P.R., and Granger, D.N. Oxidized LDL-induced microvascular dysfunction: dependence on oxidation procedure. *Arterioscler. Throm. Vasc. Biol.* 15, 2305, 1995.
32. Quinn, M.T., Parthasarathy, S., and Steinberg, D. Endothelial cell-derived chemotactic activity for mouse peritoneal macrophages and the effects of modified forms of low density lipoprotein. *Proc. Natl. Acad. Sci. U.S.A.* 82, 5949, 1985.
33. Quinn, M.T., Parthasarathy, S., Fong, L.G., and Steinberg, D. Oxidatively modified low density lipoproteins: a potential role in recruitment and retention of monocyte/macrophages during atherogenesis. *Proc. Natl. Acad. Sci. U.S.A.* 84, 2995, 1987.
34. Quinn, M.T., Parthasarathy, S., and Steinberg, D. Lysophosphatidylcholine: a chemotactic factor for human monocytes and its potential role in atherogenesis. *Proc. Natl. Acad. Sci. U.S.A.* 85, 2805, 1988.
35. Rajavashisth, T.B., Andalibi, A., Territo, M.C., Berliner, J.A., Navab, M., Fogelman, A.M., and Lusis, A.J. Induction of endothelial cell expression of granulocyte and macrophage colony-stimulating factors by modified low density lipoproteins. *Nature* (London), 344, 254, 1990.
36. Rajavashisth, T.B., Yamada, H., and Mishra, N.K. Transcription activation of the macrophage-colony stimulating factor gene by minimally modified LDL: involvement of nuclear factor-kB. *Arterioscler. Thromb. Vasc. Biol.* 15, 1591, 1995.
37. Thomas, C.E., Jackson, R.L., Ohlweiler, D.F., and Ku, G. Multiple lipid oxidation products in low density lipoproteins induce interleukin-1 beta release from human blood mononuclear cells. *J. Lipid. Res.* 35, 417, 1994.
38. Malden, L.T., Chait, A., Raines, E.W., and Ross, R. The influence of oxidatively modified low density lipoproteins on expression of platelet derived growth factor by human monocyte derived macrophages. *J. Biol. Chem.* 266, 13901, 1991.

39. Triau, J.E., Meydani, S.N., and Schaefer, E.J. Oxidized low density lipoprotein stimulates prostacyclin production by adult human vascular endothelial cells. *Arterioscler* 8, 810, 1988.

40. Ek, B. and Humble, L. Correlation between oxidation of low density lipoproteins and prostacyclin synthesis in cultured smooth muscle cells. *Biochem. Pharmacol.* 41, 695, 1991.

41. Thorin, E., Hamilton, C.A., Dominiczak, M.H., and Reid, J.L. Chronic exposure of cultured bovine endothelial cells to oxidized LDL abolishes prostacyclin release. *Arterioscler. Thromb.* 14, 453, 1994.

42. Yokode, M., Kita, T., Arai, H., Kawai, C., Narumiya, S., and Fujiwara, M. Cholesterol ester accumulation in macrophages with low density lipoprotein pretreated with cigarette smoke. *Proc. Natl. Acad. Sci. U.S.A.* 85, 2344, 1988.

43. Drake, T.A., Hanan, K., Fei, H., Levi, S., and Berliner, J.A. Minimally modified low density lipoprotein induces tissue factor expression in cultured human endothelial cells. *Am. J. Pathol.* 138, 601, 1991.

44. Latron, Y., Chautan, M., Anfosso, F., Alessi, M.C., Nalbone, G., Lafort, H., and Juhan-Vague, I. Stimulating effect of oxidized low density lipoproteins on plasminogen activator inhibitor-1 synthesis by endothelial cells. *Arterioscler. Thromb.* 11, 1821, 1991.

45. Ettelaie, C., Howell, R.M., and Bruckdorfer, D.R. The effect of lipid peroxidation and lipolysis on the ability of lipoproteins to influence thromboplastin activity. *Biochim. Biophys. Acta* 1257, 25, 1995.

46. Weidtmann, A., Scheithe, R., Hrboticky, N., Pietsch, A., Lorenz, R., and Siess, W. Mildly oxidized LDL induces platelet aggregation through activation of phospholipase A2. *Arterioscler. Thromb. Vasc. Biol.* 15, 1131, 1995.

47. Tanner, F.C., Noll, G., Boulanger, C.M., and Lüscher, T.F. Oxidized low density lipoproteins inhibit relaxations of porcine coronary arteries: role of scavenger receptor and endothelium-derived nitric oxide. *Circulation* 83, 2012, 1991.

48. He, Y., Kwan, W.C.P., and Steinbrecher, U.P. Effects of oxidized low density lipoprotein on endothelin secretion by cultured endothelial cells and macrophages. *Atheroscler.* 119, 107, 1996.

49. Jougasaki, M., Kugiyama, K., Saito, Y., Nakao, K., Imura, H., and Yasue, H. Suppression of endothelin-I secretion by lysophosphatidylcholine in oxidized low density lipoprotein in cultured vascular endothelial cells. *Circ. Res.* 71, 614, 1992.

50. Haberland, M.E., Fong, D., and Cheng, L. Malondialdehyde-altered protein occurs in atheroma of Watanabe heritable hyperlipidemic rabbits. *Science* 241, 215, 1988.

51. Ylä-Herttuala, S., Palinski, W., Rosenfeld, M.E., Parthasarathy, S., Carew, T.E., Butler, S., Witztum, J.L., and Steinberg, D. Evidence for the presence of oxidatively modified low density lipoprotein in atherosclerotic lesions of rabbit and man. *J. Clin. Invest.* 84, 1086, 1989.

52. Lecomte, E., Artur, Y., Chancerelle, Y., Herbeth, B., Galteau, M.-M., Jeandel, C., and Siest, G. Malondialdehyde adducts to, and fragmentation of, apolipoprotein B from human plasma. *Clin. Chim. Acta* 218, 39, 1993.

53. Palinski, W., Ylä-Herttuala, S., Rosenfeld, M.E., Butler, S.W., Socher, S.A., Parthasarathy, S., Curtiss, L.K., and Witztum, J.L. Antisera and monoclonal antibodies specific for epitopes generated during oxidative modification of low density lipoprotein. *Arteriosclerosis* 10, 325, 1990.

54. Salonen, J.T., Ylä-Herttuala, S., Yamamoto, R., Butler, S., Korpela, H., Salonen, R., Nyyssö, K., Palinski, W., and Witztum, J.L. Auto-antibody against oxidized LDL and progression of carotid atherosclerosis. *Lancet* 339, 883, 1992.

55. Regnström, J., Nilsson, J., Tornvall, P., Landou, C., and Hamsten, A. Susceptibility to low-density lipoprotein oxidation and coronary atherosclerosis in man. *Lancet* 339, 1183, 1992.

56. Carew, T.E., Schwenke, D.C., and Steinberg, D. Antiatherogenic effect of probucol unrelated to its hypocholesterolemic effect: Evidence that antioxidants *in vivo* can selectively inhibit low density lipoprotein degradation in macrophage-rich fatty streaks and slow the progression of atherosclerosis in the Watanabe heritable hyperlipidemic rabbit. *Proc. Natl. Acad. Sci. U.S.A.* 84, 7725, 1987.

57. Björkhem, I., Henriksson-Freyschuss, A., Breuer, O., Diczfalusy, U., Berglund, L., and Henriksson, P. The antioxidant butylated hydroxytoluene protects against atherosclerosis. *Arterioscler. Thromb.* 11, 15, 1991.

58. Sparrow, C.P., Doebber, T.W., Olszewski, J., Wu, M.S., Ventre, J., Stevens, K.A., and Chao, Y. Low density lipoprotein is protected from oxidation and the progression of atherosclerosis is slowed in cholesterol-fed rabbits by the antioxidant N,N'-diphenyl-phenylenediamine. *J. Clin. Invest.* 89, 1885, 1992.

59. Hirose, M., Shibata, M., Hagiwara, A., Imaida, K., and Ito, N. Chronic toxicity of butylated hydroxytoluene in Wistar rats. *Food Cosmet. Toxicol.* 19, 147, 1981.

60. Physicians' Desk Reference, 44th ed. Oradell, NJ: Medical Economics Company, 1990.

61. Chisolm, G.M. and Morel, D.W. Lipoprotein oxidation and cytotoxicity: Effect of probucol on streptozotocin-treated rats. *Am. J. Cardiol.* 62, 20B, 1988.

62. Parthasarathy, S., Young, S.G., Witztum, J.L., Pittman, R.C., and Steinberg, D. Probucol inhibits oxidative modification of low density lipoprotein. *J. Clin. Invest.* 77, 641, 1986.

63. Jialal, I. and Grundy, S.M. Preservation of the endogenous antioxidants in low density lipoprotein by ascorbate but not probucol during oxidative modification. *J. Clin. Invest.* 87, 597, 1991.

64. Reaven, P., Parthasarathy, S., Beltz, W., and Witztum, J. Effect of probucol dosage on plasma lipid and lipoprotein levels and on protection of low density lipoprotein against *in-vitro* oxidation in humans. *Arterioscler. Thromb.* 12, 318, 1992.

65. Walldius, G., Erikson, U., Olsson, A.G., et al. The effect of probucol on femoral atherosclerosis. *Am. J. Cardiol.* 74, 875, 1994.

66. Berliner, J.A. and Heinecke, J.W. The role of oxidized lipoproteins in atherogenesis. *Free Rad. Biol. Med.* 20, 707, 1996.

67. Walter, P. Supraphysiological dosages of vitamins and their implications in humans. *Experientia* 47, 178, 1991.

68. Kappus, H. and Diplock, A.T. Tolerance and safety of vitamin E: A toxicological position report. *Free Radical Biol. Med.* 13, 55, 1992.

69. Hathcock, J.N., Hattan, D.G., Jenkins, M.Y., McDonald, J.T., Sundaresan, P.R., and Wilkening, V.L. Evaluation of vitamin A toxicity. *Am. J. Clin. Nutr.* 52, 183, 1990.

70. Esterbauer, H., Dieber-Rotheneder, M., Waeg, G., Puhl, H., and Tatzber, F. Endogenous antioxidants and lipoprotein oxidation. *Biochem. Soc. Transact.* 18, 1059, 1990.

71. Esterbauer, H., Dieber-Rotheneder, M., Striegl, G., and Waeg, G. Role of vitamin E in preventing the oxidation of low-density lipoprotein. *Am. J. Clin. Nutr.* 53 (suppl.), 314S, 1991.

72. Westrope, K.L., Miller, R.A., and Wilson, R.B. Vitamin E in a rabbit model of endogenous hypercholesterolemia and atherosclerosis. *Nutr. Rep. Intl.* 25, 83, 1982.

73. Smith, T.L. and Kummerow, F.A. Effect of dietary vitamin E on plasma lipids and atherogenesis in restricted ovulator hens. *Atherosclerosis* 75, 105, 1989.

74. Verlangieri, A.J. and Bush, M.J. Effects of d-a-tocopherol on experimentally induced primate atherosclerosis. *J. Am. Coll. Nutr.* 11, 131, 1992.

75. Kleinveld, H.A., Demacker, P.N.M., and Stalenhoef, A.F.H. Comparative study on the effect of low-dose vitamin E and probucol on the susceptibility of LDL to oxidation and the progression of atherosclerosis in Watanabe heritable hyperlipidemic rabbits. *Arterioscler. Thromb.* 14, 1386, 1994.

76. Matz, J., Andersson, T.L.G., Ferns, G.A.A., and Ånggård, E.E. Dietary vitamin E increases the resistance to lipoprotein oxidation and attenuates endothelial dysfunction in the cholesterol-fed rabbit. *Atherosclerosis* 110, 241, 1994.

77. Dieber-Rotheneder, M., Puhl, H., Waeg, G., Striegl, G., and Esterbauer, H. Effect of oral supplementation with D-a-tocopherol on the vitamin E content of human low density lipoproteins and resistance to oxidation. *J. Lipid. Res.* 32, 1325, 1991.

78. Jialal, I. and Grundy, S.M. Effect of dietary supplementation with alpha-tocopherol on the oxidative modification of low density lipoprotein. *J. Lipid. Res.* 33, 899, 1992.

79. Jialal, I. and Scaccini, C. Antioxidants and atherosclerosis. *Curr. Opin. Lipidol.* 3, 324, 1992.

80. Princen, H.M.G., van Poppel, G., Vogelezang, C., Buytenhek, R., and Kok, F.J. Supplementation with vitamin E but not β-carotene *in vivo* protects low density lipoprotein from lipid peroxidation *in vitro*: Effect of cigarette smoking. *Arterioscler. Thromb.* 12, 554, 1992.

81. Jialal, I., Fuller, C.J., and Huet, B.A. The effect of α-tocopherol supplementation on LDL oxidation: A dose-response study. *Arterioscler. Thromb. Vasc. Dis.* 15, 190, 1995.

82. Princen, H.M.G., van Duyvenvoorde, W., Buytenhek, R., van der Laarse, A., van Poppel, G., Gevers Leuvens, J.A., and van Hinsbergh, W.W. Supplementation with low doses of vitamin E protects LDL from lipid peroxidation in men and women. *Arterioscler. Thromb. Vasc. Biol.* 15, 325, 1995.

83. Belcher, J.D., Balla, J., Jacobs, D.R., Gross, M., Jacob, H.S., and Vercellotti, G.M. Vitamin E LDL and endothelium: Brief oral vitamin supplementation prevents oxidized LDL-mediated vascular injury *in vivo. Arterioscler. Thromb.* 13, 1774, 1993.

84. Reaven, P.D., Herold, D.A., Branett, J., and Edelman, S. Effects of vitamin E on susceptibility of low-density lipoprotein and low-density lipoprotein subfractions to oxidation and on protein glycation in NIDDM. *Diabetes Care* 18, 807, 1995.

85. Fuller, C.J., Chandalia, M., Garg, A., Grundy, S.M., and Jialal, I. RRR-α-tocopheryl acetate supplementation at pharmacologic doses decreases low-density-lipoprotein oxidative susceptibility but not protein glycation in patients with diabetes mellitus. *Am. J. Clin. Nutr.* 63, 753, 1996.

86. DeMaio, S.J., King, S.B., III, Lembo, N.J., Roubin, G.S., Hearn, J.A., Bhagavan, H.N., and Sgoutas, D.S. Vitamin E supplementation, plasma lipids and incidence of restenosis after percutaneous transluminal coronary angioplasty (TCA). *J. Am. Coll. Nutr.* 11, 68, 1992.

87. Hodis, H.N., Mack, W.J., LaBree, L., et al. Serial coronary angiographic evidence that antioxidant vitamin intake reduces progression of coronary artery atherosclerosis. *J. Am. Med. Assoc.* 273, 1849, 1995.

88. Stephens, S.G., Parsons, A., Schofield, P.M., Kelly, F., Cheeseman, K., Mitchinson, M.J., and Brown, M.J. Randomized controlled trial of vitamin E in patients with coronary disease: Cambridge Heart Antioxidant Study (CHAOS). *Lancet* 347, 781, 1996.

89. The Alpha-Tocopherol, Beta-Carotene Cancer Prevention Study Group. The effect of vitamin E and beta-carotene on the incidence of lung cancer and other cancers in male smokers. *N. Engl. J. Med.* 330, 1029, 1994.

90. Machlin, L.J. and Bendich, A. Free radical tissue damage: Protective role of antioxidant nutrients. *FASEB J.* 1, 441, 1987.

91. Packer, J.E., Slater, T.F., and Willson, R.L. Direct observation of a free radical interaction between vitamin E and vitamin C. *Nature* (London) 278, 737, 1979.

92. Frei, B., England, L., and Ames, B.N. Ascorbate is an outstanding antioxidant in human blood plasma. *Proc. Natl. Acad. Sci. U.S.A.* 86, 6377, 1989.

93. Gey, K.F., Brubacher, G.B., and Stähelin, H.B. Plasma levels of antioxidant vitamins in relation to ischemic heart disease and cancer. *Am. J. Clin. Nutr.* 45, 1368, 1987.

94. Dubick, M., Hunter, G., Casey, S., and Keen, C. Aortic ascorbic acid, trace elements and superoxide dismutase activity in human aneurysmal and occlusive disease. *Proc. Soc. Exp. Biol. Med.* 184, 138, 1987.

95. Stankova, L., Riddle, M., Larned, J., Burry, K., Menashe, D., Hart, J., and Bigley, R. Plasma ascorbic concentrations and blood cell dehydroascorbate transport in patients with diabetes mellitus. *Metabolism* 33, 347, 1984.

96. Chow, C.K., Thacker, R.R., Changchit, C., Bridges, R.B., Rehm, S.R., Humble, J., and Turbok, J. Lower levels of vitamin C and carotenes in plasma of cigarette smokers. *J. Am. Coll. Nutr.* 3, 305, 1986.

97. Ramirez, J. and Flowers, N. Leukocyte ascorbic acid and its relationship to coronary artery disease in man. *Am. J. Clin. Nutr.* 33, 2079, 1980.

98. Mezzetti, A., Lapenna, D., Pierdomenico, S.D., Calafiore, A.M., Costantini, F., Riario-Sforza, G., Imbastero, T., Neri, M., and Cuccurullo, F. Vitamins E, C and lipid peroxidation in plasma and arterial tissue of smokers and non-smokers. *Atherosclerosis* 112, 91, 1995.

99. Jialal, I., Vega, G.L., and Grundy, S.M. Physiologic levels of ascorbate inhibit the oxidative modification of low density lipoprotein. *Atherosclerosis* 82, 185, 1990.

100. Retsky, K.L., Freeman, M.W., and Frei, B. Ascorbic acid oxidation product(s) protect human low density lipoprotein against atherogenic modification. *J. Biol. Chem.* 268, 1304, 1993.

101. Retsky, K.L. and Frei, B. Vitamin C prevents metal ion-dependent initiation and propagation of lipid peroxidation in human low-density lipoprotein. *Biochim. Biophys. Acta* 1257, 279, 1995.

102. Stait, S.E. and Leake, D.S. Ascorbic acid can either increase or decrease low density lipoprotein modification. *FEBS Lett.* 341, 263, 1994.

103. Frei, B. Ascorbic acid protects lipids in human plasma and low density lipoprotein against oxidative damage. *Am. J. Clin. Nutr.* 54, 1113S, 1991.
104. Jialal, I. and Grundy, S.M. Influence of antioxidant vitamins on LDL oxidation. *Ann. N.Y. Acad. Sci.* 669, 237, 1992.
105. Harats, D., Ben-Naim, M., Dabach, Y., Hollander, G., Havivi, E., Stein, O., and Stein, Y. Effect of vitamin C and E supplementation on susceptibility of plasma lipoproteins to peroxidation induced by acute smoking. *Atheroscler* 85, 47, 1990.
106. Rifici, V.A. and Khachadurian, A.K. Dietary supplementation with vitamins C and E inhibits *in vitro* oxidation of lipoproteins. *J. Am. Coll. Nutr.* 12, 631, 1993.
107. Fuller, C.J., Grundy, S.M., Norkus, E.P., and Jialal, I. Effect of ascorbate supplementation on low density lipoprotein oxidation in smokers. *Atherosclerosis* 119, 139, 1996.
108. Abbey, M., Noakes, M., and Nestel, P.J. Dietary supplementation with orange and carrot juice in cigarette smokers lowers oxidation products in copper-oxidized low density lipoprotein. *J. Am. Diet. Assoc.* 95, 671, 1995.
109. Krinsky, N.I., Cornwell, D.G., and Oncley, J.L. The transport of vitamin A and carotenoids in human plasma. *Arch. Biochem. Biophys.* 73, 233, 1958.
110. Burton, G.W. and Ingold, K.U. β-Carotene: an unusual type of lipid antioxidant. *Science* 224, 569, 1984.
111. Shaish, A., Daugherty, A., O'Sullivan, F., Schonfeld, G., and Heinecke, J.W. Beta-carotene inhibits atherosclerosis in hypercholesterolemic rabbits. *J. Clin. Invest.* 96, 2075, 1995.
112. Riemersma, R.A., Wood, D.A., MacIntyre, C.C.A., Elton, R.A., Gey, K.F., and Oliver, M.F. Risk of angina pectoris and plasma concentrations of vitamins A, C, and E and carotene. *Lancet* 337, 1, 1991.
113. Bolton-Smith, C., Casey, C.E., Gey, K.F., Smith, W.C.S., and Tunstall-Pedoe, H. Antioxidant vitamin intake assessed using a food-frequency questionnaire: Correlation with biochemical status in smokers and non-smokers. *Br. J. Nutr.* 65, 337, 1991.
114. Kardinaal, A.F.M., Kok, F.J., Ringstad, J., Gomez-Arcéna, J., Mazaev, V.P., Kohlmeier, L., Martin, B.C., Aro, A., Kark, J.D., Delgado-Rodriguez, M., Riemersma, R.A., van Veer, P., Hultunen, J.K., and Martin-Moreno, J.M. Antioxidants in adipose tissue and risk of myocardial infarction: the EURAMIC study. *Lancet* 342, 1379, 1993.
115. Jialal, I., Norkus, E.P., Cristol, L., and Grundy, S.M. β-Carotene inhibits the oxidative modification of low density lipoprotein. *Biochim. Biophys. Acta* 1086, 134, 1991.
116. Lavy, A., Ben-Amotz, A., and Aviram, M. Preferential inhibition of LDL oxidation by the all-trans isomer of β-carotene in comparison with 9-cis-β-carotene. *Eur. J. Clin. Chem. Clin. Biochem.* 31, 83, 1993.
117. Gaziano, J.M., Hatta, A., Flynn, M., Johnson, E.J., Krinsky, N.I., Ridker, P.M., Hennekens, C.H., and Frei, B. Supplementation with β-carotene *in vivo* and *in vitro* does not inhibit low density lipoprotein oxidation. *Atherosclerosis* 112, 187, 1995.
118. Jialal, I. and Fuller, C.J. Effect of vitamin E, vitamin C and beta-carotene on LDL oxidation and atherosclerosis. *Can. J. Cardiol.* 11, 97G, 1995.
119. Reaven, P.D., Ferguson, E., Navab, M., and Powell, F.L. Susceptibility of human LDL to oxidative modification: Effects of variations in β-carotene concentration and oxygen tension. *Arterioscl. Thromb.* 14, 1162, 1994.
120. Reaven, P.D., Khouw, A., Beltz, W.F., Parthasarathy, S., and Witztum, J.L. Effect of dietary antioxidant combinations in humans: Protection of LDL by vitamin E but not by β-carotene. *Arterioscler. Thromb.* 13, 590, 1993.
121. Nenseter, M.S., Volden, V., Berg, T., Drevon, C.A., Ose, L., and Tonstad, S. No effect of β-carotene supplementation on the susceptibility of low density lipoprotein to *in vitro* oxidation among hypercholesterolemic, postmenopausal women. *Scand. J. Clin. Lab. Invest.* 55, 477, 1995.
122. Abbey, M., Nestel, P.J., and Baghurst, P.A. Antioxidant vitamins and low-density-lipoprotein oxidation. *Am. J. Clin. Nutr.* 58, 525, 1993.
123. Jialal, I. and Grundy, S.M. Effect of combined supplementation with alpha-tocopherol, ascorbate and β-carotene on low-density lipoprotein oxidation. *Circulation* 88, 2780, 1993.
124. Dimascio, P., Kaiser, S., and Sies, H. Lycopene as the most efficient biological carotenoid singlet oxygen quencher. *Arch. Biochem. Biophys.* 274, 532, 1989.

125. Jandak, J., Steiner, M., and Richardson, P.D. a-Tocopherol, an effective inhibitor of platelet adhesion. *Blood* 73, 141, 1989.
126. Salonen, J.T., Salonen, R., Rinta-Kiikas, S., Kuukka, M., Korpela, H., Alfthan, G., Kantola, M., and Schalch, W. Effect of antioxidant supplementation on platelet function: A randomized pair-matched, placebo-controlled, double-blind trial in men with low antioxidant status. *Am. J. Clin. Nutr.* 53, 1222, 1991.
127. Boscoboinik, D., Szewczyk, A., Hensey, C., and Azzi, A. Inhibition of cell proliferation by a-tocopherol: Role of protein kinase C. *J. Biol. Chem.* 266, 6188, 1991.
128. Özer, N.K., Palozza, P., Boscoboinik, D., and Azzi, A. d-a-Tocopherol inhibits low density lipoprotein-induced proliferation and protein kinase C activity in vascular smooth muscle cells. *FEBS Lett.* 322, 307, 1993.
129. Faruqi, R., De La Motte, C., and DiCorleto, P.E. Alpha tocopherol inhibits agonist-induced monocytic cell adhesion to cultured human endothelial cells. *J. Clin. Invest.* 94, 592, 1994.
130. Keaney, J.F., Jr., Gaziano, J.M., Xu, A., Frei, B., Curran-Celentano, J., Shwaery, G.T., Loscalzo, J., and Vita, J.A. Low-dose a-tocopherol improves and high-dose a-tocopherol worsens endothelial vasodilator function in cholesterol-fed rabbits. *J. Clin. Invest.* 93, 844, 1994.
131. Kontush, A., Hübner, C., Finckh, B., Kohlschütter, A., and Beisiegel, U. Antioxidative activity of ubiquinol-10 at physiologic concentrations in human low density lipoprotein. *Biochim. Biophys. Acta* 1258, 177, 1995.
132. Stocker, R., Bowry, V.W., and Frei, B. Ubiquinol-10 protects human low density lipoprotein more efficiently against lipid peroxidation than does alpha-tocopherol. *Proc. Natl. Acad. Sci. U.S.A.* 88, 1646, 1991.
133. Suarna, C., Hood, R.L., Dean, R.T., and Stocker, R. Comparative antioxidant activity of tocotrienols and other natural lipid-soluble antioxidants in a homogeneous system, and in rat and human lipoproteins. *Biochim. Biophys. Acta* 1166, 163, 1993.
134. Mohr, D., Bowry, V.W., and Stocker, R. Dietary supplementation with coenzyme Q10 results in increased levels of circulating lipoproteins and increased resistance of human low-density lipoprotein to the initiation of lipid peroxidation. *Biochim. Biophys. Acta* 1126, 247, 1992.
135. Cook, N.C. and Samman, S. Flavonoids-Chemistry, metabolism, cardioprotective effects, and dietary sources. *J. Nutr. Biochem.* 7, 66, 1996.
136. Frankel, E.N., Kanner, J., German, J.B., Parks, E., and Kinsella, J.E. Inhibition of oxidation of human low-density lipoprotein by phenolic substances in red wine. *Lancet* 341, 454, 1993.
137. Fuhrman, B., Lavy, A., and Aviram, M. Consumption of red wine with meals reduces the susceptibility of human plasma and low-density lipoprotein to lipid peroxidation. *Am. J. Clin. Nutr.* 61, 549, 1995.
138. Struck, M., Watkins, T., Tomeo, A., Halley, J., and Bierenbaum, M. Effect of red and white wine on serum lipids, platelet aggregation, oxidation products and antioxidants: A preliminary report. *Nutr. Res.* 14, 1811, 1994.
139. De Rijke, Y.B., Demacker, P.N.M., Assen, N.A., Sloots, L.M., Katan, M.B., and Stalenhoef, A.F.H. Red wine consumption does not affect oxidizability of low-density lipoproteins in volunteers. *Am. J. Clin. Nutr.* 63, 329, 1996.
140. Rankin, S.M., deWhalley, C.V., Hoult, J.R.S., Jessup, W., Wilkins, G.M., Collard, J., and Leake, D.S. The modification of low density lipoprotein by the flavonoids myricetin and gossypetin. *Biochem. Pharmacol.* 45, 67, 1993.
141. Nègre-Salvayre, A. and Salvayre, R. Quercetin prevents the cytotoxicity of oxidized LDL on lymphoid cell lines. *Free Radical Biol. Med.* 12, 101, 1992.
142. Ramanathan, R., Das, N.P., and Tan, C.H. Effects of a-linolenic acid, flavonoids, and vitamins on cytotoxicity and lipid peroxidation. *Free Radical Biol. Med.* 16, 43, 1994.
143. Mazière, C., Auclair, M., Ronveaux, M.-F., Salmon, S., Santus, R., and Mazière, J.-C. Estrogens inhibit copper and cell-mediated modification of low density lipoprotein. *Atherosclerosis* 89, 175, 1991.
144. Sacks, M.N., Rader, D.J., and Cannon, R.O. Estrogen and inhibition of oxidation of LDL in postmenopausal women. *Lancet* 343, 269, 1994.

145. Wander, R.C., Du, S.-H., Ketchum, S.O., and Rowe, K.E. Effects of interaction of RRR-a-tocopheryl acetate and fish oil on low-density-lipoprotein oxidation in postmenopausal women with and without hormone-replacement therapy. *Am. J. Clin. Nutr.* 63, 184, 1996.

146. Applebaum-Bowden, D., McLean, P., Steinmetz, A., Fontana, D., Matthys, C., Warnick, G.R., Cheung, M., Albers, J.J., and Hazzard, W.R. Lipoprotein, apolipoprotein, and lipolytic enzyme changes following estrogen administration in postmenopausal women. *J. Lipid. Res.* 30, 1895, 1989.

147. Granfone, A., Campos, H., McNamara, J.R., Schaefer, M.M., Lamon-Fava, S., Ordovas, J.M., and Schaefer, E.J. Effects of estrogen replacement on plasma lipoproteins and apolipoproteins in postmenopausal, dyslipidemic women. *Metabolism* 41, 1193, 1992.

148. Denke, M.A. Effects of continuous combined hormone-replacement therapy on lipid levels in hypercholesterolemic postmenopausal women. *Am. J. Med.* 99, 29, 1995.

Chapter 10

ANTIOXIDANTS AND CORONARY ARTERY DISEASE PREVENTION

Richard M. Hoffman and Harinder S. Garewal

Contents

I. Introduction 131

II. Animal Studies 132

III. Ecologic Studies 132

IV. Cross-Sectional Studies 133

V. Nested Case-Control Studies 134

VI. Prospective Cohort Studies 135

VII. Intervention Trials 139

VIII. Discussion 143

References 144

I. INTRODUCTION

Cardiovascular disease, despite aggressive treatment of traditional risk factors, remains the leading cause of death in most developed countries. Recently, considerable attention has focused on the atherogenic risk of oxygen free radicals. These chemical entities, common byproducts of many oxidative biochemical reactions in the body, cause cellular damage. While the mechanisms for atherogenesis are not completely understood, studies suggest that free-radical modification of low-density lipoprotein (LDL) is a critical factor, creating an oxidized LDL that is more atherogenic than native LDL. Consequently, investigators have begun examining the role of free-radical scavengers, particularly dietary nutrients, in coronary artery disease prevention. Antioxidants, such as vitamin E, carotenoids, and vitamin C, are able to neutralize oxygen free radicals, inhibit LDL oxidation, and, therefore, potentially reduce the risk of coronary artery disease. This chapter will review evidence on antioxidants from animal studies, ecologic data, cross-sectional studies, case-control studies, prospective cohort studies, and intervention trials.

II. ANIMAL STUDIES

The role of antioxidants in cardiovascular disease prevention has been extensively tested in animal models. Studies using either probucol, an antioxidant lipid-lowering agent, or vitamin E have generally reported positive effects. Carew et al.[1] randomly assigned 6-week-old LDL-receptor deficient Watanabe heritable hyperlipidemic (WHHL) rabbits to treatment with either probucol or lovastatin. Lovastatin was selected to control for the lipid-lowering effect of probucol. The probucol-treated rabbits had significantly less aortic atherosclerosis, almost a 50% reduction in lesion surface area, although changes in plasma cholesterol concentrations were similar in both treatment groups. Kita et al.[2] further showed that LDL isolated from the plasma of probucol treated WHHL rabbits was highly resistant to oxidative modification. Probucol prevented the progression of atherosclerosis, but the plasma cholesterol levels were 20% higher in the untreated control group. Daugherty et al.[3] found that mature WHHL rabbits treated with probucol had less cholesterol deposited into aortic intimal lesions, although there was no regression of existing lesions.

Vitamin E supplements prevented hypercholesterolemia and decreased the incidence and severity of aortic and coronary atherosclerosis in rabbits receiving an atherogenic diet.[4] Modified WHHL rabbits receiving vitamin E supplementation for 12 weeks consistently had lower cholesterol levels than controls and a 32% reduction in aortic lesions on postmortem examination. Vitamin E also inhibited the susceptibility of LDL to oxidative modification.[5] Wójcicki et al.[6] reported that selenium and vitamin E supplements significantly reduced atherosclerotic plaque formation and suppressed the elevation of lipoprotein levels in male mongrel rabbits fed high-fat atherogenic diets. The surface area of intimal aortic plaque was 76% in control animals, but only 28% in animals receiving supplements.

Studies in other animals have also supported the protective role of vitamin E. Verlangieri and Bush[7] used carotid duplex ultrasound imaging to investigate experimentally induced atherosclerosis in primates. D-α-tocopherol supplements lessened the rate and reduced the severity of atherogenesis in primates receiving atherogenic diets. Furthermore, when primates with established atherosclerosis were treated with vitamin E supplements, the extent of existing stenoses significantly decreased from 33 to 8%. Cholesterol-fed guinea pigs supplemented with vitamin E had significantly fewer aortic intimal lesions than controls.[8] In restricted anovulatory chickens, which develop extreme hyperlipidemia and accelerated atherosclerosis, dietary vitamin E significantly reduced lipid peroxidation and aortic intimal thickening, although serum lipid levels were unaffected.[9]

III. ECOLOGIC STUDIES

Ecologic data suggest that dietary antioxidants protect against atherosclerosis. In England and Scotland, the consumption of fresh fruits and green vegetables was inversely related to mortality from cerebrovascular disease, and calculated vitamin C intake was inversely related to standardized mortality rates for coronary heart disease.[10,11] A risk factor survey in Scotland, which has an extremely high coronary artery disease mortality rate, found that a substantial proportion of men and women did not eat fresh fruit or green vegetables.[12] Randomly selected Australian Seventh Day Adventist vegetarians, whose diet is high in vitamins C and E, were found to have significantly lower blood pressures and serum cholesterol levels than a cohort of Mormon omnivores matched for consumption of caffeine, alcohol, and tobacco.[13] Department of Agriculture and vital statistics data showed that declining cardiovascular mortality rates in the U.S. from 1964 to 1978 were correlated with increased consumption of fruits and vegetables, particularly those rich in vitamin C.[14] Ginter[15] reported a similar association between coronary mortality and ascorbic acid production from 1958 to 1978 and hypothesized that the higher intake of synthetic ascorbic acid may have led to the decline in coronary mortality. Neither of these observational studies, however, adjusted for any concomitant changes in risk factors such as smoking, exercise, blood pressure, or cholesterol level.

Gey et al.[16,17] randomly sampled healthy men, aged 40 to 49 years, across 16 European populations. Each study population was representative for regions with different incidences of ischemic heart disease mortality, ranging from 66 deaths/100,000 men in Catalonia, Spain to 481 deaths/100,000 men in North Karelia, Finland. The lipid-standardized median plasma levels of vitamin E showed a strong inverse univariate correlation ($r^2 = 0.62$, $p = 0.0003$) with age-specific regional coronary disease mortality. This apparent protective effect persisted after adjusting vitamin E levels for total cholesterol, blood pressure, and smoking history. A weak inverse correlation was found for vitamin C levels ($r^2 = 0.11$, $p = 0.22$), but β-carotene and selenium levels were not associated with mortality. Bellizzi et al.[18] studied 24 developed countries, 19 European and 5 non-European, and found a strong inverse relationship between estimated α-tocopherol consumption and the rate of premature coronary heart disease mortality. A protective effect for α-tocopherol was apparent on both cross-sectional and longitudinal analyses; dietary vitamin C and β-carotene consumption had weaker correlations. Despite the consistent findings across studies, ecologic data is susceptible to important biases because the specific individuals with low antioxidant consumption or concentrations may not actually be developing cardiovascular disease (ecologic fallacy). Attributing population differences in cardiovascular disease to antioxidants also obscures the potentially confounding role of numerous other coronary risk factors. Consequently, no definitive inferences can be drawn from ecologic data about the causal relationship between antioxidants and coronary artery disease mortality.

IV. CROSS-SECTIONAL STUDIES

Cross-sectional studies, which gather concurrent data on antioxidant levels and cardiovascular disease, are not subject to the ecologic fallacy. Findings in cross-sectional studies, however, have not consistently demonstrated benefit for antioxidant consumption. Riemersma et al.[19] studied a cohort of Scottish men and found an inverse relationship between plasma concentrations of vitamins E and C and the presence of angina pectoris identified by a self-administered chest pain questionnaire.

After adjusting for age, smoking, blood pressure, lipids, and relative weight, only vitamin E remained independently associated with angina. The adjusted odds ratio between the lowest and highest quintiles of vitamin E concentration for the presence of angina was 2.68 (95% Confidence Interval [CI]: 1.07, 6.70). Ramirez et al.[20] reported that patients with angiographically proven atherosclerosis had significantly lower leukocyte ascorbic acid levels than controls. The finding was consistent across gender and smoking status.

Two other cross-sectional studies, however, found little association between antioxidant levels and coronary artery disease. Salonen et al.[21] studied 1132 middle-aged Finnish men and found that neither vitamin C nor cholesterol-adjusted vitamin E correlated with prevalent ischemic heart disease as defined by angina pectoris, previous myocardial infarction, or an ischemic response to exercise testing. Men who developed ischemic changes on exercise testing did have lower serum selenium concentrations. After adjusting for smoking, hypertension, and cholesterol levels, the association remained significant only for men with angina or previously diagnosed ischemic heart disease.

The second cross-sectional study, the European community multicenter study on antioxidants, myocardial infarction, and breast cancer (EURAMIC),[22] assayed adipose tissue antioxidant concentrations in 683 middle-aged men with a first myocardial infarction and 727 age- and geographically-matched controls. The adjusted relative risk (RR) of myocardial infarction in the lowest quintile of β-carotene concentration as compared with the highest was 1.78 (95% CI: 1.17, 2.71). When risk was stratified by smoking status, however, there was a significant increased risk only for current smokers. Vitamin E levels were not associated with the risk of myocardial infarction.[22]

Interpreting results from cross-sectional designs is difficult. Investigators cannot control for dietary changes resulting from earlier diagnoses of coronary artery disease or identification of cardiovascular risk factors. Furthermore, a single serum antioxidant level may correlate poorly with long-term levels and nutrient intake. The EURAMIC study did measure adipose levels, a biomarker of long-term antioxidant exposure, and attempted to exclude subjects with major dietary changes in the previous year. Dietary habits, however, may have already been substantially altered, because cases were much more likely to have histories of angina, hypertension, diabetes, and smoking.[22]

V. NESTED CASE-CONTROL STUDIES

Evidence from nested-case control studies is more reliable than data from cross-sectional studies because the temporal sequence of exposure and disease is clearly established. The nested-case control design also minimizes selection bias in choosing controls, because all subjects are drawn from the same cohort. Nested-case control studies have found inconsistent associations between antioxidant levels and cardiovascular disease. In a population-based study from Maryland, Street et al.[23] showed that decreased serum levels of β-carotene significantly increased the risk for incident myocardial infarction. Serum samples were stored for 16 years at –70°C. The odds ratio comparing the lowest quintile of β-carotene serum levels to the highest was

2.23 (95% CI: 1.11, 4.48), although only smokers were at increased risk. At low serum levels of α-tocopherol, there was a nonsignificant trend towards greater risk for myocardial infarction, but only in those individuals with higher total cholesterol concentrations.

Three other nested case-control studies showed no evidence for a significant inverse relationship between antioxidant levels and coronary heart disease. Salonen et al.[24] studied 12,155 men and women from eastern Finland, an area with exceptionally high coronary disease mortality, and found no consistent association between serum selenium, retinol, or tocopherol concentrations and the risk of death from coronary artery disease. The 92 cases, though, were more likely to have symptomatic coronary disease at baseline and may have already altered their dietary habits. Furthermore, the serum antioxidant concentrations were measured after being stored for 7 years at only −20°C, which can lead to oxidative degradation and erroneous measurements of baseline antioxidant levels.[25] A 9-year follow-up study from the Netherlands found no significant association between serum selenium, vitamin A, and vitamin E levels and cardiovascular mortality, even after adjusting for prevalent myocardial infarctions and stroke.[26] Antioxidant levels, however, were also assayed after prolonged serum storage at −20°C, and cases were more likely to have a baseline history of hypertension and diabetes. In Augsburg, Germany, Hense et al.[27] found no evidence that vitamin E levels protected against myocardial infarction. The adjusted relative risk for myocardial infarction in the lowest tertile of vitamin E (≤33.5 μmol/L in women, ≤27.9 μmol/L in men) compared to the upper two tertiles was 0.72, but the confidence interval included 1.0 (0.33, 1.57). Serum samples were stored at −70°C, minimizing oxidative degradation, but the study had limited power, because only 46 myocardial infarctions were diagnosed in the cohort of 4022 men and women. Furthermore, median serum concentrations of vitamin E were quite high: even the lowest tertile exceeded cardioprotective thresholds identified in epidemiologic studies.[28]

VI. PROSPECTIVE COHORT STUDIES

A number of prospective cohort studies have looked at the association between baseline dietary antioxidant status (estimating vitamin intake or measuring serum levels) and subsequent cardiovascular events. A secondary analysis of the Lipid Research Clinics Coronary Primary Prevention Trial and Follow-up Study[29] examined the relationship between baseline total serum carotenoid levels and the risk of subsequent nonfatal myocardial infarctions and coronary heart disease deaths. Subjects were the 1899 men, aged 40 to 59 years, with type IIA hyperlipidemia randomized to placebo. After 12 years of follow-up, men in the highest quartile of serum carotenoids (>3.16 mmol/L) compared with the lowest quartile (<2.33 mmol/L) had an adjusted relative risk of only 0.64 (95% CI: 0.44, 0.92) for coronary heart disease events. An even stronger protective effect was observed for never smokers in the highest quartile, RR = 0.28 (95% CI: 0.11, 0.73).

Dietary β-carotene was associated with decreased cardiovascular mortality in a prospective cohort study of 1299 elderly Massachusetts residents.[30] A food frequency questionnaire was used to derive a β-carotene vegetable intake score. During

4.75 years of follow-up, there were 161 cardiovascular deaths, including 48 due to myocardial infarction. The age- and sex-adjusted relative risk for cardiovascular death among those in the highest quartile of β-carotene vegetable scores was 0.54 (95% CI: 0.34, 0.87). For fatal myocardial infarction, the relative risk was 0.25 (95% CI: 0.09, 0.67).

Three studies correlated estimated dietary vitamin C intake with subsequent cardiovascular mortality. Data from the First National Health and Nutrition Examination Survey (NHANES I) Epidemiologic Follow-up Study[31] showed that an index of vitamin C dietary intake and vitamin supplements was inversely correlated with cardiovascular mortality. The cohort of 11,348 noninstitutionalized U.S. adults, aged 25 to 74 years, underwent extensive dietary and nutrition evaluation from 1971 to 1974 and were followed for a median of 10 years. Men with the highest vitamin C intake had a standardized mortality ratio (SMR) of 0.58 (95% CI: 0.41, 0.78) for all cardiovascular disease, while women with the highest vitamin C intake had an SMR of 0.75 (95% CI: 0.55, 0.99). This study, however, oversampled older patients, based the SMR on the white population, and did not adjust cardiovascular mortality for risk factors or other antioxidant vitamin intake. Lapidus et al.,[32] however, found no correlation between dietary intake of vitamin C and incidence of cardiovascular disease and death in a 12-year study of 1462 Swedish women. Dietary habits were estimated with 24-hour recall interviews, and no data were obtained on vitamin E or β-carotene intake. Additionally, the study lacked statistical power because only 41 cardiovascular events occurred during the study.

Gale et al.[33] studied a randomly selected British cohort of 730 elderly men and women and showed, after a 20-year follow-up, that dietary vitamin C protected against stroke mortality. Subjects in the highest tertile of vitamin C intake had an adjusted relative risk of 0.50 (95% CI: 0.3, 0.8) compared with those in the lowest tertile. There was no association between vitamin C status and coronary artery disease mortality. The nutritional survey, consisting of a 1-week food diary, provided no information on consumption of other antioxidant nutrients.

Among studies looking at multiple antioxidants, only the Basel study[17,28,34,35] measured baseline serum levels (vitamins A, C, E, and carotenes). From 1971 to 1973, investigators enrolled 2974 healthy male Swiss pharmaceutical employees and followed them for 12 years. Very few cardiovascular deaths occurred: only 132 from ischemic heart disease and 31 from cerebrovascular disease. Carotenes were protective: the relative risk for ischemic heart disease mortality, adjusted for cardiovascular risk factors and other antioxidant levels, was significantly increased among subjects in the lowest quartile (<0.23 μmol/L) of carotene concentration (RR = 1.53, 95% CI: 1.07, 2.20). Subjects generally had very high baseline levels of vitamins E and A — above the cardioprotective level found in epidemiologic studies.[16,19] Consequently, even the lowest quartiles were not associated with increased cardiovascular disease mortality.

A longitudinal population study in Finland[36] followed 2748 men and 2385 women, aged 30 to 69 years, all self-reported to be free of heart disease. Baseline food consumption, ascertained by a dietary history interview, was correlated with subsequent coronary mortality. During a mean of 14 years follow-up, there were 244 coronary deaths. A significant inverse association between dietary intake of antioxidant vitamins E and C and coronary mortality was found, but only in women. The relative risk for coronary mortality between the highest and lowest tertile of vitamin E intake, adjusted for age, smoking, hypertension, and cholesterol, was 0.35 (95% CI: 0.14, 0.88); the relative risk for vitamin C was 0.49 (95% CI: 0.24, 0.98). The study was limited because dietary and past medical history data were self-reported and changes in diet during the study were not assessed. Only 3% of subjects used antioxidant supplements.

The Zutphen cohort studies[37,38] in the Netherlands showed significant inverse correlations between consumption of flavonoids (antioxidants occurring in fruits, vegetables, wine, and tea), estimated from dietary histories, and cardiovascular disease in elderly men. The relative risk reduction for the highest level of flavonoid intake was 68% (95% CI: 29%, 85%) in coronary heart disease mortality and 73% (95% CI: 30%, 89%) in stroke incidence. High levels of β-carotene were associated with a reduced risk for stroke, but the finding was not significant.

The Western Electric Study[39] followed a cohort of 1556 middle-aged men for 24 years, correlating baseline measures of cardiovascular risk and dietary antioxidant intake with subsequent mortality. Nutritional data, obtained from structured interviews analyzed with food composition tables, estimated only vitamin C and β-carotene intake. For nonsmoking men, vitamin C was inversely related to the risk of coronary artery disease mortality; the relative risk for men in the highest tertile compared to the lowest was 0.58. No significant associations were found between β-carotene and coronary artery disease mortality.

The Cholesterol Lowering Atherosclerosis Study (CLAS)[40] followed the angiographic progression of coronary atherosclerosis in 156 men, aged 40 to 59 years, with a history of previous coronary artery bypass grafting. In the primary analysis, men randomized to treatment with colestipol-niacin had reduced coronary artery disease progression compared with placebo. A subsequent observational analysis measured the effect of vitamin E consumption on atherosclerosis. Compared to subjects with lesser vitamin E intake, men consuming ≥100 IU/day had a substantially reduced progression of coronary artery lesions. Stratified analyses, though, showed that vitamin E was beneficial only for subjects in the colestipol-niacin treatment group. There was no benefit for the placebo group or any patients classified with severe stenosis (≥50%) at baseline. No association was found between disease progression and either supplementary vitamin C or dietary intake of antioxidants. The study findings are limited because subjects were middle-aged men who survived coronary bypass surgery and antioxidant nutrient intake, based on self-report, was not validated.

Kushi et al.[41] found that dietary vitamin E was protective in a cohort of 34,486 postmenopausal women. The adjusted risk of coronary artery mortality for the highest quintile of dietary vitamin E compared to the lowest was 0.38 (95% CI: 0.18, 0.80). No benefit was seen for the highest quintile of combined dietary and supplemental vitamin E, and the intake of vitamins A and C was not related to coronary artery mortality. Women in the highest quintile of dietary vitamin E intake, however, had a more favorable cardiovascular risk profile, including more frequent use of estrogen-replacement therapy.

Two well-designed, large, prospective observational studies have suggested that antioxidant *supplementation* significantly reduced the risk of incident coronary heart disease. Beginning in 1980, The Nurses' Health Study began mailing questionnaires to a cohort of 87,245 American female nurses, aged 34 to 59 years old, who were free from known cancer or cardiovascular disease.[42] Dietary nutrients were ascertained using a semi-quantitative food frequency questionnaire. Data were also collected biennially throughout the study on use of multivitamins and specific supplements, including vitamins A, C, and E and β-carotene.

During 8 years of follow-up, 552 major coronary events were documented: 437 nonfatal myocardial infarctions and 115 coronary deaths. The major finding of the study was a significantly reduced risk of coronary disease in women using vitamin E supplements. After adjustment for age and smoking, the relative risk among the highest quintile of vitamin E supplement users, compared with the lowest quintile, was 0.66 (95% CI: 0.50, 0.87). The significant protective effect persisted after further adjusting for obesity, exercise level, dietary vitamin intake, hypertension, hypercholesterolemia, diabetes, menopausal status, alcohol intake, and use of aspirin, postmenopausal estrogen replacement, multivitamins, β-carotene, and vitamin C. Risk was not decreased if vitamin E supplements were taken for less than 2 years or at doses <100 IU/day, and no protective effect was observed for dietary sources of vitamin E alone. A trend towards decreasing risk of coronary heart disease was observed for higher levels of β-carotene consumption, adjusted RR = 0.78 (95% CI: 0.59, 1.03.[43] Among women in the highest quintile of antioxidant vitamin scores (a quantitative measure based on a pooled intake of β-carotene, vitamins E and C), the adjusted relative risk of coronary heart disease compared with those in the lowest quintile was 0.54 (95% CI: 0.40, 0.73).[44]

Vitamin E supplementation also significantly reduced the risk of coronary heart disease in the prospective Health Professionals Follow-up Study. In 1988, Rimm et al.[45] began following 39,910 male health professionals, aged 40 to 75 years, with no history of previous cardiovascular disease. During 139,883 person-years of follow-up, 201 nonfatal myocardial infarctions, 106 fatal myocardial infarctions, and 360 bypass surgeries or angioplasties were documented. Self-reported food frequency questionnaires were used to assess dietary and supplemental nutrient intake. Relative risks for study endpoints were adjusted for age, coronary risk factors, and intake of vitamin C and β-carotene. The adjusted relative risk of coronary heart disease in men taking at least 100 IU of vitamin E supplements for at least 2 years, compared with men not taking vitamin E supplements, was 0.63 (95% CI: 0.47, 0.84). Vitamin C was not associated with any protective effect from coronary disease, but higher quintiles of β-carotene intake were protective for current and former smokers.

Data from Stampfer[42] and Rimm[45] provided strong support for the hypothesis that antioxidant supplementation reduced the risk of coronary heart disease. The inverse association between antioxidant consumption and coronary events was strong. The prospective design established a temporal relationship between exposure and outcome and minimized recall bias. A dose response was observed, with benefit associated only with supplement levels ≥100 IU/day and supplement duration of at least 2 years. Finally, a protective role for antioxidants is biologically plausible, based on research linking oxidation of LDL and atherosclerosis.

Observational studies, however suggestive the findings, are still susceptible to important biases. Self-selection bias can occur when assembling a volunteer cohort, especially one comprised of health professionals. Additionally, identifying and measuring the appropriate exposure can be difficult. Antioxidant intake could be just a marker for another, more protective, dietary practice. Assessing long-term antioxidant status from dietary interviews is extremely difficult, leading to potential exposure misclassification. Observational studies also can never completely adjust for confounding factors; for example, neither of the vitamin E supplement studies controlled for lipoprotein levels. Serum levels were not measured, and the only available data were self-reported histories of "high cholesterol."[42,45] Results from observational studies, therefore, cannot provide definitive evidence of causality. Only data from randomized controlled trials can prove that antioxidants reduce the risk of coronary artery disease events.

VII. INTERVENTION TRIALS

Results from intervention trials, including randomized controlled trials, have not conclusively proven a benefit for antioxidant supplements. Three small randomized controlled trials of subjects with intermittent claudication showed that exercise capacity significantly improved with vitamin E therapy.[46-48] A randomized Canadian trial[49] found that vitamin E was no more effective than placebo in relieving angina. Outcome measures, however, were totally subjective, and the 9-week study enrolled only 40 subjects. A double-blind crossover trial of vitamin E[50] found that daily doses of 1600 mg did not subjectively improve anginal symptoms nor improve exercise performance or left ventricular function. The study, though, enrolled just 52 subjects, and the duration of vitamin E therapy was only 6 months.

Other studies, however, using larger sample sizes, longer treatment durations, and/or more rigorous endpoints, have also had inconsistent findings. (Table 10.1) Evidence that β-carotene protects against coronary events came from a subgroup analysis of the Physicians' Health Study,[30,51] a study enrolling 22,071 U.S. male physicians, aged 40 to 84 years. Among the 333 men with angina pectoris and/or coronary revascularization before randomization, those assigned to 50 mg of β-carotene on alternate days had a 44% reduction in all major coronary events defined as myocardial infarction, revascularization, or cardiac death (RR = 0.56, 95% CI: 0.31, 0.99). Subjects taking β-carotene also had a 49% reduction in all major vascular events, defined as stroke, myocardial infarction, revascularization, or cardiovascular death (RR = 0.51, 95% CI: 0.29, 0.88) after adjusting for age and aspirin assignment. The beneficial effect of β-carotene did not appear until the second year of follow-up, consistent with the hypothesis that antioxidants prevent progression of atherosclerosis. Although the Physicians' Health Study randomly assigned treatments, β-carotene was not randomly assigned within this subgroup of men with previous coronary disease.[30,51]

DeMaio et al.[52] followed 100 subjects who were randomly assigned to receive either 1200 mg of vitamin E or placebo after successful percutaneous transluminal angioplasty. The endpoint was restenosis, defined as ≥50% loss of the initial gain

TABLE 10.1
Completed Randomized Trials of Antioxidant Supplements: Cardiovascular and Total Mortality[a]

Study	Population	Intervention	Duration	Endpoints:	Relative risk (95% CI)
Alpha-Tocopherol Beta Carotene Prevention Study[53]	29,133 high-risk male Finnish smokers	β-carotene: 20 mg/day vitamin E: 50 mg/day	6.1 years	CVD mortality[68]	β-carotene: 1.11 (0.99, 1.23)
					vitamin E: 0.98 (0.89, 1.08)
				Total mortality	β-carotene: 1.08 (1.01, 1.16)
					vitamin E: 1.02 (0.95, 1.09)
Skin Cancer Prevention Study[59]	1720 patients with nonmelanoma skin cancer	β-carotene: 50 mg/day	8.2 years	CVD mortality	1.16 (0.82, 1.64)
				Total mortality	1.03 (0.82, 1.30)
Linxian, China[58]	29,584 Chinese persons at low risk for cardiovascular disease	Daily combination: β-carotene: 15 mg, vitamin E: 30 mg, selenium: 50 μg	5.25 years	CVA mortality	0.90 (0.76, 1.07)
				Total mortality	0.91 (0.84, 0.99)
Cambridge Heart Antioxidant Study[60]	2,002 patients with angiographically proven coronary artery disease	Vitamin E: 400–800 IU/day	510 days	CVD mortality	1.18 (0.62, 2.27)
Physicians' Health Study[62]	22,071 male physicians at usual risk	β-carotene: 50 mg every other day	12 years	CVD mortality	1.09 (0.93, 1.27)
				Total mortality	1.02 (0.93, 1.11)
Beta-Carotene and Retinol Efficacy Trial[61]	18,314 patients with tobacco and/or asbestos exposure	β-carotene: 30 mg/day	4 years	CVD mortality	1.26 (0.99, 1.61)
				Total mortality	1.17 (1.03, 1.33)

[a] CVD, cardiovascular disease; CVA, cerebrovascular accident.

in luminal diameter. After 4 months of follow-up, subjects receiving vitamin E had a 34.6% incidence of restenosis compared with a 50% incidence in subjects receiving placebo. The 31% risk reduction did not reach statistical significance, but the small sample size and short follow-up duration limited the study's statistical power.

Unexpectedly, however, a major randomized trial of antioxidants found that β-carotene supplements were associated with significant increases in total mortality, although neither β-carotene nor α-tocopherol had a significant effect on cardiovascular mortality.[53] The Alpha-Tocopherol, Beta Carotene Cancer Prevention Study (ATBC) enrolled a total of 29,133 Finnish male smokers, aged 50 to 69 years, and randomly assigned them to either α-tocopherol (50 mg/day) alone, β-carotene (20 mg/day) alone, both supplements together, or placebo. During a median of 6.1 years of follow-up, the investigators found a significant 8% increase in total mortality and an 18% increase in lung cancer among men who received β-carotene. While incidence of lung cancer was the primary study endpoint, and no cardiovascular hypotheses were specified, cardiovascular mortality data were collected. Mortality rates from ischemic heart disease (71.0 vs. 75.0/10,000 person-years) and ischemic stroke (6.6 vs. 7.9/10,000 person-years) were decreased in men who received α-tocopherol compared with no α-tocopherol, though neither finding achieved statistical significance. Subjects receiving β-carotene showed a nonsignificant trend towards higher mortality rates from ischemic heart disease (77.1 vs. 68.9/10,000 person-years) and from ischemic stroke (8.0 vs. 6.5/10,000 person-years) compared with subjects not receiving β-carotene.

A further analysis of the ATBC data was performed on the 22,269 men with no evidence of coronary heart disease at baseline to determine whether antioxidant supplementation reduced the incidence of angina pectoris.[54] A case was defined as typical angina pectoris reported on the World Health Organization (Rose) Chest Pain Questionnaire. During a median 4.7 years of follow-up, 1983 new cases of angina were detected. Subjects receiving α-tocopherol had a significantly decreased risk of angina pectoris (RR = 0.91, 95% CI: 0.83, 0.99) compared with subjects not receiving α-tocopherol. However, when subjects receiving α-tocopherol were compared with the placebo group, there was only a minor, nonsignificant decrease in the relative risk. Subjects supplemented with only β-carotene had an increased risk of angina compared with placebo, though this finding was of borderline statistical significance (RR = 1.13, 95% CI: 1.00, 1.27).

Several methodologic concerns surround the ATBC study. The synthetic preparation of α-tocopherol used in the study had low bioavailability and the daily dosage was low; increasing median blood levels by only about 50%. Observational studies have suggested that daily supplements of at least 100 mg of α-tocopherol are needed to decrease cardiovascular risk.[42,45] Currently, over-the-counter dietary supplements contain about 200 mg or more of α-tocopherol, and taking one or two capsules daily often doubles blood levels.[55] While the Rose questionnaire has been widely used in epidemiologic research, findings do not correlate well with angiographic or scintigraphic testing.[56,57] Finally, the study enrolled only middle-aged and elderly male smokers (who also consumed an average of 11 grams of alcohol daily), making the results less applicable to other populations.

A nutrient intervention study in Linxian, China randomized 29,584 adults, aged 40 to 69 years, to one of four vitamin and mineral combinations.[58] The study was designed to reduce the risk of cancer, especially esophageal and gastric, because the people of Linxian have one of the highest incidence rates in the world for these cancers and consistently low micronutrient intake. Subjects supplemented with β-carotene (15 mg), vitamin E (30 mg), and selenium (50 μg) had significantly lower total mortality (RR = 0.91, 95% CI = 0.84 to 0.99) compared with the placebo group and a trend towards lower cerebrovascular mortality (RR = 0.90, 95% CI = 0.76 to 1.07). With the combination treatment, however, the individual role of the nutrients in reducing cerebrovascular mortality could not be determined. No overall reduction in cardiovascular disease was found, but only 1% of deaths among trial participants were attributed to ischemic heart disease. Results may not apply to Western populations, which have much higher rates of cardiovascular mortality.

The Skin Cancer Prevention Study (SCPS) originally evaluated the role of β-carotene supplements in preventing nonmelanoma skin cancer. Data were recently reanalyzed to examine the relationship between β-carotene and the risk of death from major disease causes.[59] The SCPS randomized 1805 adults (mean age of 63.2 years old, 18% smokers) with biopsy-proven basal cell or squamous cell skin cancer to receive either daily β-carotene (50 mg) or placebo. Subjects were treated with supplements for a median time of 4.3 years and then followed for a median time of 8.2 years. No differences in overall mortality were detected between the β-carotene and placebo groups, though there was a trend towards increased cardiovascular mortality (RR = 1.16; 95% CI: 0.82, 1.64) in the β-carotene group. Results were unchanged after adjusting for smoking, demographics, and Quetelet index. Baseline β-carotene, however, was significantly correlated with subsequent cardiovascular mortality. Persons whose initial plasma β-carotene level was in the upper quartile (>0.52 μmol/L) had a reduced adjusted risk of cardiovascular mortality (RR = 0.57; 95% CI: 0.34, 0.95) compared with persons in the lowest quartile (<0.21 μmol/L).

The first data reported from a completed randomized study designed to measure clinical cardiovascular endpoints came from the Cambridge Heart Antioxidant Study (CHAOS).[60] This study randomized patients with angiographically proven coronary artery disease to receive either α-tocopherol (400 or 800 mg daily) or placebo. The primary endpoints were cardiovascular death and nonfatal myocardial infarction. The study enrolled 2002 subjects, 1690 men, with a mean age of 61.8 years. During a median follow-up time of 510 days, the α-tocopherol group had significantly fewer nonfatal myocardial infarctions. The relative risk for the α-tocopherol group, adjusted for age, diabetes, smoking, NYHA class, and use of beta-blockers, was 0.23, 95% CI: 0.11, 0.47. However, the α-tocopherol group had an excess of cardiovascular death (RR = 1.18; 95% CI: 0.62, 2.27), and all cause mortality, 3.5% vs. 2.7%, p = 0.31. Most deaths occurred during the first 200 days. Despite randomized treatment assignment, the α-tocopherol group was at increased risk for cardiovascular events because it had more smokers and diabetics, higher cholesterol levels, and more extensive coronary disease.

The most recently published randomized studies, including one designed to assess the role of antioxidants in preventing incident cardiovascular events, have

TABLE 10.2
Ongoing Randomized Trials of Antioxidant Supplements[a]

Trial	Population	Intervention	Endpoints
Women's Health Study (U.S.)[64]	40,000 female nurses at usual risk	β-carotene, vitamin E, low-dose aspirin	Cardiovascular death, MI, CVA, revascularization
Supplementation en Vitamines et Mineraux Antioxydants Trial (Europe)[65]	15,000 persons at usual risk	β-carotene, vitamin E, vitamin C, selenium, zinc	Cardiovascular events
Women's Antioxidant and Cardiovascular Study (U.S.)[66]	8,000 high-risk female nurses (past history of cardiovascular disease)	β-carotene, vitamin C, vitamin E	Cardiovascular death, MI, CVA, revascularization
Heart Outcomes Prevention Evaluation Study (Canada)[67]	9,000 high-risk patients (cardiovascular disease, diabetes)	Vitamin E, ramipril	Cardiovascular death, MI, CVA
Heart Protection Study (Europe)[65,68]	20,000 high-risk patients (coronary and peripheral vascular disease, diabetes)	β-carotene, vitamin E, vitamin C, simvastatin	Total mortality
GISSI prevention (Europe)[68]	12,000 high-risk patients (recent MI)	Vitamin E	Total mortality

[a] MI, myocardial infarction; CVA, cerebrovascular accident.

both reported negative findings. The Beta-Carotene and Retinol Efficacy Trial (CARET),[61] which randomized 18,314 smokers and people exposed to high levels of asbestos to daily doses of vitamin A (25,000 IU), β-carotene (30 mg), or placebo, was stopped 21 months early. The β-carotene group had 28% more lung cancer cases (95% CI: 47%, 57%) and 17% more deaths (95% CI: 3%, 33%) than the control group. Cardiovascular mortality was also increased in the β-carotene group, with relative risk of 1.26 (95% CI: 0.99, 1.61). In the Physicians' Health Study, 12 years of β-carotene supplementation had no effect on the incidence of cardiovascular disease (myocardial infarction, stroke, cardiovascular mortality) or death from all causes. When the study began, 11% of the subjects were current smokers and 39% were former smokers. No increased risk for lung cancer, cardiovascular mortality, or total mortality was observed for current or former smokers taking β-carotene.

There are still many ongoing primary and secondary prevention trials. (Table 10.2) All of these studies are using vitamin E supplementation in addition to other antioxidants, lipid lowering agents, and/or ACE inhibitors. Studies are enrolling women health professionals, diabetics, and patients with myocardial infarctions and peripheral vascular disease. By the end of the decade, study data will be available on more than 100,000 additional subjects.

VIII. DISCUSSION

The epidemiologic data suggested that antioxidant intake, especially vitamin E, substantially reduced the risk of cardiovascular events. Study findings were widely publicized, creating a clamor for antioxidant supplements. Editorialists felt obliged to urge restraint in public policy recommendations regarding the wide-spread use of antioxidants until convincing data from randomized trials became available. Steinberg further cautioned against potential unknown risks from long-term intake of antioxidants, and warned that patients taking vitamin supplements could neglect other better-established coronary disease preventive measures.[63]

The data from the randomized trials, however, are becoming available, and the unexpectedly disappointing results have considerably dampened the enthusiasm for antioxidant supplements. When the ATBC results were published, the negative findings were downplayed because supplement doses were suboptimal, and the Finnish men were not considered a representative population. The results now, though, seem less anomalous after the CARET again found higher mortality and cancer rates in smokers randomized to β-carotene. β-carotene was apparently harmful in smokers, and showed no benefit in low-risk populations,[59,62] even after 12 years of supplementation.

Vitamin E, the most promising antioxidant in observational studies, is currently being evaluated in large-scale primary and secondary prevention trials. However, the results from the CHAOS were disturbing. Even though the investigators emphasized the decreased risk for nonfatal myocardial infarction, cardiovascular and overall mortality were increased. Whether antioxidant supplementation actually increases the risk of cardiovascular mortality is uncertain. Results from larger studies with longer follow-up will help resolve this question.

How can the epidemiologic data and clinical trial results be incorporated into clinical practice? Clearly, the current evidence does not support any public policy recommendations favoring antioxidant supplements, especially β-carotene. The results from ongoing trials may eventually lead to treatment guidelines, perhaps targeting high-risk populations and identifying beneficial antioxidant regimens. Until then, however, the public, who is spending millions of dollars on vitamin supplements, should be educated that antioxidants are not a panacea. Practitioners should strongly encourage dietary intake of fruits and vegetables and continue proven prevention strategies directed at proven cardiovascular risk factors.

REFERENCES

1. Carew, T. E., Schwenke, D. C., and Steinberg, D., Antiatherogenic effect of probucol unrelated to its hypocholesterolemic effect: evidence that antioxidants *in vivo* can selectively inhibit low density lipoprotein degradation in macrophage-rich fatty streaks and slow the progression of atherosclerosis in the Watanabe heritable hyperlipidemic rabbit, *Proc. Natl. Acad. Sci. U.S.A.,* 84, 7725, 1987.
2. Kita, T., Nagano, Y., Yokode, M., et al., Probucol prevents the progression of atherosclerosis in Watanabe heritable hyperlipidemic rabbit, an animal model for familial hypercholesterolemia, *Proc. Natl. Acad. Sci. U.S.A.,* 84, 5928, 1987.
3. Daugherty, A., Zweifel, B. S., and Schonfeld, G., The effects of probucol on the progression of atherosclerosis in mature Watanabe heritable hyperlipidaemic rabbits, *Br. J. Pharmacol.,* 103, 1013, 1991.

4. Wilson, R. B., Middleton, C. C., and Sun, G. Y., Vitamin E, antioxidants and lipid peroxidation in experimental atherosclerosis of rabbits, *J. Nutr.,* 108, 1858, 1978.

5. Williams, R. J., Motteram, J. M., Sharp, C. H., and Gallagher, P. J., Dietary vitamin E and the attenuation of early lesion development in modified Watanabe rabbits, *Atherosclerosis*, 94, 153, 1992.

6. Wójcicki, J., Różewicka, L., Barcew-Wiszniewska, B., et al., Effect of selenium and vitamin E on the development of experimental atherosclerosis in rabbits, *Atherosclerosis*, 87, 9, 1991.

7. Verlangieri, A. J. and Bush, M. J., Effects of d-α-tocopherol supplementation on experimentally induced primate atherosclerosis, *J. Am. Coll. Nutr.,* 11, 131, 1992.

8. Qiao, Y., Yokoyama, M., Kameyama, K., and Asano, G., Effect of vitamin E on vascular integrity in cholesterol-fed guinea pigs, *Arterioscler. Thromb.*, 13, 1885, 1993.

9. Smith, T. L. and Kummerow, F. A., Effect of dietary vitamin E on plasma lipids and atherogenesis in restricted ovulator chickens, *Atherosclerosis*, 75, 105, 1989.

10. Acheson, R. M. and Williams, D. R. R., Does consumption of fruit and vegetables protect against stroke?, *Lancet*, 1, 1191, 1983.

11. Armstrong, B. K., Mann, J. I., Adelstein, A. M., and Eskin, F., Commodity consumption and ischemic heart disease mortality, with special reference to dietary practices, *J. Chron. Dis.,* 28, 455, 1975.

12. Smith, W. C. S., Tunstall-Pedoe, H., Crombie, I. K., and Tavendale, R., Concomitants of excess coronary deaths — major risk factor and lifestyle findings from 10, 359 men and women in the Scottish Heart Health Study, *Scot. Med. J.,* 34, 550, 1989.

13. Rouse, I. L., Armstrong, B. K., Beilin, L. J., and Vandongen, R., Vegetarian diet, blood pressure and cardiovascular risk, *Aust. N.Z. J. Med.,* 14, 439, 1984.

14. Verlangieri, A. J., Kapeghian, J. C., el-Dean, S., and Bush, M., Fruit and vegetable consumption and cardiovascular mortality, *Med. Hypotheses*, 16, 7, 1985.

15. Ginter, E., Decline of coronary mortality in United States and vitamin C [letter], *Am. J. Clin. Nutr.,* 32, 511, 1979.

16. Gey, K. F., Puska, P., Jordan, P., and Moser, U. K., Inverse correlation between plasma vitamin E and mortality from ischemic heart disease in cross-cultural epidemiology, *Am. J. Clin. Nutr.,* 53 (Suppl), 326S, 1991.

17. Gey, K. F., Moser, U. K., Jordan, P., et al., Increased risk of cardiovascular disease at suboptimal plasma concentrations of essential antioxidants: an epidemiological update with special attention to carotene and vitamin C, *Am. J. Clin. Nutr.,* 57 (suppl), 787S, 1993.

18. Bellizzi, M. C., Franklin, M. F., Duthie, G. G., and James, W. P. T., Vitamin E and coronary heart disease: the European paradox, *Eur. J. Clin. Nutr.,* 48, 822, 1994.

19. Riemersma, R. A., Wood, D. A., MacIntyre, C. C. A., et al., Risk of angina pectoris and plasma concentration of vitamins A, C, and E and carotene, *Lancet*, 337, 1, 1991.

20. Ramirez, J. and Flowers, N. C., Leukocyte ascorbic acid and its relationship to coronary artery disease in man, *Am. J. Clin. Nutr.,* 33, 2079, 1980.

21. Salonen, J. T., Salonen, R., Seppänen, K., et al., Relationship of serum selenium and antioxidants to plasma lipoproteins, platelet aggregability and prevalent ischaemic heart disease in Eastern Finnish men, *Atherosclerosis*, 70, 155, 1988.

22. Kardinaal, A. F. M., Kok, F. J., Ringstad, J., et al., Antioxidants in adipose tissue and risk of myocardial infarction: the EURAMIC study, *Lancet*, 342, 1379, 1993.

23. Street, D. A., Comstock, G. W., Salkeld, R. M., Schüep, W., and Klag, M. J., Serum antioxidants and myocardial infarction. Are low levels of carotenoids and α-tocopherol risk factors for myocardial infarction?, *Circulation*, 90, 1154, 1994.

24. Salonen, J. T., Salonen, R., Penttilä, I., et al., Serum fatty acids, apolipoproteins, selenium and vitamin antioxidants and the risk of death from coronary artery disease, *Am. J. Cardiol.*, 56, 226, 1985.

25. Gunter, W. E., Driskell, W. J., and Yeager, P. R., Stability of vitamin E in long-term stored serum serum, *Clin. Chim. Acta*, 175, 329, 1988.

26. Kok, F. J., de Bruijn, A. M., Vermeeren, R., et al., Serum selenium, vitamin antioxidants, and cardiovascular mortality: a 9-year follow-up study in the Netherlands, *Am. J. Clin. Nutr.,* 45, 462, 1987.

27. Hense, H. W., Stender, M., Bors, W., and Keil, U., Lack of an association between serum vitamin E and myocardial infarction in a population with high vitamin E levels, *Atherosclerosis*, 103, 21, 1993.

28. Gey, K. F., Stähelin, H. B., and Eichholzer, M., Poor plasma status of carotene and vitamin C is associated with higher mortality from ischemic heart disease and stroke: Basel prospective study, *Clin Investig.*, 71, 3, 1993.
29. Morris, D. L., Kritchevsky, S. B., and Davis, C. E., Serum carotenoids and coronary heart disease. The Lipid Research Clinics Coronary Primary Prevention Trial and Follow-up Study, *J. Am. Med. Assoc.*, 272, 1439, 1994.
30. Gaziano, J. M., Manson, J. E., Branch, L. G., et al., Dietary beta carotene and decreased cardiovascular mortality in an elderly cohort, *J. Am. Coll. Cardiol.*, 19, 377A, 1992.
31. Enstrom, J. E., Kanim, L. E., and Klein, M. A., Vitamin C intake and mortality among a sample of the United States population, *Epidemiology*, 3, 194, 1992.
32. Lapidus, L., Andersson, H., Bengtsson, C., and Bosaeus, I., Dietary habits in relation to incidence of cardiovascular disease and death in women: a 12-year follow-up of participants in the population study of women in Gothenburg, Sweden, *Am. J. Clin. Nutr.*, 44, 444, 1986.
33. Gale, C. R., Martyn, C. N., Winter, P. D., and Cooper, C., Vitamin C and risk of death from stroke and coronary heart disease in cohort of elderly people, *Br. Med. J.*, 310, 1563, 1995.
34. Stähelin, H. B., Eichholzer, M., and Gey, K. F., Nutritional factors correlating with cardiovascular disease: results of the Basel Study, *Bibl. Nutr. Dieta.*, 49, 24, 1992.
35. Eichholzer, M., Stähelin, H. B., and Gey, K. F., Inverse correlation between essential antioxidants in plasma and subsequent risk to develop cancer, ischemic heart disease and stroke respectively: 12-year follow-up of the Prospective Basel Study, *EXS*, 62, 398, 1992.
36. Knekt, P., Reunanen, A., Järvinen, R., et al., Antioxidant vitamin intake and coronary mortality in a longitudinal population study, *Am. J. Epidemiol.*, 139, 1180, 1994.
37. Keli, S. O., Hertog, M. G. L., Feskens, E. J. M., and Kromhout, D., Dietary flavonoids, antioxidant vitamins, and incidence of stroke. The Zutphen study, *Arch. Intern. Med.*, 154, 637, 1996.
38. Hertog, M. G. L., Feskens, E. J. M., Hollman, P. C. H., Katan, M. B., and Kromhout, D., Dietary antioxidant flavonoids and risk of coronary heart disease: the Zutphen Elderly Study, *Lancet*, 342, 1007, 1993.
39. Pandey, D. K., Shekelle, R., Selwyn, B. J., Tangney, C., and Stamler, J., Dietary vitamin C and β-carotene and risk of death in middle-aged men, The Western Electric Study, *Am. J. Epidemiol.*, 142, 1269, 1995.
40. Hodis, H. N., Mack, W. J., LaBree, L., et al., Serial coronary angiographic evidence that antioxidant vitamin intake reduces progression of coronary artery atherosclerosis, *J. Am. Med. Assoc.*, 273, 1849, 1995.
41. Kushi, L. H., Folsom, A. R., Prineas, R. J., et al., Dietary antioxidant vitamins and death from coronary heart disease in postmenopausal women, *N. Engl. J. Med.*, 334, 1156, 1996.
42. Stampfer, M. J., Hennekens, C. H., Manson, J. E., Colditz, G. A., Rosner, B., and Willett, W. C., Vitamin E consumption and the risk of coronary disease in women, *N. Engl. J. Med.*, 328, 1444, 1993.
43. Manson, J. E., Stampfer, M. J., Willett, W. C., et al., A prospective study of antioxidant vitamins and incidence of coronary heart disease in women [Abstract], *Circulation*, 84 (Suppl 2), 546, 1991.
44. Manson, J. E., Stampfer, M. J., Willett, W. C., et al., Antioxidant vitamin score and incidence of coronary heart disease in women [Abstract], *Circulation*, 86 (Suppl 1), 675, 1992.
45. Rimm, E. B., Stampfer, M. J., Ascherio, A., Giovannucci, E., Colditz, G. A., and Willett, W. C., Vitamin E consumption and the risk of coronary heart disease in men, *N. Engl. J. Med.*, 328, 1450, 1993.
46. Haeger, K., Long-time treatment of intermittent claudication with vitamin E, *Am. J. Clin. Nutr.*, 27, 1179, 1974.
47. Livingstone, P. D. and Jones, C., Treatment of intermittent claudication with vitamin E, *Lancet*, 2, 602, 1958.
48. Williams, H. T. G., Fenna, D., and Macbeth, R. A., Alpha tocopherol in the treatment of intermittent claudication, *Surg. Gynecol. Obstet.*, 132, 662, 1971.
49. Anderson, T. W., Vitamin E in angina pectoris, *Can. Med. Assoc. J.*, 110, 401, 1974.
50. Gillilan, R. E., Mondell, B., and Warbasse, J. R., Quantitative evaluation of vitamin E in the treatment of angina pectoris, *Am. Heart J.*, 93, 444, 1977.

51. Gaziano, J. M., Manson, J. E., Ridker, P. M., Buring, J. E., and Hennekens, C. H., Beta carotene therapy for chronic stable angina [Abstract], *Circulation*, 82 (Suppl 3), 201, 1990.

52. DeMaio, S. J., King, S. B., Lembo, N. J., et al., Vitamin E supplementation, plasma lipids and incidence of restenosis after percutaneous transluminal coronary angioplasty (PTCA), *J. Am. Coll. Nutr.,* 11, 68, 1992.

53. The Alpha-Tocopherol, Beta Carotene Cancer Prevention Study Group, The effect of vitamin E and beta carotene on the incidence of lung cancer and other cancers in male smokers, *N. Engl. J. Med.,* 330, 1029, 1994.

54. Rapola, J. M., Virtamo, J., Haukka, J. K., et al., Effect of vitamin E and beta carotene on the incidence of angina pectoris. A randomized, double-blind, controlled trial, *J. Am. Med. Assoc.,* 275, 693, 1996.

55. Hennekens, C. H., Buring, J. E., and Peto, R., Antioxidant vitamins — benefits not yet proved, *N. Engl. J. Med.,* 330, 1080, 1994.

56. Erikssen, J., Enge, I., Forfang, K., and Storstein, O., False positive diagnostic tests and coronary angiographic findings in 105 presumably healthy males, *Circulation*, 54, 371, 1976.

57. Garber, C. E., Carleton, R. A., and Heller, G. V., Comparison of "Rose Questionnaire Angina" to exercise thallium scintigraphy: different findings in males and females, *J. Clin. Epidemiol.,* 45, 715, 1992.

58. Blot, W. J., Li, J.-Y., Taylor, P. R., et al., Nutrition intervention trials in Linxian, China: supplementation with specific vitamin/mineral combinations, cancer incidence, and disease-specific mortality in the general population, *J. Natl. Cancer Inst.,* 85, 1483, 1993.

59. Greenberg, E. R., Baron, J. A., Karagas, M. R., et al., . Mortality associated with low plasma concentration of beta carotene and the effect of oral supplementation, *J. Am. Med. Assoc.,* 275, 699, 1996.

60. Stephens, N. G., Parsons, A., Schofield, P. M., et al., Randomised controlled trial of vitamin E in patients with coronary disease: Cambridge Heart Antioxidant Study (CHAOS), *Lancet*, 347, 781, 1996.

61. Omenn, G. S., Goodman, G. E., Thornquist, M. D., et al., Effects of a combination of beta carotene and vitamin A on lung cancer and cardiovascular disease, *N. Engl. J. Med.,* 334, 1150, 1996.

62. Hennekens, C. H., Buring, J. E., Manson, J. E., et al., Lack of effect of long-term supplementation with beta carotene on the incidence of malignant neoplasms and cardiovascular disease, *N. Engl. J. Med.,* 334, 1145, 1996.

63. Steinberg, D., Antioxidant vitamins and coronary heart disease [Editorial], *N. Engl. J. Med.,* 328, 1487, 1993.

64. Buring, J. E. and Hennekens, C. H., The Women's Health Study: summary of the study design, *J. Myocardial Ischemia*, 4, 27, 1992.

65. Hennekens, C. H., Gaziano, J. M., Manson, J. E., and Buring, J. E., Antioxidant vitamin-cardiovascular disease hypothesis is still promising, but still unproven: the need for randomized trials, *Am. J. Clin. Nutr.,* 62 (suppl), 1377S, 1995.

66. Manson, J. E., Gaziano, J. M., Spelsberg, A., et al., A secondary prevention trial of antioxidant vitamins and cardiovascular disease in women: rationale, design and methods, *Ann. Epidemiol.,* 5, 261, 1995.

67. The HOPE (Heart Outcomes Prevention Evaluation) Study: the design for a large, simple randomized trial of an angiotensin-converting enzyme inhibitor (ramipril) and vitamin E in patients at high risk of cardiovascular events, *Can. J. Cardiol.,* 12, 127, 1996.

68. Jha, P., Flather, M., Lonn, E., Farkouh, M., and Yusuf, S., The antioxidant vitamins and cardiovascular disease. A critical review of epidemiologic and clinical trial data, *Ann Intern Med.,* 123, 860, 1995.

Chapter 11

NUTRITIONAL ANTIOXIDANTS AND PREVENTION OF AGE-RELATED EYE DISEASE

Paul F. Jacques

Contents

I. Age-Related Changes in the Eye 150

II. Prevalence and Public Health Impact of Age-Related Cataract
and AMD 153

III. Overview of the Experimental Evidence for Nutritional Antioxidants
in Cataract and AMD 153
   A. Vitamin C 154
   B. Vitamin E 154
   C. Carotenoids 155
   D. Riboflavin 155

IV. Epidemiologic Evidence for Nutritional Antioxidants in Age-Related
Cataract 156
   A. Vitamin C 157
   B. Vitamin E 159
   C. Carotenoids 161
   D. Riboflavin 163
   E. Multivitamin Supplements 164
   F. Intervention Trials 165

V. Epidemiologic Evidence for Nutritional Antioxidants in AMD 167
   A. Vitamin C 167
   B. Vitamin E 169
   C. Carotenoids 169

VI. Summary 170

Acknowledgments 173

References 173

I. AGE-RELATED CHANGES IN THE EYE

The eye lens is a transparent, avascular tissue that transmits and focuses light on the retina[1,2] (Figure 11.1). It is located behind the iris and aqueous humor and is covered by a collagenous capsule. Beneath the anterior (outward facing) surface of the capsule is a single layer of epithelial cells. This is the major site of metabolic activity in the lens and the source of new lens cells. Epithelial cells in the germinative zone actively divide and are displaced from this region toward the lens equator where they differentiate and elongate to form lens fiber cells. As these cells differentiate, they lose their nuclei and organelles. The mature fiber cells are packed with protein, which comprises more than one third of the wet weight and 98% of the dry weight of the lens. Most lens proteins are structural proteins called crystallins. New cells are formed throughout life and laid down on older cells, but older cells are not lost. Rather, they are compressed into the center (nucleus) of the lens. The weight and volume of the lens continue to increase throughout life, although the rate of growth diminishes with age.

Because there is little or no protein synthesis in the center of an adult lens, fiber cell structural proteins must remain unaltered for decades in order to properly transmit light to the photosensitive retina. However, the lens is exposed to oxidative stress from light and high energy oxygen species,[3,4] and there is evidence that oxidation can modify and damage lens proteins, although processes other than oxidation may also be important causes of lens protein damage.[4-8] Because lens proteins undergo minimal turnover as the lens ages, the damaged proteins accumulate. This may ultimately impede transmission of light and result in opacification of the lens. Opacification of the lens is referred to as cataract, although clinically this designation is sometimes reserved for opacities associated with visual disfunction. Cataracts are commonly classified by their location within the lens as nuclear, cortical, or posterior subcapsular (Figure 11.1).

The retina is the neural tissue lining the back of the eye.[9] It consists of multiple layers containing the rod and cone photoreceptors and their neural connections (Figure 11.1). The front or inner layers, nearest the vitreous, contain the ganglion cells and nerve fibers, which form the optic nerve. The middle layers are comprised of integrative, supportive, and nutritive cells. The back or outer layers of the retina contain the photoreceptors. The outermost layer of the neural retina consists of the photoreceptor outer segments, which contain the photosensitive pigments. Consequently, this is the site where light is transformed into a neural signal. The outer segments are in contact with the retinal pigment epithelium (RPE), which has many functions involved in controlling the local environment of the outer layers of the retina. The vascular needs of the outer neural retina and the RPE are supplied by the choriocapillaris, which is just external to the RPE and separated from it by a thin layer of collagenous tissue called Bruch's membrane.

Located near the center of the retina is a specialized region called the fovea or macula lutea, which contains the highest concentration of cone photoreceptors (Figure 11.1). There are conspicuous changes in the macula with age.[10,11] Most notable are the development of drusen (small focal lesions visible as pale yellow

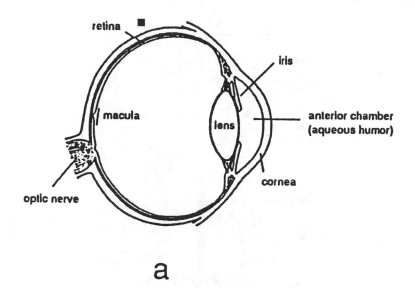

a

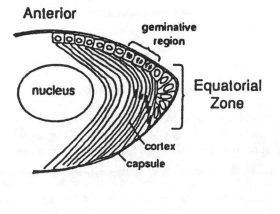

b

Figure 11.1. Diagram of the structures of (a) the human eye, (b) lens, and (c) retina. (a) The lens of the human eye is a transparent, avascular, biconvex structure located behind the pupil. (b) It is surrounded by a mucopolysaccharide capsule. Beneath the anterior capsule is a single layer of epithelial cells, which is the major site of metabolic activity in the lens. The epithelial cells form a germative region near the lens equator. As the epithelial cells migrate toward the equator, they differentiate and elongate to form fiber (cortical) cells. Throughout life, new fiber cells are formed. As they differentiate, these cells lose their nuclei and many organelles, limiting their capacity for protein synthesis. Old fibers are not lost as they age, but are compressed to form the lens nucleus. Cataracts are commonly characterized by location in the lens: nuclear cataract is found in the lens nuclear, cortical in the lens cortex, and posterior subcapsular in the back of the lens adjacent to the lens capsule. A mixed cataract might involve opacities in two or three of these regions of the lens. (c) Diagram of the main cellular elements of the human retina.

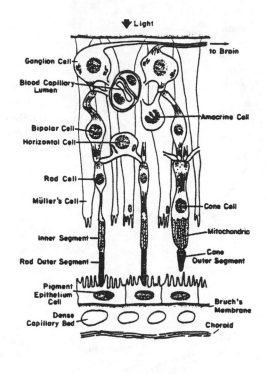

C

Figure 11.1. (continued)

spots), accumulation of lipofuscin, loss of pigment in the RPE, and sclerotic changes in the choroid vessels. These changes occur typically with no impact on visual function. The relation between these age-associated changes and macular damage associated with visual loss is not established.

Damage to the photoreceptors in the macula can have devastating effects on visual function because this is the region of the retina responsible for the keenest visual acuity. Moreover, cone photoreceptors, which are the exclusive photoreceptor in the macula, appear to be more susceptible to damage from visible light than rod photoreceptors. Accumulation of damage to the macula with age can have clinical manifestations referred to age-related macular degeneration (AMD). There are two distinct stages or forms of AMD.[12] The predominant atrophic or "dry" form is characterized by a slow atrophy of photoreceptors, the RPE, and the choriocapillaris. The more advanced or severe form, exudative or "wet" AMD, is characterized by an aggressive growth of blood vessels from the choriocapillaris (subretinal neovascularization), which results in hemorrhaging and scarring of the retina. The pathogenesis of AMD remains uncertain, but it is believed to result from a disorder of the RPE cells that may disrupt the normal interaction between the photoreceptors and the underlying tissues.[13,14] As in the development of lens opacification, available evidence implicates exposure to light and active forms of oxygen as a cause of damage leading to AMD.[11,15,16]

II. PREVALENCE AND PUBLIC HEALTH IMPACT OF AGE-RELATED CATARACT AND AMD

Age-related cataract is a significant public health problem throughout the world.[17-19] Although visual impairment and blindness caused by cataract can be surgically corrected, it is estimated that approximately 50% of the 30 to 50 million cases of blindness worldwide result from unoperated cataract.[17,18] The impact of cataract-related disability is much greater in less developed countries where more than 90% of the cases of blindness and visual impairment are found.[18] There are two reasons that cataract presents a greater burden in less developed countries: cataracts are more common and develop earlier in life than in more developed countries,[20-22] and cataract is more likely to result in blindness because there are too few ophthalmologists to perform lens extractions.[17,18]

In the U.S. and other developed countries, AMD is the leading cause of severe visual loss and blindness,[12] but age-related cataract remains the leading cause of visual disability, accounting for 40 to 60% of visual disability among adults.[23-26] The lack of standard diagnostic criteria have previously hindered the estimation of prevalence of both cataract and maculopathy. Diagnostic criteria used in earlier studies tended to be variable and included some degree of visual impairment. Recent studies have used more uniform grading systems without consideration of visual function. Estimates of prevalence of age-related macular changes in population-based samples of Americans ranged from approximately 8% for men and women aged 43 to 54 years to 30% for those age 75 years or older.[27,28] Maculopathy associated with degenerative changes were seen in less than 1% of individuals between the ages of 43 and 64 years, but increased dramatically to 7% in those age 75 years or older. The prevalence of age-related lens cataract associated with impaired vision increases from approximately 1% by age 54 years to approximately 5% at age 65 and about 40% for persons older than 75 years in the U.S., whereas prevalence of cataract defined without consideration of visual acuity increased from approximately 10% to greater than 80% across this age range.[28,29]

In addition to the associated visual disability, age-related cataract and AMD represent an enormous economic burden. For example, in the U.S. more than 1.3 million cataract extractions are performed annually at a cost of approximately $3.5 billion.[30] Cataract extraction is the most frequently performed surgery among elderly Americans and accounts for the largest single item in Medicare expenditures.[31] Unlike cataract, there is no treatment available for most cases of AMD.[12]

III. OVERVIEW OF THE EXPERIMENTAL EVIDENCE FOR NUTRITIONAL ANTIOXIDANTS IN CATARACT AND AMD

Much of the experimental research on the etiology of cataract and AMD has focused on the role of nutritional antioxidants (vitamin C, vitamin E, and carotenoids) because of the evidence that oxidative damage is involved in the pathogenesis of these disorders and because of the presence of high concentrations of specific antioxidants in the lens and macula. A brief overview of the evidence from animal, *in vitro,* and cell free experiments relating antioxidants to cataract and AMD is presented as background to assist in the review and interpretation of the epidemiologic data, which follows.

A. VITAMIN C

Vitamin C (ascorbic acid) is probably the most effective, least toxic, water-soluble antioxidant identified in mammalian systems.[32,33] Vitamin C is present at high levels in the human lens[34] and macula.[35] The levels in the lens, which concentrates vitamin C to over 3 mmol/L, is 20 to 60 fold higher than plasma.[34] It has also been demonstrated that the concentration of vitamin C in the lens can be increased with vitamin C supplements beyond levels achieved in persons who already consumed more than 120 mg/day, which is two times the RDA for vitamin C.[34] The amount of vitamin C in the central retina is reported to be approximately 40 nmol/cm^2 or 20 nmol/mg protein.[35]

Animal experiments provided the first evidence that vitamin C might play a role in the prevention of cataract formation. Feeding increased amounts of vitamin C delayed progress of or prevented galactose-induced cataract in guinea pigs[36] and rats,[37] selenite-induced cataract in rats,[38] and cataract in glutathione-depleted chick embryos.[39] In addition to delaying cataract in these experimental models, vitamin C has also been shown to protect lens constituents from earlier stages of damage. Vitamin C prevented (1) *in vitro* light-induced lens lipid peroxidation assessed by malonaldehyde,[40] (2) UV-induced high molecular weight lens protein aggregate formation and reduced protease activity in guinea pigs *in vivo*[41] and in lens homogenates,[42] and (3) lens cell membrane damage or impaired cation pump activity by *in vitro* exposure to light and active oxygen species.[43-45]

There are few experimental observations relating vitamin C to the protection of the macula. Vitamin C appeared to protect against the loss of rhodopsin and the integrity of the photoreceptor cell nuclei in rats exposed to damaging light.[46] Exposure to light also reduced concentrations of vitamin C in the rat retina[47] and resulted in lower levels of the reduced form of vitamin C and higher levels of the oxidized form of vitamin C in the guinea pig[48] and primate[49] retina. Vitamin C supplementation also appeared to protect against light-induced damage of retina in dark-reared rats.[47,50] Damage to the retina from bright light was also reported in scorbutic guinea pigs reared in normal cyclic room light.[51]

B. VITAMIN E

Vitamin E (α-tocopherol), a natural lipid-soluble antioxidant, can inhibit lipid peroxidation, which helps to preserve membrane integrity and critical membrane functions.[52] The amount of α-tocopherol in normal human lenses were recently demonstrated to be approximately 1.6 µg/g wet weight of lens tissue.[53] Vitamin E levels in the human retina have also been recently characterized.[54] Total tocopherol was 2.0 and 1.2 nmol/mg protein in the peripheral retina and macula, respectively. Levels in the RPE averaged 3.2 nmol/mg protein in both the macular and peripheral regions. Stephens et al.[55] also demonstrated that vitamin E concentration in rat photoreceptors was responsive to vitamin E intake.

There is limited evidence from experimental studies in animals relating vitamin E and development of cataract. Vitamin E is reported to be effective in delaying galactose-induced[56] and aminothiazole-induced[57] cataracts in rabbits. Vitamin E also protects against photo-peroxidation of lens lipids.[58] It has also been shown to retard the development of cataract-like lens changes induced *in vitro* by a large number of cataractogenic agents including glucose,[59,60] galactose,[61] ionizing radiation,[62] heat,[63] steroids, and other cataractogenic drugs.[64,65]

There is also little experimental evidence relating vitamin E and AMD. Evidence of a vitamin E effect on macular degeneration is derived from dogs fed rations without vitamin E for up to 3 years,[66] and from monkeys fed a vitamin E-deficient diet for 2 years.[67] These animals developed macular degeneration characterized by disruption and loss of photoreceptors. This was most pronounced in the macula of the monkeys. There was also extensive accumulation of lipofuscin in the RPE in these animals. Although the role of lipofuscin in AMD is not established, it is hypothesized that it contributes to pathogenesis.[11,68]

C. CAROTENOIDS

The carotenoids are among the most common pigments in nature[69] and, like vitamin E, are natural lipid-soluble antioxidants.[52] β-Carotene is the best known carotenoid because of its importance as a vitamin A precursor. However, it is only one of the approximately 400 naturally occurring carotenoids.[70] In addition to β-carotene, α-carotene, lutein, and lycopene are important carotenoid components of the human diet.[71] The antioxidant potential of these other carotenoids may be similar or greater than that of β-carotene.[72,73]

Amounts of xanthophylls, lutein, and zeaxanthin in normal adult lenses were shown to be 13.8 ng/g wet weight of tissue, but β-carotene and lycopene, which are the predominant carotenoids in human plasma,[74] were not detected in human lenses.[53] The retina, particularly the macula, have very high quantities of carotenoids.[75,76] Like the lens, the predominant carotenoids in the macula are the polar carotenoids lutein and zeaxanthin, while other nonpolar carotenoids, including β-carotene, are absent. The levels of lutein and zeaxanthin both average approximately 35 ng/macula.[76] The high concentration of the xanthophylls are responsible for the yellowish color of this region of the retina as well as its designation as the macula lutea or "yellow spot." The hydroxy groups of the xanthophylls may allow these carotenoids to incorporate into cell membranes in an orderly orientation that stabilizes the membrane.[11]

There are no experimental animal data and relating carotenoids to cataract formation and little data relating carotenoids to AMD. It has been noted that the macular pigment is depleted in monkeys fed diets without xanthophylls,[77] and maintenance on such a diet for up to 14 years resulted in retinal changes including a loss of RPE cells and increased photoreceptor cell death.[78] The retinal changes were more notable in areas where lutein and zeaxanthin were absent.

D. RIBOFLAVIN

Riboflavin (vitamin B2) is one of a number of nutrients that does not function directly as antioxidants, but serve as cofactors for antioxidant enzymes in the eye.[79]

Riboflavin is a cofactor for the FAD-dependent enzyme, glutathione reductase, which restores oxidized glutathione to its reduced form. The earliest studies of nutrition in development of cataract focused on riboflavin. In 1928, it was reported that cataracts developed in rats fed diets free of the "B-complex."[80] Since that time, numerous studies have observed that riboflavin deficiency results in experimental cataract in many species including rats, mice, cats, pigs, chickens, salmon, and trout.[81] No experimental or human studies have considered riboflavin as a potential determinant of AMD.

IV. EPIDEMIOLOGIC EVIDENCE FOR NUTRITIONAL ANTIOXIDANTS IN AGE-RELATED CATARACT

Eleven epidemiologic studies examined the associations between cataract and antioxidant nutrients.[82-95] Although each of these studies has specific limitations, several limitations are common to many of these studies because of similarities in design. These include the retrospective assessment of nutrient intake or status (i.e., after the diagnosis of cataract), the measurement of antioxidant nutrient intake or status at only one point in time to characterize usual intake or status, and the failure to account for the correlations between intake (or status) of the individual antioxidant nutrients.

Eight of the studies were retrospective case-control or cross-sectional studies comparing the nutrient levels of cataract patients with that of similarly aged individuals with clear lenses.[82-92] Our ability to interpret data from retrospective studies, such as these, is limited by the concurrent assessment of lens status and nutrient levels. Prior diagnosis of cataract might influence diet or bias reporting of usual diet. In two other studies,[84,90] nutrient status was determined prior to lens assessment. However, like the other retrospective studies, these studies measured prevalent (existing) cataract, and it is possible that diet or participation in the study might have been based on knowledge of the existing cataract. To further limit the potential for such bias, the investigators in one of these studies[84] excluded individuals with a diagnosis of cataract prior to enrollment to insure that actual intake or the report of intake was not altered by knowledge of lens status.

As cataracts develop over a period of decades, the most relevant measure of antioxidant intake or status would be that measured over a comparable time interval. Most of these studies used only one measure of nutrient intake or status, which may not accurately reflect usual, long-term intake or status of antioxidant nutrients. One of the studies[84] addressed the issue of long-term intake by selecting women from an existing cohort with multiple measurement of nutrient intake over the previous 10 years prior to determining lens status. A second study asked participants to recall their usual diet 10 years before entry into the study in an attempt to assess diet at a more appropriate point in time.[88]

Three other studies assessed nutrient levels and then followed individuals with intact lenses for 5,[95] 8,[94] and 15 years,[93] respectively. Prospective studies such as these are less prone to bias because assessment of exposure is performed before the outcome is present. These studies did not directly assess lens status, but used cataract extraction[93-95] or self-reported diagnosis confirmed by ophthalmologist reports or medical records[95] as measures of cataract risk. Extraction may not be a good measure of cataract incidence (development of new cataract) in some populations, because it incorporates components of both incidence and progression in severity of existing cataract. Access to medical services also has the potential to bias this endpoint, but unequal access to medical care is unlikely in any of these cohorts. In addition, the distribution of cataract types in extracted lenses is not representative of the distribution of prevalent cataract in the general population.[96,97] In spite of these factors, extraction is the result of visually disabling cataract and is the endpoint that one ultimately wants to prevent. Hankinson et al.[94] measured nutrient intake over a 4-year period, while Knekt et al.[93] used only one measure of serum antioxidant status. As noted above, one measure may not provide an accurate assessment of usual, long-term nutrient levels. Hankinson et al.[94] and Seddon et al.[95] examined the relation between supplement use and extraction using reports of current and past supplement use. This allowed for determination of duration of use as an estimate of usual supplement consumption.

Finally, the antioxidant nutrients in the diet, and therefore also in the blood, tend to be correlated with each other. Failure to account for these correlations make it difficult to identify the independent contribution of the different nutrients. For example, if associations are observed between prevalence of cataract and both vitamin C and carotenoid intake, it is not possible to attribute the association to either of these nutrients without statistical adjustment for the correlation between these nutrients.

Results are summarized by nutrient to aid in consideration of the coherence of the relations between each antioxidant nutrient and risk of cataract. Figures 11.2 to 11.7 display the risk ratios (RR) and 95% confidence intervals (CI) for individuals with high intake, supplemental, and blood levels of antioxidant nutrients relative to those with low levels. High and low levels are defined differently for most studies and the criteria for high and low are described in the text. Most of these studies determined the high and low categories on the basis of percentile categories, i.e., those individuals with intakes or blood levels above a given percentile were categorized as high and those below a given percentile were categorized as low. The most commonly used percentile categories were based on quintiles, which divide the sample into fifths and result in a comparison between the highest fifth or quintile category and the lowest fifth or quintile category.

A. VITAMIN C

The relation of vitamin C and cataract was considered in nine studies,[82-86,88,90-92,94] and observed to be inversely associated with at least one type of cataract in six of these studies (Figure 11.2). Jacques and Chylack[83] observed that the prevalence of cataract was about 75% lower (RR: 0.25; 95% CI: 0.06 to 1.09) in persons with high vitamin C intakes (>490 mg/day), which constituted the highest quintile category, than in those with intakes in the lowest quintile category (<125 mg/day) after adjustment for age, sex, race, and diabetes in a small case-control study (n = 112). They observed a similar relation between high and low quintiles of plasma vitamin C and cataract prevalence. Persons with high plasma vitamin C levels (>90 μmol/L) had less than one third the prevalence of early cataract as persons with low plasma vitamin C (<40 μmol/L) (RR: 0.29; 95% CI: 0.06 to 1.32).[83] These same investigators

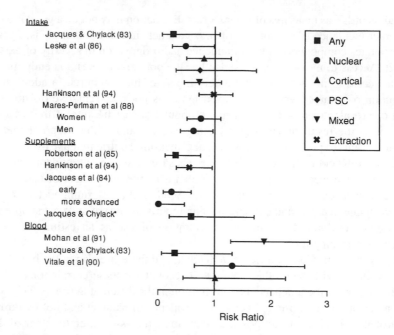

Figure 11.2.   Summary of studies of vitamin C and age-related cataract: risk ratio and 95% confidence intervals. *unpublished observation.

considered the relation between vitamin C supplement use and cataract prevalence and observed a modestly lower prevalence of cataract among a small number of supplement users (RR: 0.58; 95% CI: 0.20 to 1.70) compared with those who did not use vitamin C supplements (unpublished).

Lower risk of cataract was also observed in four other studies that considered either vitamin C intake or supplement use. Leske and co-workers[86] observed that persons with vitamin C intake in the highest quintile category had a 52% lower prevalence for nuclear cataract (RR: 0.48; 95% CI: 0.24 to 0.99) compared with persons who had intakes in the lowest quintile category after controlling for age and sex. Weaker inverse associations were noted between those in the highest and lowest fifths of this sample for other types of cataract. Mares-Perlman and colleagues[88] also observed that the prevalence of nuclear cataract was lower for men (RR: 0.62; 95% CI: 0.39 to 0.97) and women (RR: 0.75; 95%: 0.51 to 1.11) with total vitamin C intakes in the highest quintile category relative to the lowest intake quintile after adjusting for age, smoking, and alcohol consumption. Median intakes in the lowest and highest intake quintile categories were 33 and 104 mg/day for men and 34 and 171 mg/day for women. Hankinson and co-workers[94] did not observe an association between total vitamin C intake assessed at baseline and rate of cataract surgery (RR: 0.98; 95% CI: 0.72 to 1.32) in a large prospective study of women when they compared women with intakes in the highest quintile category (median = 705 mg/day) to women with intakes in the lowest quintile category (median = 70 mg/day) after controlling for nine potential confounders including age, diabetes, smoking, and energy intake. However, they did note an association between cataract

surgery and sustained higher vitamin C intakes from supplements. Women who reported use of vitamin C supplements for ≥10 years had a 45% reduction in rate of cataract surgery (RR: 0.55; 95% CI: 0.32 to 0.96). This inverse relation between vitamin C supplement use and cataract risk is the most consistently observed among the vitamin C measures. Robertson and co-workers[85] compared cases with cataracts that impaired vision to age- and sex-matched controls who were either free of cataract or had minimal opacities that did not impair vision. Their results indicated that the prevalence of cataract in persons who consumed daily vitamin C supplements of >300 mg was approximately one third the prevalence in persons who did not consume vitamin C supplements (RR: 0.30; 95% CI: 0.12 to 0.75). Jacques et al.[84] observed that vitamin C supplement use for ≥10 years was related to a greater than 75% lower prevalence of early nuclear opacities (RR: 0.23; 95% CI: 0.09 to 0.59). None of the 26 women who used vitamin C supplements for ≥10 years had a more advanced nuclear cataract (RR: 0.0; 95% CI: 0.00 to 0.47).

Not all studies suggest a benefit of higher vitamin C. A study conducted in India[91] noted an 87% (RR: 1.87; 95% CI: 1.29 to 2.69) increased prevalence of mixed cataract with posterior subcapsular and nuclear involvement for each standard deviation increase in plasma vitamin C levels after controlling for 11 possible confounders including age, sex, body mass index, blood pressure, dietary protein, and education. Vitale and co-workers[90] considered the relations between both plasma vitamin C and vitamin C intake and risk of nuclear and cortical cataract. Persons with plasma levels in the highest quartile category (or fourth) of their sample (greater than 80 μmol/L) and those with plasma levels in the lowest quartile (below 60 μmol/L) had a similar prevalence of both nuclear (RR: 1.31; 95% CI: 0.65 to 2.60) and cortical (RR: 1.01; 95% CI: 0.45 to 2.26) cataract after controlling for age, sex, and diabetes. They also reported no differences in cataract prevalence between persons with high (>261 mg/day) and low (<115 mg/day) vitamin C intakes. One other study[92] did not observe any association between prevalence of cataract and vitamin C intake.

B. VITAMIN E

Vitamin E intake was inversely correlated with cataract risk in three of the four studies in which it was considered (Figure 11.3). Jacques and Chylack[83] observed an inverse association when they related total vitamin E intake (combined dietary and supplemental intake) to cataract prevalence in their small case-control study. Persons with vitamin E intake greater than 35.7 mg/day (highest quintile) had a 55% lower prevalence of cataract (RR: 0.46; 95% CI: 0.12 to 1.79) than did persons with intakes less than 8.4 mg/day (lowest quintile), but this association was not statistically significant. Leske and colleagues[86] also observed that vitamin E intake was inversely associated with prevalence of cataract after controlling for age and sex. Persons with vitamin E intakes in the highest quintile category had an approximately 40% lower prevalence of cortical (RR: 0.59; 95% CI: 0.35 to 0.99) and mixed (RR: 0.58; 95% CI: 0.37 to 0.93) cataract relative to persons with intakes in the lowest quintile category. Mares-Perlman and co-workers[88] reported a lower prevalence of nuclear cataract in men (RR: 0.67; 95% CI: 0.43 to 1.03) and women (RR: 0.78; 95% CI: 0.53 to 1.14) in the highest quintile category of total vitamin E intake

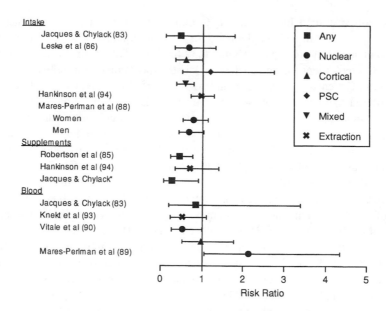

Figure 11.3.   Summary of studies of vitamin E and age-related cataract: risk ratio and 95% confidence intervals. *unpublished observation.

(median intake = 12.8 and 19.9 mg/day for men and women, respectively) relative to those in the lowest vitamin E intake quintile (median intake = 4.0 mg/day for men and 5.0 mg/day for women). This relation was not statistically significant in women, but the trend for risk across intake quintiles was statistically significant ($p = 0.03$) in men. In contrast to these studies, Hankinson et al.[94] observed no association between total vitamin E intake and cataract surgery after adjustment for a variety of potential confounders. Women with vitamin E intakes in the highest quintile (median = 210 mg/day) had a similar rate of cataract surgery (RR: 0.96; 95% CI: 0.72 to 1.29) as women with intakes in the lowest quintile category (median = 3.3 mg/day).

Three studies considered the relation between supplemental vitamin E use and risk of cataract. Robertson and co-workers[85] found that among age- and sex-matched cases and controls the prevalence of cataract was 56% lower (RR: 0.44; 95% CI: 0.24 to 0.77) in persons who consumed vitamin E supplements (>400 IU/day) than in persons not consuming supplements. Jacques and Chylack (unpublished) also observed a 67% (RR: 0.26: 95% CI: 0.08 to 0.90) reduction in prevalence of cataract for vitamin E supplement users after adjusting for age, sex, race, and diabetes. Hankinson et al.[94] reported that women who had consumed vitamin E supplements for ≥10 years had a nonsignificant 30% lower risk of cataract surgery (RR: 0.70; 95% CI: 0.35 to 1.41) compared with women who did not use vitamin E supplements. This observation was based on a relatively small proportion of women (approximately 2%) who had consumed vitamin E supplements for this period of time.

Two of the six studies that assessed plasma vitamin E reported inverse associations with cataract (Figure 11.3). Knekt and co-workers[93] followed a cohort of 1419 Finns for 15 years and identified 47 patients admitted to ophthalmological wards

for mature cataract. They selected two controls per patient matched for age, sex, and municipality. These investigators reported that persons with serum vitamin E concentrations above approximately 20 µmol/L (the upper two thirds of the sample) had about one half the rate of subsequent cataract surgery (RR: 0.52; 95% CI: 0.24 to 1.1) compared with persons with vitamin E concentrations below this concentration (i.e., in the lowest third). Vitale and co-workers[90] observed the age-, sex-, and diabetes-adjusted prevalence of nuclear cataract to be about 50% less (RR: 0.52; 95% CI: 0.27 to 0.99) among persons with plasma vitamin E concentrations in the highest quartile (>30 µmol/L) compared to persons in the lowest quintile (<19 µmol/L). A similar comparison showed that the prevalence of cortical cataract did not differ between those with high and low plasma vitamin E levels (RR: 0.96; 95% CI: 0.52 to 0.1.78). Plasma vitamin E was inversely associated with prevalence of cataract in a large Italian study after adjusting for age and sex, but the relationship was no longer statistically significant after adjusting for other factors such as education, sunlight exposure, and family history of cataract.[93] Jacques and Chylack[83] reported that the prevalence of any cataract did not differ substantially (RR: 0.83; 95% CI: 0.20 to 3.40) between those in the highest (>35 µmol/L) and lowest (below 21 µmol/L) quintiles of plasma vitamin E. One other study failed to observe any association between cataract and plasma vitamin E levels.[91] In contrast to these studies and to the intake data from the same population-based sample, Mares-Perlman and colleagues[89] demonstrated a significantly increased prevalence of nuclear cataract (RR: 2.1; 95% CI: 1.1 to 4.3) among individuals in the highest serum vitamin E quintile (median levels 37.8 µmol/L for men and 46.5 µmol/L for women) relative to those in the lowest quintile (median levels 16.9 µmol/L for men and 18.2 µmol/L for women).

C. CAROTENOIDS

Three studies[83,88,94] considered the relations between cataract risk and carotenoid intake (Figure 11.4). Jacques and Chylack[83] were unable to detect any association between carotene intake and cataract prevalence. Persons with carotene intakes in the highest quintile (>18,700 IU/day) had the same prevalence of cataract (RR: 0.94; 95% CI: 0.23 to 3.78) as those with intakes in the lowest quintile (<5677 IU/day). Hankinson and co-workers[94] reported that the multivariate-adjusted rate of cataract surgery was about 30% lower (RR: 0.73; 95% CI: 0.55 to 0.97) for women in the highest quintile of carotene intake (median = 14,558 IU/day) compared with women in the lowest quintile (median = 2935 IU/day). However, while cataract surgery was inversely associated with total carotene intake, it was not strongly associated with consumption of carotene-rich foods, such as carrots. Rather, cataract surgery was associated with lower intakes of foods, such as spinach and other greens, that are rich in the xanthophyll lutein. These authors suggested that the observed association with carotene intake might be due to the correlation between carotene and lutein in the diet. Mares-Perlman and co-workers[88] conducted a detailed examination of the intake of individual carotenoids and nuclear cataract. Their intake data was based on recall of usual diet 10 years before their eye examination. In women, they observed a significant inverse trend (*p*-trend = 0.02) across quintiles of lutein intake and a significant positive trend (*p*-trend = 0.03) across quintiles of lycopene intake.

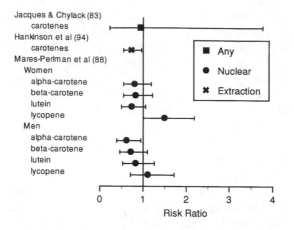

Figure 11.4. Summary of studies of carotenoid intake and age-related cataract: risk ratio and 95% confidence intervals.

Women in the highest quintile of lutein intake (median = 949 μg/day) and a 27% lower prevalence of nuclear cataract (RR: 0.73; 95% CI: 0.50 to 1.06) than women in the lowest lutein intake quintile (median = 282 μg/day). The women with lycopene intakes in the upper fifth (median = 203 μg/day) had almost a 50% increase risk of nuclear cataract (RR: 1.49; 95% CI: 1.01 to 2.19) relative to those in the lowest fifth (median = 66 μg/day). Although the trends were in the same direction in men, neither of these carotenoids were significantly related to cataract prevalence. Rather, intakes of two other carotenoids α-carotene (*p*-trend = 0.04) and β-carotene (*p*-trend = 0.07), were inversely associated with cataract risk. Men in the highest α-carotene intake quintile (median = 268 μg/day) had a 39% lower prevalence of nuclear cataract (RR: 0.61; 95% CI: 0.39 to 0.95) compared with men in the lowest intake quintile (median = 87 μg/day). The risk ratio comparing men in the highest (median = 1113 μg/day) and lowest (median = 372 μg/day) β-carotene quintiles was 0.71 (95% CI: 0.46 to 1.10). There were no observational studies that considered carotenoid supplement intake.

Four studies[83,89,90,93] considered the relations between cataract risk and blood carotenoid measures (Figure 11.5). In contrast to the lack of association between dietary carotene and cataract prevalence in the study of Jacques and Chylack,[83] they observed that persons with plasma total carotenoid concentrations in the highest quintile (>3.3 μmol/L) had less than one fifth the prevalence of any cataract (RR: 0.18; 95% CI: 0.03 to 1.03) compared to persons with low plasma carotenoid levels (<1.7 μmol/L). Knekt and co-workers[93] reported that among age- and sex-matched cases and controls, persons with serum β-carotene concentrations above approximately 0.1 μmol/L (the upper two thirds of this sample) had a 40% reduction in the rate of cataract surgery compared with persons with concentrations below this level (RR: 0.59; 95% CI: 0.26 to 1.25). Vitale and colleagues[90] also examined the relationships between plasma β-carotene levels and age-, sex-, and diabetes-adjusted prevalence of cortical and nuclear cataract. Although the data suggested a weak inverse association between plasma β-carotene and cortical cataract and a weak

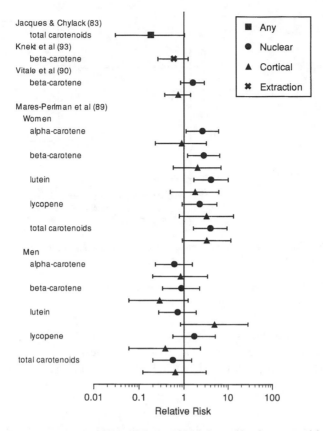

Figure 11.5.   Summary of studies of blood carotenoids and age-related cataract: risk ratio and 95% confidence intervals.

positive association between this nutrient and nuclear cataract, neither association was statistically significant. Persons with plasma β-carotene concentrations in the highest quartile (>0.9 μmol/L) had a 28% lower prevalence of cortical cataract (RR: 0.72; 95% CI: 0.37 to 1.42) and a 57% (RR: 1.57; 95% CI: 0.84 to 2.93) higher prevalence of nuclear cataract compared to persons with levels in the lowest quartile (<0.3 μmol/L). As with intake, Mares-Perlman and colleagues[89] examined the relation between cataract risk and a number of individual serum carotenoids, but their observations based serum carotenoids measured at the time of the eye examination differed from those based on recall of diet from 10 years earlier. Except for lycopene, the intake data suggested a protective relation between nuclear cataract and the carotenoids,[88] but the serum data were consistent with either no association in men or an increased prevalence of nuclear cataract with higher serum carotenoid concentrations in women. Women with total serum carotenoid concentrations in the highest quintile (median = 2.2 μmol/L) had a fourfold greater prevalence of nuclear cataract (RR: 3.95; 95% CI: 1.65 to 9.47) than those in the lowest quintile (median = 0.79 μmol/L), where as men in the highest quintile of total serum carotenoids (median = 1.93 μmol/L) had a lower prevalence of nuclear cataract (RR: 0.55; 95%

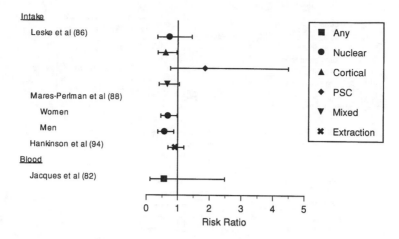

Figure 11.6. Summary of studies of riboflavin and age-related cataract: risk ratio and 95% confidence intervals.

CI: 0.20 to 1.49) than those in the lowest quintile (median = 0.69 μmol/L). Similar relations were reported between serum carotenoids and cortical cataract. For total serum carotenoids, women in the highest quintile again demonstrated an elevated prevalence of cortical cataract compared with those in the lowest quintile (RR: 3.26; 95% CI: 0.92 to 11.5), while the data for men suggested a lower prevalence of cortical cataract for those in the highest relative to the lowest quintile (RR: 0.62; 95% CI 0.12 to 3.20).

D. RIBOFLAVIN

Riboflavin deficiency was considered a risk factor for age-related cataract in humans prior to the current focus on antioxidant nutrients.[98] Four studies[82,86,88,94] that measured intake or blood markers of riboflavin are summarized here (Figure 11.6). Jacques et al.[82] considered the relation between cataract and riboflavin status measured by erythrocyte glutathione reductase activation. They observed that individuals in the highest quintile category of status (activity coefficients <1.01) had approximately one half the prevalence of cataract (RR: 0.54; 95% CI: 0.12 to 2.49) compared with those in the lowest status quintile category (activity coefficients >1.22), but the very wide confidence interval does not allow for a clear interpretation of this association. Leske and colleagues[86] observed a lower prevalence of cortical cataract (RR: 0.59; 95% CI: 0.36 to 0.97), mixed cataract (RR: 0.65: 95% CI: 0.40 to 1.05), and nuclear cataract (RR: 0.72; 95% CI: 0.35 to 1.45), and a higher prevalence of posterior subcapsular cataract (RR: 1.85; 95% CI: 0.76 to 4.49) in persons with riboflavin intake in the highest quintile compared with those in the lowest intake quintile. Mares-Perlman and co-workers[88] reported that women in the highest ribo-flavin intake quintile category (median = 2.2 mg/day) had a 33% lower prevalence of nuclear cataract (RR: 0.67; 95% CI: 0.46 to 0.98) than women in the lowest quintile intake category (median = 0.8 mg/day). The prevalence of nuclear cataract was also lower (RR: 0.56; 95% CI: 0.36 to 0.87) for men in the highest intake quintile category (median = 1.6 mg/day) compared with those in the lowest category

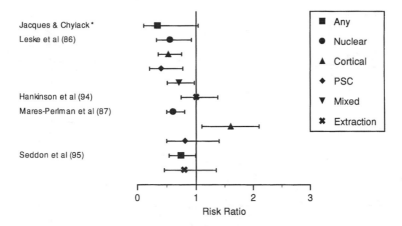

Figure 11.7. Summary of studies of multivitamin supplement use and age-related cataract: risk ratio and 95% confidence intervals.

(median = 0.8 mg/day). Hankinson and colleagues[94] did not observe any difference between rates of cataract extraction (RR: 0.91; 95% CI: 0.69 to 1.20) in the highest quintile of total riboflavin intake (median = 1.5 mg/day) and the lowest (median = 1.2 mg/day).

E. MULTIVITAMIN SUPPLEMENTS

One unpublished and four published reports[86,87,94,95] have examined the relation between multivitamin supplement use and risk of cataract (Figure 11.7). Although multivitamins are a source of antioxidant nutrients and riboflavin, they also include many other nutrients. Therefore, it is not possible to directly attribute the associations between multivitamins and cataract risk to any individual component. Jacques and Chylack (unpublished) observed a reduced prevalence of any cataract among multivitamin supplement users (RR: 0.34; 95% CI: 0.11 to 1.04) in their small case-control study. Leske and co-workers[86] reported that multivitamin supplement users had a lower prevalence of each type of cataract: nuclear (RR: 0.55; 95% CI: 0.33 to 0.92), cortical (RR: 0.52; 95% CI: 0.36 to 0.75), posterior subcapsular (RR: 0.40; 95% CI: 0.21 to 0.77), and mixed (RR: 0.70; 95% CI: 0.51 to 0.97). Mares-Perlman and colleagues[87] reported a lower prevalence of nuclear cataract (RR: 0.6; 95% CI: 0.5 to 0.8) and a higher prevalence of cortical cataract (RR: 1.6; 95% CI: 1.1 to 2.1) based on reported multivitamin supplement use 10 years before the eye examination. They saw no significant association between multivitamin supplement use and posterior subcapsular cataract (RR: 0.8; 95% CI: 0.5-1.4). Seddon and colleagues[95] observed that incidence of cataract was 27% lower (RR: 0.73; 95% CI: 0.54 to 0.99) and the rate of cataract extraction was 21% lower (RR: 0.79; 95% CI: 0.46 to 1.35) in male physicians that used multivitamin supplements compared with those who did not. These investigators also reported that the strength of these associations increased with the duration of supplement use. However, Hankinson et al.[94] fail to see any relation between multivitamin use and cataract extraction, even among women who used these supplements for ≥10 years (RR: 1.00; 95% CI: 0.74 to 1.38).

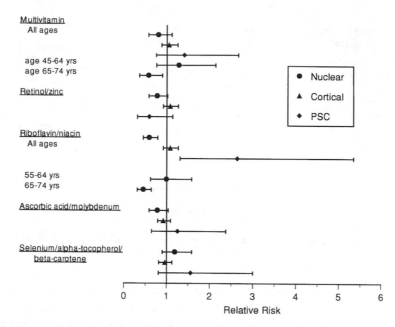

Figure 11.8.   Summary of Linxian cataract trials:[99] risk ratio and 95% confidence intervals.

F. INTERVENTION TRIALS

To date there has been only one intervention study completed that assessed the effect of vitamin supplements on cataract risk. Sperduto and co-workers[99] took advantage of two ongoing randomized, double-blinded cancer trials to assess the impact of vitamin supplements on cataract prevalence among surviving participants. The trials were conducted among almost 4000 participants aged 45 to 74 years from rural communes in Linxian, China. Participants in one trial received either a multivitamin supplement or placebo. In the second trial, a more complex factorial design was used to evaluate the effects of four different vitamin/mineral combinations: retinol (5000 IU) and zinc (22 mg); riboflavin (3 mg) and niacin (40 mg); vitamin C (120 mg) and molybdenum (30 μg); and vitamin E (30 mg), β-carotene (15 mg), and selenium (50 μg). At the end of the 5 to 6 year followup, the investigators conducted eye examinations to determine the prevalence of cataract. The results are summarized in Figure 11.8.

In the first trial, there was a significant 43% reduction in the prevalence of nuclear cataract for persons aged 65 to 74 years who received the multivitamin supplement (RR: 0.57; 95% CI: 0.36 to 0.90). The second trial demonstrated a significantly reduced prevalence of nuclear cataract in persons receiving the riboflavin/niacin supplement relative to those persons not receiving this supplement (RR: 0.59; 95% CI: 0.45 to 0.79). The effect was due entirely to the reduced risk in those aged 65 to 74 years (RR: 0.45; 95% CI: 0.31 to 0.64). The riboflavin/niacin supplement also appeared to increase the risk of posterior subcapsular cataract (RR: 2.64; 95% CI: 1.31 to 5.35). The results further suggested a protective effect of the retinol/zinc supplement (RR: 0.77; 95% CI: 0.58 to 1.02) and the vitamin C/molybdenum supplement

(RR: 0.78; 95% CI: 0.59 to 1.04) on prevalence of nuclear cataract. The selenium/α-tocopherol/β-carotene supplement appeared unrelated to cataract at any site.

This trial does suggest a role for nutrition in development of cataract, but these findings must be interpreted cautiously. These trials were conducted in a population with a fair amount of nutritional deprivation making it difficult to apply these results to other populations. Furthermore, lens status was not assessed in the study sample at baseline; these results are based on the prevalence of cataract among survivors of these trials. Finally, duration of treatment is questionable based on three observational studies[84,94,95] that demonstrated no or little reduction in risk of cataract until vitamin supplements had been used for ≥10 years.

V. EPIDEMIOLOGIC EVIDENCE FOR NUTRITIONAL ANTIOXIDANTS IN AMD

The relation between antioxidant nutrients and AMD has been examined in three large retrospective studies[100-103] and one smaller case-control study.[104] A fifth study[105] examined early maculopathy in 65 cases and age-matched controls, and unlike the other studies considered here, fewer than 15% of the cases had evidence of macular degeneration, and cases and controls had a similar distribution of visual acuity. These studies have many of the same limitations previously described for the studies of cataract and antioxidant nutrients. These studies are all retrospective with concurrent assessment of the retina and nutrient levels, and they are based on single measurements of nutrient levels, and most of these studies failed to account for the correlation between antioxidant nutrients.

Figures 11.9 and 11.10 display the risk ratios and 95% confidence intervals for individuals with high intakes or blood levels of vitamin C, vitamin E, and carotenoids compared with those with low intakes or blood levels. As with the cataract studies, these studies defined high and low nutrient categories based on percentiles, except for Tsang et al.[104] and Sanders et al.[105] who compared mean plasma nutrient concentrations in cases to controls.

A. VITAMIN C

Three studies examined the relation between AMD and intake or blood levels of vitamin C (Figure 11.9). Seddon et al.[101] examined the relation between advanced AMD and vitamin C intake. Individuals in the highest (median = 1039 mg/day) and lowest (65 mg/day) intake quintiles had the same prevalence of advanced (exudative) AMD (RR: 1.01; 95% CI: 0.60 to 1.70). These investigators reported that the prevalence of AMD in persons who consumed vitamin C supplements for ≥2 years was similar to those who never took vitamin C supplements (RR: 0.89; 95% CI: 0.6 to 1.3). Serum vitamin C was also measured in this same sample.[100] Individuals with serum vitamin C concentrations in the highest quintile (≥91 μmol/L) had a 30% lower prevalence of AMD (RR: 0.7; 95% CI: 0.5 to 1.2) compared with those in the lowest quintile (≤40 μmol/L). Although the risk ratio comparing the high and low quintile categories was not statistically significant, that comparing the middle three quintile categories to the lowest quintile category was significantly reduced (RR: 0.6; 95% CI: 0.4 to 0.9). West and colleagues[102] reported that individuals in the

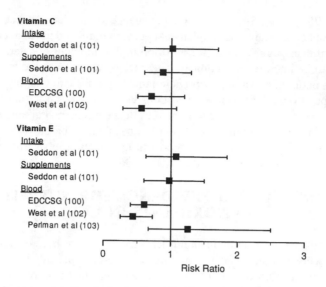

Figure 11.9. Summary of studies of vitamins C and E and age-related maculopathy: risk ratio and 95% confidence intervals.

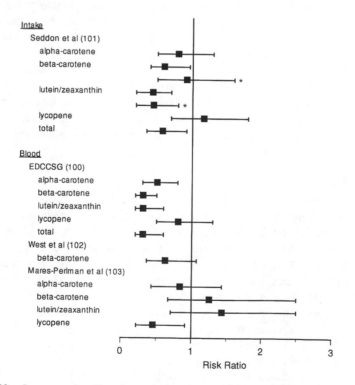

Figure 11.10. Summary of studies of carotenoids and age-related maculopathy: risk ratio and 95% confidence intervals. (* indicates that the risk ratios were mutually adjusted.)

highest plasma vitamin C quartile (>80 μmol/L) had a 45% lower prevalence of AMD (RR: 0.55; 95% CI: 0.28 to 1.08) compared with individuals in the lowest plasma vitamin C quartile (<60 μmol/L).

B. VITAMIN E

Four studies that examined the relation between AMD and intake or blood levels of vitamin E are summarized in Figure 11.9. Seddon et al.[101] observed no difference in prevalence of advanced AMD (RR: 1.07; 95% CI: 0.63 to 1.84) between individuals in the highest (median = 405 mg/day) and lowest vitamin E intake quintiles (median = 3.4 mg/day). Prevalence of AMD was also similar in those who took vitamin E supplements for ≥2 years and those who never took vitamin E supplements (RR: 0.97; 95% CI: 0.6 to 1.5). In this sample,[100] the prevalence of AMD among those with serum vitamin E concentrations in the highest quintile (≥43 μmol/L) was 40% lower (RR: 0.6; 95% CI: 0.4 to 1.0) than the prevalence among those in the lowest quintile (≤25 μmol/L). West and colleagues[102] observed a strong inverse association between plasma vitamin E concentration and prevalence of AMD. Individuals in the highest plasma vitamin E quartile (>30 μmol/L) had a 57% lower prevalence of AMD (RR: 0.43; 95% CI: 0.25 to 0.73) compared with individuals in the lowest plasma vitamin E quartile (<19 μmol/L). Mares-Perlman et al.[103] reported that the mean serum α-tocopherol concentrations were significantly lower in cases with AMD (29.9 μmol/L) than controls (34.1 μmol/L). This difference was no longer statistically significant when presented as the ratio of serum α-tocopherol to cholesterol concentrations. Also, the risk of AMD among individuals with serum α-tocopherol above the 20th percentile (23 μmol/L) was similar to the risk among those with serum levels below the 20th percentile (RR: 1.3; 95% CI: 0.7 to 2.5). There was also no significant difference in risk (RR: 0.8; 95% CI: 0.4 to 1.4) for individuals with γ-tocopherol levels above and below the 20th percentile (4.5 μmol/L). Tsang et al.[104] and Sanders et al.[105] did not observe any difference in mean plasma vitamin E concentrations between cases with AMD or maculopathy and controls.

C. CAROTENOIDS

Four studies that examined the relation between AMD and intake or blood levels of carotenoids are summarized in Figure 11.10. Seddon et al.[101] determined the intake of total carotenoid and the individual carotenoids. They observed that individuals in the highest total carotenoid quintile (median = 19,250 IU/day) had a >40% lower prevalence of advanced AMD (RR: 0.57; 95% CI: 0.35 to 0.92) compared with those with intakes in the lowest quintile (median = 3154). Inverse associations were seen with the individual carotenoids lutein/zeaxanthin (RR = 0.4; 95% CI: 0.2 to 0.7) and β-carotene (RR = 0.6; 95% CI: 0.4 to 1.0). However, when they examined the independent associations of these two carotenoids with AMD, lutein/zeaxanthin remained related to risk of AMD (RR: 0.4; 95% CI: 0.2 to 0.8), but β-carotene did not (RR: 0.9; 95% CI: 0.5 to 1.6). The relation of individual and total serum carotenoids to AMD was also considered in this sample.[100] Prevalence of AMD among those with total serum carotenoid concentrations in the highest quintile (≥2.39 μmol/L) was 66% lower (RR: 0.34; 95% CI: 0.21 to 0.55) than the prevalence among those in the lowest quintile (≤1.02 μmol/L). With the exception of lycopene (RR: 0.8; 95% CI: 0.5 to 1.3), AMD prevalence was significantly lower among those in the highest quintile of each individual serum carotenoid relative to those in the lowest quintile: α-carotene (RR: 0.5; 95% CI: 0.3 to 0.8); β-carotene (RR: 0.3; 95% CI: 0.2 to 0.5), and lutein/zeaxanthin (RR: 0.3; 95% CI: 0.2 to 0.6). Although these investigators did not identify the independent contribution for the individual carotenoids, they did demonstrate the generally high correlations between them and cautioned their readers to focus on the total rather than individual carotenoids. The study of West and colleagues[102] also suggested an inverse association between plasma β-carotene concentration and prevalence of AMD. Individuals in the highest plasma β-carotene quartile (>0.9 μmol/L) had a 38% lower prevalence of AMD (RR: 0.62; 95% CI: 0.36 to 1.07) compared with individuals in the lowest plasma β-carotene quartile (<0.3 μmol/L). Mares-Perlman et al.[103] observed a significant, inverse association between serum lycopene concentrations and prevalence of AMD, but they did not see any relations between AMD risk and other carotenoids including lutein and zeaxanthin. Individuals with lycopene concentrations above 294 nmol/L were 50% less likely to have AMD than individuals with concentrations above this level (RR: 0.5: 95% CI: 0.2 to 0.9), whereas the prevalence of AMD in those with the sum of lutein and zeaxanthin above 169 nmol/L was not significantly different from that among individuals with concentrations below this level (RR: 1.4; 95% CI: 0.7 to 2.5). Sanders et al.[105] did not observe any difference in mean plasma β-carotene concentrations between cases with maculopathy and controls and Mares-Perlman et al.[106] reported that intake of dietary carotenoids was not related to maculopathy.

VI. SUMMARY

Epidemiologic studies provide support for a protective role of nutritional antioxidants in prevention of age-related cataract and macular degeneration. Nine[82-87,90,93-95] of the eleven[82-95] studies of antioxidant nutrients and risk of cataract described above show inverse associations between at least one type of cataract and at least one antioxidant nutrient. Three[100-103] of the five[100-105] studies of antioxidant nutrients and risk of AMD described above show inverse associations with at least one antioxidant nutrient. However, the epidemiologic studies also present many inconsistencies.

For example, the studies of antioxidant nutrients and cataract do not demonstrate consistent associations with any one antioxidant nutrient or with a specific type of cataract. Many of these inconsistencies might be explained by differences in the populations studied and the methods used. For example, the populations studied might explain some of these differences because of unique dietary patterns and underlying nutritional differences, or unmeasured competing risk factors or confounders affecting specific populations. It is of interest that the nine studies in which relations with antioxidant nutrients were observed were conducted in the U.S.,[82-84,86-88,90,94,95] Canada,[85] and Finland,[93] while the two in which no associations were noted were conducted in Italy[92] and India.[91] Both sunlight exposure and diet, as well as many other factors, would differ somewhat between these later populations and those in North America and Northern Europe.

The lack of specificity in these studies for relations between type of cataract and individual antioxidant nutrients might be the result of different definitions of cataract from one study to the next. Some studies did not create mutually exclusive categories of cataract type, while other studies based cataract categories on opacities exclusive to one lens region and classifying individuals with opacities in more than one region of the lens as mixed cataract. In addition, studies using cataract extraction as an endpoint have not presented information on location of cataract, and posterior sub-capsular cataract is usually over-represented among surgically-removed cataract relative to prevalent cataract.[96,97]

The lack of specificity of antioxidant nutrients associated with cataract might be due to the failure to consider the correlations between intake and status of these antioxidant nutrients. The correlation between nutrients is caused by use of multi-vitamin supplements (which contain both vitamin C and E) and dietary patterns (e.g., a diet high in fruits and vegetables with be high in both carotenoids and vitamin C whereas a diet low in these foods will be low in both of these nutrients). This is particularly problematic for the recent studies that have focused on individual carotenoids. Lack of specificity of nutrients might also result from population differences in nutrient intake and status. The ability to detect associations and the strength of those associations depends on the prevalence of low levels and the variability of intake and status of these nutrients in a population.

The most daunting problem in the study of antioxidant nutrients and cataract is the measurement of long-term nutrient intake or status. The epidemiological studies presented above are based almost exclusively on one concurrent or past measure of nutrient status or intake. As cataracts develop over a period of decades, one measure is not likely to be sufficient to classify an individual's long-term intake for a specific nutrient; thus, these studies would tend to underestimate the strength of the association between that nutrient and cataract risk, or even fail to note any association. To date, only studies that have considered vitamin supplements have been able to assess usual intake over an extended period of time by examining duration of supplement use.[84,94,95] These studies all suggest that little or no benefit of vitamin supplementation is seen until it was used for at least 5 to 9 years and no substantial reduction in cataract is risk observed until it is used for ≥10 years. In addition, the studies of Mares-Perlman and co-workers[88] demonstrated apparent protective associations with individual carotenoids based on reported diet recall of intake 10 years before lens assessment, but using serum measures derived concurrently with lens assessment observed an increased risk with certain individual carotenoids.[89] It is possible that the inconsistency of this observation could be a consequence of the timing and not the adequacy of the carotenoid measures, because results based on intakes of these carotenoids at the time of the eye examination were largely consistent with the results based on the serum carotenoid measures.[89]

The Linxian intervention trials have not clarified the role of antioxidant nutrients in prevention of cataract.[99] The multivitamin trial demonstrated that nutrition can modify the risk of nuclear cataract, but these results do not address the specific nutrients involved. The second trial examined specific nutrient combinations and indicated a beneficial effect of riboflavin/niacin on nuclear cataract, but a detrimental effect on posterior subcapsular cataract. Although nuclear cataract is the most common type of cataract and posterior subcapsular cataract the least common type, posterior subcapsular cataracts comprise the greatest proportion of surgical cases.[96,97] Thus, it is difficult to project the overall benefit of this intervention. Although there is little evidence from this trial to support an effect of the supplement containing vitamin E, β-carotene, and selenium, a modest effect of vitamin C/molybdenum or retinol/zinc cannot be ruled out. In addition to the uncertainty of the results, these trials were conducted in a population with a fair amount of nutritional deprivation, making it difficult to apply these results to other populations, and duration of the trial might have been insufficient to overcome a lifelong deficiency of these nutrients.

Goldberg and co-workers[107] presented the first evidence for a relation between nutrition and AMD in humans. They reported an inverse association between AMD and consumption of fruits and vegetables high in vitamin A and vitamin C. Vitamin A intake, but not vitamin C intake, was associated with prevalent AMD. The more recent studies provide some support for these observations.[100,101,102] Vitamin C was weakly, but inconsistently, associated with AMD in the studies described above. Carotenoids were strongly related to AMD in one sample, but unrelated or only weakly related in others. Blood levels of vitamin E were associated with AMD risk in two of these studies.[100,102] These studies relating antioxidant nutrients to AMD have many of the potential problems with interpretation that are discussed above for studies of cataract such as the use of a single retrospective assessment of nutrient intake and status to characterize usual intake and status, differences in definition of AMD, and lack of specificity of the nutrient-AMD relations. Seddon and colleagues[101] addressed this latter methodologic problem demonstrating that lutein and zeaxanthin were responsible for the relation between overall carotenoid intake and AMD.

Based on the observations summarized here, it would seem prudent to consume diets high in vitamins C and E and carotenoids, particularly the xanthophylls, and to use multivitamin supplements as insurance against the development of cataract and AMD. However, it is not yet possible to conclude for or against a role of antioxidant nutrients in formation of cataract or AMD, nor is it possible to identify the nutrients that are the most likely candidates to be involved in development of these disorders. Based on the recent report that β-carotene is not detectable in the lens, and that lutein and zeaxanthin are present,[53] it seems reasonable that the latter, and not the former, carotenoids should be the focus of any research relating carotenoids and cataract risk. Given the specificity of uptake of these carotenoids in the macula, this is also true for studies of AMD. Future studies must also address the independent contribution of each antioxidant nutrient and must strive to identify means of assessing usual, long-term intake of these nutrients.

Finally, in designing new trials to assess the role of antioxidant nutrients in development of cataract and macular degeneration, the distinction between treatment and prevention paradigms must be considered. The features that would characterize a nutritional treatment paradigm are an intervention that is effective over a relatively short period, and a study population that has early or treatable cataract or AMD and that has average intakes of the nutrient(s) under study. The prevention paradigm is derived from observational studies and is characterized by a population at risk that is free of cataract or AMD at the initiation of the intervention, and a comparison between those with the highest and lowest (not average) intakes. Moreover, in a preventive paradigm we would not expect to overcome decades of adverse exposure and resulting tissue damage with an intervention of only 5 to 10 years. If we are proposing that antioxidant nutrients have therapeutic effects on existing cataract or AMD, then a treatment model is appropriate. However, if we are proposing that these nutrients can prevent or delay the development of cataract or AMD, we need to consider long-term interventions in people who are initially free of these eye disorders and who have low intakes. Such an undertaking would be formidable, but may be the only means of determining the true relation between antioxidant nutrients and prevention of these age-related visual disorders.

ACKNOWLEDGMENTS

I would like to thank Garry Handelman for this thoughtful review and comments. This project has been funded at least in part with Federal funds from the U.S. Department of Agriculture, Agricultural Research Service, under contract number 53-3K06-01. The contents of this publication do not necessarily reflect the views or policies of the U.S. Department of Agriculture, nor does mention of trade names, commercial products, or organizations imply endorsement by the U.S. Government.

REFERENCES

1. Harding, J. J. and Crabbe, M. J. C., The lens: development, proteins, metabolism and cataract, in *The Eye*, vol. 1B, 3rd edition, Davson, H., Eds., Academic Press, New York, 1984, chap. 3.
2. Worgul, B. V., Lens, in *Biochemical Foundations of Ophthalmology*, Duane, T. D., and Jaeger, E. A., Eds., J.B. Lippincott Co., Philadelphia, 1988, vol. 1, chap. 15, 1.
3. Fridovich, I., Oxygen: Aspects of its toxicity and elements of defense, *Curr. Eye Res.*, 3, 1, 1984.
4. Augusteyn, R. C., Protein modification in cataract: possible oxidative mechanisms, *Mechanisms of Cataract Formation in the Human Lens*, Duncan, G., Ed., Academic Press, New York, 1981, 71.
5. Hoenders, H. J. and Bloemendal, H., Aging of lens proteins, in *Molecular and Cellular Biology of the Eye Lens*, Bloemendal, H., Ed., John Wiley and Sons, New York, 1981, 279.
6. Jahngen-Hodge, J., Taylor, A., Shang, F., Huang, L. L., and Mura, C., Oxidative stress to lens crystallins, *Methods Enzymol.*, 233, 512, 1994.
7. Varma, S. D., Chand, O., Sharma, Y. R., Kuck, J. F., and Richards, K. D., Oxidative stress on lens and cataract formation. Role of light and oxygen, *Curr. Eye Res.*, 3, 35, 1984.
8. Harding, J. J., Changes in lens proteins in cataract, in *Molecular and Cellular Biology of the Eye Lens*, Bloemendal, H., Ed., John Wiley and Sons, New York, 1981, 327.
9. Sigelman, J. and Ozanics, V., Retina, in *Biochemical Foundations of Ophthalmology*, Duane, T. D., and Jaeger, E.A., Eds., J.B. Lippincott Co., Philadelphia, 1988, vol. 1, chap. 19, 1.
10. Marmor, M. F., Aging and the retina, in *Aging and Human Visual Function*, Sekuler, R., Kline, D., Pismukes, K., Eds., Alan R Liss, Inc., New York, NY, 1982, 59.
11. Snodderly, M. D., Evidence for protection against age-related macular degeneration by carotenoids and antioxidant vitamins, *Am. J. Clin. Nutr.*, 62(suppl), 1448S, 1995.
12. Bressler, N. M., Bressler, S. B., and Fine, S. L., Age-related macular degeneration, *Surv. Ophthalmol. Vis. Sci.*, 32, 375, 1988.
13. Green, W. R., McDonnell, P. J., and Yeo, J.H., Pathologic features of senile macular degeneration, *Ophthalmology*, 92, 615, 1985.

14. Young, R. Pathophysiology of age-related macular degeneration, *Surv. Ophthalmol.*, 31, 291, 1987.
15. Young, R. W., Solar radiation and age-related macular degeneration, *Surv. Ophthalmol.*, 32, 252, 1988.
16. Handelman, G. J. and Dratz, E. A., The role of antioxidants in the retina and retinal pigment epithelium and the nature of prooxidant-induced damage, *Adv. Free Rad. Biol. Med.*, 2, 1, 1986.
17. Schwab, L., Cataract blindness in developing nations, *Internat. Ophthalmol. Clinics*, 30, 16, 1990.
18. World Health Organization, Use of intraocular lenses in cataract surgery in developing countries, *Bull. World Health Organ.*, 69, 657, 1991.
19. Kupfer, C., The conquest of cataract: a global challenge, *Trans. Ophthal. Soc. U.K.*, 104, 1, 1984.
20. Chatterjee, A., Milton, R. C., and Thyle, S., Prevalence and etiology of cataract in Punjab, *Br. J. Ophthalmol.*, 66, 35, 1982.
21. Wang, G. M., Spector, A., Luo, C. Q., Tang, L. Q., Xu, L. H., Guo, W. Y., and Huang, Y. Q., Prevalence of age-related cataract in Ganzi and Shanghai. The Epidemiological Study Group, *Chinese Med. J.*, 103, 945, 1990.
22. Whitfield, R., Schwab, L., Ross-Degnan, D., Steinkuller, P., and Swartwood J., Blindness and eye disease in Kenya: ocular status survey results from the Kenya Rural Blindness Prevention Project, *Br. J. Ophthalmol.*, 74, 333, 1990.
23. Chan, C.W. and Billson, F.A., Visual disability and major causes of blindness in NSW: a study of people aged 50 and over attending the Royal Blind Society 1984 to 1989, *Aust. N. Zealand J. Ophthalmol.*, 19, 321, 1991.
24. Dana, M. R., Tielsh, J. M., Enger, C., Joyce, E., Santoli, J. M., and Taylor, H. R., Visual impairment in a rural Appalachian community: Prevalence and causes, *J. Am. Med. Assoc.*, 264, 2400. 1990.
25. Salive, M. E., Guralnik, J., Christian, W., Glynn, R. J., Colsher, P., and Ostfeld, A. M., Functional blindness and visual impairment in older adults from three communities, *Ophthalmol.*, 99, 1840, 1992.
26. Wormald, R. P. L., Wright, L. A., Courtney, P., Beaumont, B., and Haines, A. P., Visual problems in the elderly population and implications for services, *Br. Med. J.*, 304, 1226, 1992.
27. Klein, B.E.K., Klein, R., and Linton, K. L. P., Prevalence of age-related maculopathy: The Beaver Dam Eye Study, *Ophthalmol.*, 99, 933, 1992.
28. Leibowitz, H., Krueger, D., Maunder, C., Milton, R. C., Kini, M. M., Kahn, H. A., Nickerson, R. J., Pool, J., Colton, T. L., Ganley, J. P., Loewenstein, J. I., and Dawber, T. R., The Framingham Eye Study Monograph, *Surv. Ophthalmol.*, 24 (suppl.), 335, 1980.
29. Klein, B. E. K., Klein, R., and Linton, K. L. P., Prevalence of age-related lens opacities in a population: The Beaver Dam Eye Study, *Ophthalmol.*, 99, 546, 1992.
30. Steinberg, E. P., Javitt, J. C., Sharkey, P. D., Zuckerman, A., Legro, M. W., Anderson, G. F., Bass, E. B., and O'Day, D., The content and cost of cataract surgery, *Arch. Ophthalmol.*, 111, 1041, 1993.
31. Stark, W. J., Sommer, A., and Smith, R. E., Changing trends in intraocular lens implantation, *Arch. Ophthalmol.*, 107, 1441, 1989.
32. Frei, B., Stocker, R., and Ames, B. N., Antioxidant defenses and lipid peroxidation in human blood plasma., *Proc. Nat. Acad. Sci. U.S.A.*, 85, 9748, 1988.
33. Levine, M., New concepts in the biology and biochemistry of ascorbic acid, *New Engl. J. Med.*, 314, 892, 1986.
34. Taylor, A., Jacques, P. F., Nadler, D., Morrow, F., Sulsky, S. I., and Shepard, D., Relationship in humans between ascorbic acid consumption and levels of total and reduced ascorbic acid in lens, aqueous humor, and plasma, *Curr. Eye Res.*, 10, 751, 1991.
35. Nielsen, J. C., Naash, M. I., and Anderson, R. E., The retinal distribution of vitamins E and C in mature and premature human retinas, *Invest. Ophthalmol. Vis. Sci.*, 29, 22, 1988.
36. Kosegarten, D. C. and Mayer, T. J., Use of guinea pigs as model to study galactose-induced cataract formation, *J. Pharm. Sci.*, 67, 1478, 1978.
37. Vinson, J. A., Possanza, C. J., and Drack, A. V., The effect of ascorbic acid on galactose-induced cataracts, *Nutr. Reports Internat.*, 33, 665, 1986.
38. Devamanoharan, P.S., Henein, M., Morris, S., Ramachandran, S., Richards, R.D., and Varma, S.D. (1991). Prevention of selenite cataract by vitamin C. *Exp. Eye Res.* 52, 563.
39. Nishigori, H., Lee, J. W., Yamauchi, Y., and Iwatsuru, M., The alteration of lipid peroxide in glucocorticoid-induced cataract of developing chick embryos and the effect of ascorbic acid, *Curr. Eye Res.*, 5, 37, 1986.

40. Varma, S. D., Srivastava, V. K., and Richards, R. D., Photoperoxidation in lens and cataract formation: Preventive role of superoxide dismutase, catalase and vitamin C, *Ophthalmic Res.*, 14, 167, 1982.
41. Blondin, J., Baragi, V. J., Schwartz, E., Sadowski, J., and Taylor, A., Delay of UV-induced eye lens protein damage in guinea pigs by dietary ascorbate, *Free Radic. Biol. Med.*, 2, 275, 1986.
42. Blondin, J. and Taylor, A., Measures of leucine aminopeptidase can be used to anticipate UV-induced age-related damage to lens proteins: ascorbate can delay this damage, *Mech. Aging Dev.*, 41, 39, 1987.
43. Varma, S. D., Kumar, S., and Richards, R. D., Light-induced damage to ocular lens cation pump: Prevention by vitamin C, *Proc. Natl. Acad. Sci. U.S.A.*, 76, 3504, 1979.
44. Varma, S. D., Morris, S. M., Bauer, S. A., and Koppenol, W. H., *In vitro* damage to rat lens by xanthine-xanthine oxidase: Protection by ascorbate, *Exp. Eye Res.*, 43, 1067, 1986.
45. Varma, S. D., Ascorbic acid and the eye with special reference to the lens, *Ann. N.Y. Acad. Sci.*, 498, 280, 1987.
46. Organisciak, D. T., Wang, H.-M., Li, Z.-Y., and Tso, M. O. M., The protective effect of ascorbate in retinal light damage of rats, *Invest. Ophthalmol. Vis. Sci.*, 26, 1580, 1985.
47. Organisciak, D. T., Jiang, Y.-L., Wang, H.-M., and Bicknell, I., The protective effect of ascorbic acid in retinal light damage of rats exposed to itermittent light, *Invest. Ophthalmol. Vis. Sci.*, 31, 1195, 1990.
48. Woodford, B. J., Tso, M. O. M., and Lam, K.-W., Reduced and oxidized ascorbates in guinea pig retina under normal and light-exposed conditions, *Invest. Ophthalmol. Vis. Sci.*, 24, 862, 1983.
49. Tso, M. O. M., Woodford, B. J., and Lam, K. W., Distribution of ascorbate in normal primate retine and after photic injury: a biochemical, morphological correlated study, *Curr. Eye Res.*, 3, 181, 1984.
50. Noel, W. K., Organisciak, D. T., Ando, H., Braniecki, M. A., and Durlin, C., Ascorbate and dietary protective mechanisms in retinal light damage of rats: electrophysiological, histological and DNA measurements, *Prog. Clin. Biol. Res.*, 247, 469, 1987.
51. Woodford, B. J. and Tso, M. O. M., Exaggeration of photic injury in scorbutic guinea pig retinas, *Invest. Ophthalmol. Vis. Sci.*, 25 (suppl), 90, 1984.
52. Machlin, L. J. and Bendich, A., Free radical tissue damage: Protective role of antioxidant nutrients, *FASEB J.*, 1, 441, 1987.
53. Yeum, K.-J., Taylor, A., Tang, G., and Russell, R. M., Measurement of carotenoids, retinoids and tocopherols in human lenses, *Invest. Ophthalmol. Vis. Sci.*, 36, 2756, 1995.
54. Friedrichson, T., Kalbach, H. L., Buck, R., and van Kuijk, F. J. G. M., . Vitamin E in macular and peripheral tissues of the human eye, *Curr. Eye Res.*, 14, 693, 1995.
55. Stephens, R. J., Negi, D. S., Short, S. M., van Kuijk, F. J. G. M., Dratz, E. A., and Thomas, D. W., Vitamin E distribution in ocular tissues following long-term dietary depletion and supplementation as determined by microdissection and gas chromatography-mass spectrometry, *Exp. Eye Res.*, 47, 237, 1988.
56. Bhuyan, D. K., Podos, S. M., Machlin, L. T., Bhagavan, H. N., Chondhury, D. N., Soja, W. S., and Bhuyan, K. C., Antioxidant in therapy of cataract II: Effect of all-roc-alpha-tocopherol (vitamin E) in sugar-induced cataract in rabbits, *Invest. Ophthalmol. Vis. Sci.*, 24, 74, 1983.
57. Bhuyan, K. C. and Bhuyan, D. K., Molecular mechanism of cataractogenesis: III. Toxic metabolites of oxygen as initiators of lipid peroxidation and cataract, *Curr. Eye Res.*, 3, 67, 1984.
58. Varma, S. D., Beachy N. A., and Richards, R. D., Photoperoxidation of lens lipids: prevention by vitamin E, *Photochem. Photobiol.*, 36, 623, 1982.
59. Trevithick, J. R., Creighton, M. O., Ross, W. M., Stewart-DeHaan, P. J., and Sanwal, M., Modeling cortical cataractogenesis: 2. *In vitro* effects on the lens of agents preventing glucose- and sorbitol-induced cataracts, *Can. J. Ophthalmol.*, 16, 32, 1981.
60. Creighton, M. O. and Trevithick, J. R., (1979). Cortical cataract formation prevented by vitamin E and glutathione, *Exp. Eye Res.*, 29, 689, 1979.
61. Creighton, M. O., Ross, W. M., Stewart-DeHaan, P. J., Sanwai, M., and Trevithick, J. R., Modeling cortical cataractogenesis. VII: Effects of vitamin E treatment on galactose-induced cataracts, *Exp. Eye Res.*, 40, 213, 1985.
62. Ross, W. M., Creighton, M. O., Inch, W. R., and Trevithick, J. R., Radiation cataract formation diminished by vitamin E in rat lenses *in vitro*, *Exp. Eye Res.*, 36, 645, 1983.

63. Stewart-DeHaan, P. J., Creighton, M. O., Sanwal, M., Ross, W. M., and Trevithick, J. R., Effects of vitamin E on cortical cataractogenesis induced by elevated temperature in intact rat lenses in medium 199, *Exp. Eye Res.*, 32, 51, 1981.

64. Creighton, M. O., Trevithick, J. R., Sanford, S. E., and Dukes, T. W., Modeling cortical cataractogenesis. IV. Induction by Hygromycin B *in vivo* (swine) and *in vitro* (rat lens), *Exp. Eye Res.*, 34, 467, 1982.

65. Creighton, M. O., Sanwai, M., Stewart-DeHaan, P. J., and Trevithick, J. R., Modeling cortical cataractogenesis. V: Steroid cataracts induced by solumedrol partially prevented by vitamin E *in vitro*, *Exp. Eye Res.*, 37, 65, 1983.

66. Hayes, K. C., Rousseau, J. E., and Hegsted, D. M., Plasma tocopherol concentrations and vitamin E deficiency in dogs, *J. Am.Vet. Med. Assoc.*, 157, 64, 1970.

67. Hayes, K. C., Retinal degeneration in monkeys induced by deficiencies of vitamin E or A, *Invest. Ophthalmol. Vis. Sci.*, 13, 499, 1974.

68. Dorey, C. K., Staurenghi, G., and Delori, F. C., Lipofuscin in aged and AMD eyes, in *Retinal Degeneration*, Hollyfield, J. G., LaVail, M. M., and Anderson, R. E., Eds., Plenum Press, New York, 1993, 3.

69. Daun, H., The chemistry of carotenoids and their importance in food, *Clin. Nutr.*, 7, 97, 1988.

70. Erdman, J., The physiologic chemistry of carotenes in man, *Clin. Nutr.*, 7, 101, 1988.

71. Micozzi, M. S., Beecher, G. R., Taylor, P. R., and Khachik, F., Carotenoid analyses of selected raw and cooked foods associated with a lower risk for cancer, *J.N.C.I.* 82, 282, 1990.

72. Krinsky, N. I. and Deneke, S. S., Interaction of oxygen and oxy-radicals with carotenoids, *J. N. C. I.*, 69, 205, 1982.

73. DiMascio, P., Murphy, M. E., and Seis, H., Antioxidant defense systems: the role of carotenoids, tocopherols and thiols, *Am. J. Clin. Nutr.*, 53, 194S, 1991.

74. Krinsky, N. I., Russett, M. D., Handelman, G. J., and Snodderly, D. M., Structural and geometric isomers of carotenoids in human plasma, *J. Nutr.*, 120, 1654, 1990.

75. Bone, R. A., Landrum, J. T., Fernandez, L., and Tarsis, S. L., Analysis of the macular pigment by HPLC: retinal distribution and age study, *Invest. Ophthalmol. Vis. Sci.*, 29, 843, 1988.

76. Handelman, G. J., Dratz, E.A., Reay, C. C., and van Kuijk, F. J. G. M., Carotenoids in the human macula and whole retina, *Invest. Ophthalmol. Vis. Sci.*, 29, 850, 1988.

77. Malinow, M. R., Feeney-Burns, L., Peterson, L. H., Klien, M. L., and Neuringer, M., Diet-related macular abnormalities in monkeys, *Invest. Ophthalmol. Vis. Sci.*, 19, 857, 1980.

78. Feeney-Burns, L., Neuringer, M., and Gao, C.L., Macular pathology in monkeys fed semipurified diets, *Prog. Clin. Biol. Res.*, 314, 601, 1989.

79. Bunce, G. E., Nutrition and eye disease of the elderly, *J. Nutr. Biochem.*, 5, 66, 1994.

80. Salmon, W. D., Hayes, I. M., and Guerrant, N. D., Etiology of dermatitis of experimental pellagra in rats, *J. Infect. Dis.*, 43, 426, 1928.

81. Jacques, P. F. and Chylack, L. T., Nutritional factors in senile cataract genesis, in *Biomedical Foundations of Ophthalmology*, Duane, T. D. and Jaeger, E. A., Eds., J. B. Lippincott Co., Philadelphia, 1988, vol. 3, chap. 12A.

82. Jacques, P. F., Hartz, S. C., Chylack, L. T., McGandy, R. B., and Sadowski, J. Nutritional status in persons with and without senile cataract: Blood vitamin and mineral levels, *Am. J. Clin. Nutr.*, 48, 152, 1988.

83. Jacques, P. F. and Chylack, L. T. Jr., Epidemiologic evidence of a role for the antioxidant vitamins and carotenoids in cataract prevention, *Am. J. Clin. Nutr.*, 53, 352S, 1991.

84. Jacques, P. F., Taylor, A., Hankinson, S. E., Lahav, M., Mahnken, B., Lee, Y., Vaid, K., and Willett, W. C., Long-term vitamin C supplement use and prevalence of age-related lens opacities, *Am. J. Clin. Nutr.*, submitted.

85. Robertson, J. McD., Donner, A.P., and Trevithick, J. R., Vitamin E intake and risk for cataracts in humans, *Ann. N.Y. Acad. Sci.*, 570, 372, 1989.

86. Leske, M. C., Chylack, L. T. Jr., and Wu, S., The lens opacities case-control study risk factors for cataract, *Arch. Ophthalmol.*, 109, 244, 1991.

87. Mares-Perlman, J. A., Klein, B. E. K., Klein, R., and Ritter, L. L., Relationship between lens opacities and vitamin and mineral supplement use, *Ophthalmology*, 101, 315, 1994.

88. Mares-Perlman, J. A., Brady, W. E., Klein, B. E. K., Klein, R., Haus, G.J., Palta, M., Ritter, L.L., and Shoff, S. M., Diet and nuclear lens opacities, *Am. J. Epidemiol.*, 141, 322, 1995.

89. Mares-Perlman, J. A., Brady, W. E., Klein, B. E. K., Klein, R., Palta, M., Bowen, P., and Stacewicz-Sapuntzakis, M., Serum carotenoids and tocopherols and severity of nuclear and cortical opacities, *Invest. Ophthalmol. Vis. Sci.,* 36, 276, 1995.

90. Vitale, S., West, S., Hallfrisch, J., Alston, C., Wang, F., Moorman, C., Muller, D., Singh, V., and Taylor, H. R., Plasma antioxidants and risk of cortical and nuclear cataract, *Epidemiology*, 4, 195, 1993.

91. Mohan, M., Sperduto, R. D., Angra, S. K., Milton, R. C., Mathur, R. L., Underwood, B., Jaffery, N., and Pandya, C. B., India-US case-control study of age-related cataracts, *Arch. Ophthalmol.*, 107, 670, 1989.

92. The Italian-American Cataract Study Group, Risk factors for age-related cortical, nuclear, and posterior subcapsular cataracts, *Am. J. Epidemiol.*, 133, 541, 1991.

93. Knekt, P., Heliovaara, M., Rissanen, A., Aromaa, A., and Aaran, R., Serum antioxidant vitamins and risk of cataract, *Br. Med. J.*, 305, 1392, 1992.

94. Hankinson, S. E., Stampfer, M. J., Seddon, J. M., Colditz, G. A., Rosner, B., Speizer, F. E., and Willett, W. C., Nutrient intake and cataract extraction in women: a prospective study, *Br. Med. J.*, 305, 335, 1992.

95. Seddon, J. M., Christen, W. G., Manson, J. E., LaMotte, F. S., Glynn, R. J., Buring, J. E. and Hennekens, C. H., The use of vitamin supplements and risk of cataract among U.S. male physicians, *Am. J. Public Health*, 84, 788, 1994.

96. Hiller, R., Sperduto, R. D., and Ederer, F., Epidemiologic associations with nuclear, cortical, and posterior subcapsular cataracts, *Am. J. Epidemiol.*, 124, 916, 1986.

97. Adamsons, I., Munoz, B., Enger, C., and Taylor, H. R., Prevalence of lens opacities in surgical and general populations, *Arch. Ophthalmol.*, 109, 993, 1991.

98. Skalka, H. W. and Prchal, J. T., Cataracts and riboflavin deficiency, *Am. J. Clin. Nutr.*, 34, 861, 1981.

99. Sperduto, R. D., Hu, T.-S., Milton, R. C., Zhao, J.-L., Everett, D. F., Cheng, Q.-F., Blot, W. J., Bing, L., Taylor, P. R., Jun-Yao, L., Dawsey, S., and Guo, W.-D., The Linxian Cataract Studies: Two nutrition intervention trials, *Arch. Ophthalmol.*, 111, 1246, 1993.

100. Eye Disease Case-control Study Group, Antioxidant status and neovascular age-related macular degeneration, *Arch.Ophthalmol.*, 11:104, 1993.

101. Seddon, J.M., Ajani, U. A., Sperduto, R. D., Hiller, R., Blair, N., Burton, T. C., Farber, M. D., Gragoudas, E. S., Haller, J., Miller, D. T., Yannuzzi, L. A. and Willett, W., Dietary carotenoids, vitamins A, C, and E, and advanced age-related macular degeneration, *J. Am. Med. Assoc.*, 272, 1413, 1994.

102. West, S. K., Vitale S., Hallfrisch, J., Munoz, B., Muller, D., Bressler, S., and Bressler, N. M., Are antioxidants or supplements protective for age-related macular degeneration? *Arch. Ophthalmol.*, 112, 222, 1994.

103. Mares-Perlman, J. A., Brady, W. E., Klein, R., Klein, B. E. K., Bowen, P., Stacewicz-Sapuntzakis, M., and Palta, M., Serum antioxidants and age-related macular degeneration in a population-based case-control study, *Arch. Ophthalmol.*, 113, 1518, 1995.

104. Tsang, N. C. K., Penfold, P. L., Snitch, P. J., and Billson, F., Serum levels of antioxidants and age-related macular degeneration, *Documenta Ophthalmologica*, 81, 387, 1992.

105. Sanders, T. A. B., Haines, A. P., Wormald, R., Wright, L. A., and Obeid, O., Essential fatty acids, plasma cholesterol, and fat-soluble vitamins in subjects with age-related maculopathy and matched control subjects, *Am. J. Clin. Nutr.*, 57, 428, 1993.

106. Mares-Perlman, J. A., Brady, W. E., Klein, R., VandenLangenberg, G. M., Klein, B. E. K., and Palta, M., Dietary fat and age-related maculopathy, *Arch. Ophthalmol.*, 113, 743, 1995.

107. Goldberg, J., Flowerdrew, G., Smith, E., Brody, J. A., and Tso, M. O. M., Factors associated with age-related macular degeneration. An analysis of data from the First National Health and Nutrition Examination Survey, *Am. J. Epidemiol.*, 128:700, 1988.

INDEX

A

Acetyhydrolase, 118
2-Acetylaminofluorene, 104
Acquired immunodeficiency syndrome
    (AIDS), 32–39
Aflatoxins, 104
Age-related macular degeneration (AMD)
    carotenoids and, 153, 155, 168–170
    epidemiological studies of, 167–173
    overview of, 152–153
    riboflavin and, 156
    vitamin A and, 172
    vitamin C and, 153–154, 167–169
    vitamin E and, 153, 155, 168–169
Aging, effects of, 20–21, 26, 150–153
AIDS (acquired immunodeficiency
    syndrome), 32–39
AIDS-related complex (ARC), 36–38
Air pollution and lung cancer, 68
Alcohol and free radicals, 20
Alpha-Tocopherol Beta-Carotene (ATBC)
    Cancer Prevention Study
    cardiovascular disease results, 119,
        140–141
    lung cancer results, 6, 8, 73, 80, 82–83,
        144
AMD. *See* Age-related macular
    degeneration
Angina pectoris
    [β-]carotene and, 139, 141
    vitamin C and, 133–134
    vitamin E/[α-]tocopherol and, 13,
        133–134, 139, 141
Animal model studies, 102–103, 132
Anticlastogenesis and vitamin E, 11
Antigen presenting cells (APC), 22
Antioxidants
    AIDS and, 32–39
    ascorbic acid, 24, 26, 34–35, 77, 115,
        120–121
    carotenoids. *See* Carotenoids;
        [α-]Carotene; [β-]Carotene
    enzymes, 21
    epidemiological studies of. *See*
        Epidemiological studies

flavonoids, 3, 38, 115, 122, 137
    immune function and, 19–26
    index of, 84
    mechanism of, 20, 103–106
    overview of, 1–4
    role in disease prevention, 3–4
    [α-]tocopherol. *See* [α-]Tocopherol
    vitamin A. *See* Vitamin A
    vitamin C. *See* Vitamin C
    vitamin E. *See* Vitamin E
AP-1, 23
APC (Antigen presenting cells), 22
Apolipoprotein B (apoB), 116, 118
Apoptosis, 32–33, 35, 106
ARC (AIDS-related complex), 36–38
Arginine, 38
Arthritis, 26
Asbestos-exposure, 7, 68–69, 75, 80–81,
    140, 143
Ascorbic acid, 24, 26, 34–35, 77, 115,
    120–121. *See also* Vitamin C
Aspirin, 80, 139, 143
ATBC (Alpha-Tocopherol Beta-Carotene)
    Cancer Prevention Study
    cardiovascular disease results, 119,
        140–141
    lung cancer results, 6, 8, 73, 80, 82–83,
        144
Atherosclerosis, 20, 115–120, 132,
    137–138

B

Benzo(a)pyrene, 104
Benzopyrones, 38
Beta-Carotene and Retinol Efficacy Trial,
    140
Betel nuts, 91
BHA (Butylated hydroxy anisole), 23
BHT (Butylated hydroxytoluene), 118
Biomarkers, oxidation, 84
Bladder cancer, 98, 100–102
Blindness, 153
Blood clotting and vitamin E, 12–14
Blood pressure, 133
Brain cancer, 99

179

Brain disorders and free radicals, 20
Breast cancer, 24, 47–54, 97–99, 103, 134
Butylated hydroxy anisole (BHA), 23
Butylated hydroxytoluene (BHT), 118

C

Cadaverine, 38
Calcium, 20, 23, 35
Cambridge Heart Antioxidant Study
   (CHAOS), 119, 140, 142, 144
Cancer
   aging and, 20–21
   animal model studies of, 102–103
   bladder, 98, 100–102
   brain, 99
   breast, 47–54, 97–99, 103, 134
   cervical, 48, 54–55, 98–99
   colon. *See* Colon cancer
   endometrial, 99
   epidemiological studies of. *See*
      Epidemiological studies
   esophageal, 77, 98, 100, 107
   etiology of, 87–88
   gastric, 47, 49–54, 77, 97, 142
   head and neck, 47, 49–55, 93
   liver, 98, 100, 102
   lung. *See* Lung cancer
   melanoma, 24, 77, 98, 100, 140, 142
   oral cavity. *See* Oral cavity cancer
   ovarian, 24, 98–99
   pancreatic, 24, 48, 54, 98, 100
   peritoneal, 97
   prostate, 5, 47, 49–54, 107
   rectal, 47–54, 98–99, 101–102, 105,
      107
   renal, 100, 102
   stomach, 98–99, 101–102
   thyroid, 102
Cardiovascular disease
   animal model studies of, 132
   [β-]carotene and, 134–143
   diet and, 132–133, 137, 144
   epidemiological studies of, 132–143
   estrogens and, 137
   flavonoids and, 137
   low-density lipoproteins (LDL) and, 132
   prevention of, 87, 133
   retinol and, 135
   selenium and, 140, 143

[α-]tocopherol/vitamin A and, 119–121,
      133, 135–136, 141–142
   vitamin C and, 120, 132–134, 136–138,
      143
   vitamin E and, 13–14, 132–141,
      143–144
   zinc and, 143
CARET (Carotene and Retinol Efficacy Trial),
      4, 6, 75–76, 80, 82–83, 143–144
[α-]Carotene, 69, 155, 162–163, 168,
      170
[β-]Carotene. *See also* Carotenoids
   as antioxidant, 3, 85
   asbestos exposure and, 7, 69, 140,
      143
   atherosclerosis and, 121
   bioavailable dose, 82–83
   cardiovascular disease and, 134–143
   epidemiological studies of, 47–55, 68–69,
      72–79
   eye disorders and, 155, 162–163,
      166–170, 172
   immune system function and, 26
   LDL oxidation and, 115, 121
   lung cancer and, 4, 6–8, 49–54, 68–69,
      72–83, 141
   oral cavity disease and, 91–93
   prostate cancer and, 5
   recommended intake levels of, 8
   safety of, 4–8, 144. *See also* CARET
   skin cancer and, 140, 142
   smoking and, 6–8, 83. *See also* CARET
   vitamin E and, 5–6
Carotene and Retinol Efficacy Trial
   (CARET) Study, 4, 6, 75–76, 80,
      82–83, 143–144
Carotenoids. *See also* [α-]Carotene;
      [β-]Carotene
   AIDS and, 35
   database on, 69
   eye disorders and, 155, 161–164,
      168–170, 172
   lung cancer and, 68–73
Catalase (CT), 21, 26, 36, 38
Cataracts, age-related
   carotenoids and, 153, 155, 161–164,
      171–172
   description of, 150–151
   epidemiological studies of, 156–167,
      170–173

multivitamin supplements and, 165–166
riboflavin and, 156, 164–165, 171
selenium and, 172
vitamin C and, 153–154, 157–159,
171–172
vitamin E and, 153, 155, 159–161, 171–172
Catechins, 38
Ceruloplasmin, 36
Cervical cancer, 48, 54–55, 98–99
c-fos, 24
CHAOS (Cambridge Heart Antioxidant
Study), 119, 140, 142, 144
Chemoprevention, 1–2, 80–81
Chinese cataract trials (Linxian County),
166, 171
Chinese lung cancer trial (Linxian County),
77, 80, 82–84, 140, 142
Cholesterol, 13, 116–117, 132–133
Cholesterol Lowering Atherosclerosis Study
(CLAS), 137
c-myc, 24
Coenzyme Q_{10} (ubiquinone) and AIDS,
37–38
Colestipol-niacin treatment, 137
Colon cancer
epidemiological studies of, 47–54
familial polyposis and, 1
free radicals and, 20, 24
selenium and, 98–99, 101–102, 104–105,
107
Colonic adenomas, 90, 98–99
ConA, 23
Concanavalin, 35
Copper (Cu), 21, 36
CoQ_{10} (ubiquinone) and AIDS, 37–38
Coronary artery disease, 14, 119, 122, 131–144.
See also Cardiovascular disease
Coumarins, 38
CT (Catalase), 21, 26, 36, 38
Cu (Copper), 21, 36
Cystamine amino thiol compounds, 23
Cysteine and AIDS, 33
Cytochrome P450, 21
Cytokines, 22–25, 36

D

DCFH, 23
DDTC (Diethyldithiocarbamate), 37
Desferrioxamine (DES; DFX), 23, 37

Desferrithiocin (DFT), 23
DFX (Desferrioxamine), 23, 37
DHLA (Dihydrolipoic acid), 34
Diabetes, 119–120, 143
Diamid, 25
Diamide, 24
2′5′-Dideoxyadenosine, 24
Diet and cancer, 45, 47, 68–71. *See also*
Fruits and vegetables
Diethyldithiocarbamate (DDTC), 37
Dihydrolipoic acid (DHLA), 34
N,N-Dimethylanaline, 104
Dimethylbenzanthracene, 104
Dimethyl sulfoxide (DMSO), 22
Dimethyl urea, 22
N,N′-Diphenyl-phenylenediamine (DPPD),
118
Disease risk, 3
DMSO (Dimethyl sulfoxide), 22
DPPD (N,N′-Diphenyl-phenylenediamine),
118

E

Endometrial cancer, 99
Endothelins and LDL oxidation, 118
Epidemiological studies
case-cohort, 46, 68
cross-sectional, 133–134, 156
difficulties with, 2, 4, 46, 54–55, 92–93,
171
ecological, 46, 132–133
intervention, 47, 55, 68–82, 85,
139–143
nested case-control, 46, 134–135
prospective dietary, 46, 50–51, 68,
70–71
prospective serum, 46, 52–53, 78–79
publication bias in, 54–55
randomized, 141–144
retrospective dietary, 46, 48–50, 68,
156
retrospective serum, 46, 50–52
Erlich ascites tumors, 105
Erythroplakia, 90
Erythropoietic protoporphyria, 85,
118
Esophageal cancer, 77, 98, 100, 107
Estrogens, 104, 115, 122, 137
Etretinate, 93

European community multicenter study
    (EURAMIC), 134
EUROSCAN, 81
Exercise and free radicals, 20
Eye disorders. *See* Age-related macular
    degeneration; Cataracts, age-related
Eyes and aging, 150–152

F

Fat intake and free radicals, 20
Fiber and lung cancer, 75
Field cancerization, 89, 93
Flavonoids, 3, 38, 115, 122, 137
Folic acid, 35, 47, 75
Free radicals
    action of, 19–21
    AIDS and, 32
    antioxidant enzymes and, 21
    atherosclerosis and, 118, 122
    carcinogenicity of, 20
    cardiovascular disease and, 132
    immune function and, 22–26
    sources of, 19–20
    vitamin C and, 26
Fruits and vegetables
    cardiovascular disease and, 132–133, 137,
        144
    effect of cooking, 69
    epidemiological studies of, 48–51, 54–56,
        70–71
    eye disorders and, 171–172
    importance of, 3, 7–8
    lung cancer and, 68–75, 82, 84
    oral cavity cancer and, 89

G

Gastric cancer, 47, 49–54, 77, 97, 142
Glutathione (GSH), 26, 33–34, 37, 105
Glutathione peroxidase (GSHPx;GPx), 21,
    36, 38, 104–105
Glutathione reductase, 22, 156
Glutathione-S-transferase (GS-T), 21
Gossypetin, 122
Gout, 9
GPx (Glutathione peroxidase), 21, 36, 38,
    104–105
Granulomas, 26
GSH (Glutathione), 26, 33–34, 37, 105

GSHPx (Glutathione peroxidase), 21, 36,
    38, 104–105
GSSeSG (Selenodiglutathione), 105
GSSG, 105
GS-T (Glutathione-S-transferase), 21

H

HDL (High-density lipoproteins), 118
Head and neck cancer, 47, 49–55, 93
Health Professionals Follow-up Study,
    138
Heart disease. *See* Cardiovascular disease;
    Coronary artery disease
Heart Protection Study, 81, 83
Hemochromatosis and Vitamin C, 9
Hepatoma, 98, 100, 102
HIC-5 gene, 24
High-density lipoproteins (HDL), 118
HIV (Human immunodeficiency virus), 32,
    35, 39. *See also* AIDS
Hodgkin's disease, 98
Hormone levels, 104, 115, 122, 137
Human immunodeficiency virus (HIV-1;
    HIV-2), 32, 35, 39. *See also* AIDS
Hydrogen peroxide, 23–24, 36
Hypercarotenemia, 5
Hypercholesterolemia, 132
Hypertension, 100

I

IL (Interleukins), 22–25, 35, 36, 117
Immune function, 19–26, 32–35, 104
Inflammation, 20, 26, 36
Insulin, 25
Interleukins (IL), 22–25, 35, 36, 117
Iron, 9, 20, 23

K

7-Ketocholesterol, 116
Kidney cancer, 100, 102

L

LDL (Low-density lipoproteins), 115–123,
    132
Lens of the eye, 150–151. *See also*
    Cataracts, age-related

Leukemia, 25, 98, 100
Leukoplakia, 55, 90, 91–93
Linoleic acid, 105
Linxian cataract trials, 166, 171
Linxian lung cancer trials, 77, 80, 82–84,
      140, 142
Lipid peroxidation
   action of, 20, 22, 116
   arthritis and, 26
   flavonoids and, 38
   selenium and, 105
   ubiquinone and, 37
   vitamin C and, 154
   vitamin E and, 132, 154
Lipid Research Clinics Coronary Primary
      Prevention Trial and Follow-up Study,
      135
[α-]Lipoic acid and AIDS, 34
Lipoxygenase (LO), 23–24
Liver cancer, 98, 100, 102
LO (Lipoxygenase), 23–24
Long terminal repeat (LTR) and AIDS,
      32
Lovastatin, 132
Low-density lipoproteins (LDL), 115–123,
      132
Lung cancer
   air pollution and, 68
   asbestos and, 68, 75, 80–81
   carotenes and, 4, 6–8, 49–54, 68–69,
      72–83, 141
   diet and, 68–76, 82, 84
   epidemiological studies of, 47–55, 68–69,
      77, 80–84, 140, 142
   N-acetylcysteine (NAC) and, 81
   nutritional agent interactions and, 101
   overview of, 67–68, 84–85
   retinol and, 69, 71, 73, 77, 82
   selenium and, 49–54, 69, 77–81, 83–84,
      97–102, 107
   smoking and, 67–68, 77
   [α-]tocopherol and, 77, 82
   vitamin A and, 50–54, 71, 75, 78–79
   vitamin C and, 49–54, 68, 71, 75,
      78–79
   vitamin E and, 49–54, 68, 71, 74–81
   vitamin supplements and, 72
Lutein, 69, 155, 161–163, 168–170,
      172
Lycopene, 121, 155, 161–163, 168, 170

Lymphoblasts, 105
Lymphocytes, 22–24, 26
Lymphomas, 97

M

[β$_2$-]Macroglobulin, 22
Macula, 150–152. *See also* Age-related
      macular degeneration (AMD)
Major Histocompatibility Complex (MHC)
      molecules, 22
Malonyldialdehyde (MDA), 104, 116, 154
Manganese (Mn), 21
Mannitol, 22
MEDLINE database, 46
Melanoma (skin cancer), 24, 77, 98, 100,
      140, 142
MHC (Major Histocompatibility Complex)
      molecules, 22
Mn (Manganese), 21
Molybdenum (Mo), 77, 166, 172
Mutagenesis, 10, 11
Myocardial infarction, 119, 134–136,
      138–139, 143–144. *See also*
      Cardiovascular disease
Myricetin, 122

N

N-Acetylcysteine (NAC), 24–25, 33–34, 81
NADPH oxidase, 23–24
Nass, 92
National Cancer Institute of the U.S., 4, 6
National Health and Nutrition Examination
      Survey (NHANES I), 136
NDGA, 24
Neomycin sulfate, 24
Neuroblastoma, 24
NHANES I (National Health and Nutrition
      Examination Survey), 136
Niacin, 77, 166, 171
Nuclear factor [κ]B (NF-[κ]B), 23–25, 32,
      34, 117
Nurses' Health Study, 138

O

Oncogenes and free radicals, 24
Oral cavity cancer
   [β-]carotene and, 91–93

etiology of, 88
    leukoplakia and, 90
    nutritional agents and, 89–94
    premalignant lesions, 55, 90–93
    prevention of, 1, 81, 89
    13-cis-retinoic acid and, 89, 91, 93
    retinol and, 92
    selenium and, 91, 93, 100–101
    smoking and, 88
    vitamin A and, 89, 91, 93
    vitamin C and, 91, 93
    vitamin E and, 55, 90–93
OTC (L-2-Oxothiazolidine 4-carboxylate)
    and AIDS, 33–34
Ovarian cancer, 24, 98–99
Oxidative stress, 32, 38, 87, 104
8-Oxo-7,8-dihydro-2′deoxyguanosine,
    73
L-2-Oxothiazolidine 4-carboxylate (OTC)
    and AIDS, 33–34
Ozone and lung cancer, 68

P

PAI-1 (Plasminogen activator inhibitor-1),
    117
Pancreatic cancer, 24, 48, 54, 98, 100
Papillomas and selenium, 102
Paraoxanase, 118
PDGF (Platelet-derived growth factor) and
    LDL oxidation, 117
2,2,5,7,8-Pentamethyl-6-hydroxychromane
    (PMC), 34
Peritoneal cancer, 97
Phagocytosis disorders, 26
PHA (Phytohaemoagglutinin), 23–24
1,4-Phenylenebis [methylene] selenocyanate,
    106
Phorbol myristate acetate (PMA), 23, 25,
    33
Phospholipid hydroperoxide glutathione
    peroxidase (PLGSHPx), 21
Photosensitivity and [β-]carotene, 5
Physicians' Health Study, 77, 80, 82–83,
    139–140, 143
Phytohaemoagglutinin (PHA), 23–24
PKC (Protein kinase C), 23–24
Plant metabolites as antioxidants, 37–38
Plasminogen activator inhibitor-1 (PAI-1),
    117

Platelet-derived growth factor (PDGF) and
    LDL oxidation, 117
PLGSHPx (Phospholipid hydroperoxide
    glutathione peroxidase), 21
PMA (Phorbol myristate acetate), 23, 25,
    33
PMC (2,2,5,7,8-Pentamethyl-6-
    hydroxychromane), 34
Polyphenols and lung cancer, 68
Polyp Prevention Study, 6
Polyunsaturated fatty acids (PUFA), 20, 22,
    116
Pregnancy and free radicals, 21
Primary prevention, 80–81
Probucol, 118, 120, 132
Procysteine and AIDS, 34
Programmed cell death and AIDS, 32
Prostacyclin, 117
Prostate cancer, 5, 47, 49–54, 107
Protein kinase C (PKC), 23–24
Putrescine, 38
Pyridoxal (vitamin B6), 35
Pyrolidine dithiocarbamate, 24

Q

Quercitin, 38, 122

R

Radiation and free radicals, 20
Ramipril, 143
Reactive oxygen species (ROS). *See* Free
    radicals
Rectal cancer, 47–54, 98–99, 101–102, 105,
    107
Renal cancer, 100, 102
Reproductive function, 5, 10–11
Retina, 150–152
13-cis-Retinoic acid, 89, 91, 93
Retinoids, synthetic, 55, 89
Retinol
    cardiovascular disease and, 135
    eye disorders and, 166, 172
    lung cancer and, 69, 71, 73, 77, 82
    oral cavity disease and, 92
Retinopathy and [β-]carotene, 5
Rheumatoid arthritis, 26
Riboflavin, 22, 35, 77, 91, 155–156,
    164–166

ROS (Reactive oxygen species). *See* Free
 radicals
Rutin, 122

S

SCPS (Skin Cancer Prevention Study), 140,
 142
Secondary prevention, 81
Selenium (Se)
 AIDS and, 36
 animal model studies of, 102–103
 as antioxidant, 21
 cancer prevention and, 77, 97,
  103–107
 cardiovascular disease and, 140,
  143
 cataracts and, 166–167, 172
 coronary artery disease and, 135
 epidemiological studies of, 47–54, 77–81,
  97–102
 hormone levels and, 104
 intake levels of, 103–105, 107
 lung cancer and, 49–54, 69, 77–81,
  83–84, 97–102, 107
 oral cavity disease and, 91, 93
 in toenails, 101
Selenodiglutathione (GSSeSG), 105
Signal transduction and oxidative stress, 24,
 33
Simvastatin, 143
Skin cancer (melanoma), 24, 77, 98, 100,
 140, 142
Skin Cancer Prevention Study (SCPS), 140,
 142
Smoking. *See also* CARET; Lung
  cancer
 cancer and, 67–68, 77, 88, 93
 [β-]carotene and, 6–8, 83
 free radicals and, 20
 "reverse," 88, 91
 selenium status and, 101
SOD (Superoxide dismutase), 21, 26,
 36–38
Spermine, 38
Sputum atypia, 69, 72, 80
Stomach cancer, 98–99, 101–102
Strokes, 136, 137, 143. *See also*
  Cardiovascular disease
Superoxide dismutase (SOD), 21, 26, 36–38

T

T-cells, 22–23, 25, 32–33, 35
Tea, 137
Testosterone, 122
TGF, 24
Thiamin (vitamin B1), 35
Thiobarbituric acid-reactive substances
  (TBARS) assay, 116–117, 120, 122
Thiouren, 22
Thrombosis, 117
Thymulin and zinc, 35
Thyroid cancer, 102
Thyroid function, 13
TNF, 24–25, 32, 36
[α-]Tocopherol. *See also* Vitamin E
 cardiovascular disease and, 119–121, 133,
  135, 141–142
 HDL and, 118
 intake levels of, 141
 LDL oxidation and, 115, 118–119
 lung cancer and, 77, 82
 vasodilation and, 121
[α-]Tocopheryl succinate, 34
Trolox, 24
Tumors. *See also* Cancer
 [β-]carotene and, 5
 hydrogen peroxide and, 24
 selenium and, 102–103
 vitamin E and, 11
Tyler (Texas) Chemoprevention Trial, 69

U

Ubiquinol-10, 115, 121–122
Ubiquinone and AIDS, 37–38
Ultraviolet light, 20, 154
Urinary oxalate stones, 8–9

V

Vasodilation, 121
Verapamil, 24
Vitamin A. *See also* [α-]Carotene;
  [β-]Carotene; Carotenoids
 AIDS and, 35
 AMD and, 172
 cardiovascular disease and, 136
 epidemiological studies of, 47–54,
  78–81

lung cancer and, 50–54, 71, 75,
  78–79
oral cavity disease and, 89, 91, 93
Vitamin B complex, 156
Vitamin B1 (thiamin), 35
Vitamin B2, 22, 35, 77, 91, 155–156,
  164–166
Vitamin B6 (pyridoxal), 35
Vitamin B12, 9, 35
Vitamin C. *See also* Ascorbic acid
  absorption of, 8
  AIDS and, 34–35, 38
  as antioxidant, 3
  atherosclerosis and, 118
  cardiovascular disease and, 120, 132–134,
    136–138, 143
  epidemiological studies of, 47–54,
    78–79
  eye disorders and, 153–154, 157–159,
    166, 167–169, 171–172
  free radicals and, 26
  gout and, 9
  hemochromatosis and, 9
  intake levels of, 154, 157, 159
  iron absorption and, 9
  lipid peroxidation and, 154
  lung cancer and, 49–54, 68, 71, 75, 78–79
  oral cavity disease and, 91, 93
  safety of, 4, 8–10
  urinary oxalate stones and, 8–9
  vitamin B12 and, 9
Vitamin E. *See also* [α-]Tocopherol
  AIDS and, 34–35, 38
  as antioxidant, 3
  atherosclerosis and, 118–119, 137
  blood clotting and, 12–14
  cardiovascular disease and, 13–14, 119,
    132–141, 143–144

[β-]carotene and, 5–6
cholesterol and, 13
epidemiological studies of, 47–54, 78–81
eye disorders and, 153–155, 159–161,
  166–169, 171–172
free radicals and, 26
gastric cancer and, 142
intake levels of, 14, 138
lipid peroxidation and, 132, 154
lung cancer and, 49–54, 68, 71, 74–81
lymphocytes and, 26
oral cavity disease and, 55, 90–93
safety of, 4, 10–15
vitamin K levels and, 12–14
Warfarin anticoagulant therapy and,
  12–13
Vitamin K, 12–14
Vitamin supplements, 55, 72, 165–172

W

Warfarin anticoagulant therapy, 12–13
Wine, 122, 137
Women's Antioxidant Cardiovascular Study,
  81, 83

X

Xanthophylls, 155, 161, 172

Z

Zeaxanthin, 155, 168–170, 172
Zinc (Zn)
  AIDS and, 35
  antioxidants and, 21, 24
  cancer prevention and, 77, 91
  eye disorders and, 166, 172